# Medical Emerg
# in General Practice

# Medical Emergencies in General Practice

**Tenth Edition**

**SP Gupta**
MD FAMS FCCP (USA) FICA (USA) FIAMS
Formerly, Professor and Head, Department of Medicine, and
Dean, School of Medicine and Allied Sciences
Maharishi Dayanand University and Medical College
Rohtak, Haryana, India
Senior Consultant, Department of Medicine
Moolchand Medcity, New Delhi, India

**Dinesh K Gupta**
MBBS (Hons) MD (AIIMS) MD (USA) FACC FACP
Consultant Cardiologist
Tennessee, USA

*Foreword*
PN Chhuttani

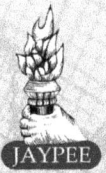

**JAYPEE BROTHERS MEDICAL PUBLISHERS**
*The Health Sciences Publisher*
New Delhi | London

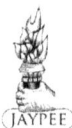 **Jaypee Brothers Medical Publishers (P) Ltd.**

### Headquarters
Jaypee Brothers Medical Publishers (P) Ltd.
EMCA House
23/23-B, Ansari Road, Daryaganj
New Delhi - 110 002, India
Landline: +91-11-23272143, +91-11-23272703
+91-11-23282021, +91-11-23245672
Email: jaypee@jaypeebrothers.com

### Corporate Office
Jaypee Brothers Medical Publishers (P) Ltd.
4838/24, Ansari Road, Daryaganj
New Delhi 110 002, India
Phone: +91-11-43574357
Fax: +91-11-43574314
Email: jaypee@jaypeebrothers.com

### Overseas Office
J.P. Medical Ltd.
83 Victoria Street, London
SW1H 0HW (UK)
Phone: +44 20 3170 8910
Fax: +44 (0)20 3008 6180
Email: info@jpmedpub.com

Website: www.jaypeebrothers.com
Website: www.jaypeedigital.com

© 2023, Jaypee Brothers Medical Publishers

The views and opinions expressed in this book are solely those of the original contributor(s)/author(s) and do not necessarily represent those of editor(s) and publisher of the book.

All rights reserved. No part of this publication may be reproduced, stored or transmitted in any form or by any means, electronic, mechanical, photocopying, recording or otherwise, without the prior permission in writing of the publishers.

All brand names and product names used in this book are trade names, service marks, trademarks or registered trademarks of their respective owners. The publisher is not associated with any product or vendor mentioned in this book.

Medical knowledge and practice change constantly. This book is designed to provide accurate, authoritative information about the subject matter in question. However, readers are advised to check the most current information available on procedures included and check information from the manufacturer of each product to be administered, to verify the recommended dose, formula, method and duration of administration, adverse effects and contraindications. It is the responsibility of the practitioner to take all appropriate safety precautions. Neither the publisher nor the author(s)/editor(s) assume any liability for any injury and/or damage to persons or property arising from or related to use of material in this book.

This book is sold on the understanding that the publisher is not engaged in providing professional medical services. If such advice or services are required, the services of a competent medical professional should be sought.

Every effort has been made where necessary to contact holders of copyright to obtain permission to reproduce copyright material. If any have been inadvertently overlooked, the publisher will be pleased to make the necessary arrangements at the first opportunity.

Inquiries for bulk sales may be solicited at: jaypee@jaypeebrothers.com

*Medical Emergencies in General Practice*

First Edition: 1978;
   Reprinted: 1979
Second Edition: 1981;
   Reprinted: 1981, 1983
Third Edition: 1984;
   Reprinted: 1986
Fourth Edition: 1988;
   Reprinted: 1989, 1990, 1991, 1992
Fifth Edition: 1993;
   Reprinted: 1994, 1996, 1997, 1998

Sixth Edition: 1999;
   Reprinted: 2000, 2001, 2002
Seventh Edition: 2005;
   Reprinted: 2007, 2008
Eighth Edition: 2010;
   Reprinted: 2011
Ninth Edition: 2016

Tenth Edition: **2023**

ISBN: 978-93-5465-663-7

# Dedicated to

My wife, Raj Gupta for her continual help, encouragement and endurance during all these years.
*and*
Generations of students who inspired me to pen down this text.

# Foreword

A simple authoritative book on management of medical emergencies in general practice in India, has been overdue, as the texts available are mostly from sources outside the country and therefore somewhat out of context. Professor Shanti Gupta has done service to the profession by bringing out a very readable and an accurate treatise to guide those who meet the emergencies first. Whether it is the individual doctor or a hospital, emergencies constitute a major challenge which must be met with speed, sympathy and the best science can offer. No book can teach the former two but transmission of latest knowledge is its principal objective which Dr Gupta has achieved with admirable success. My colleagues and I have read the contents with pleasure and Professor Gupta was gracious to accept the minor suggestions we made. I have no doubt this volume does credit to the author and would be of immense benefit to the general practitioners everywhere. The standard of excellence achieved is consistent throughout the book.

**PN Chhuttani**
President, National Academy of Medical Sciences
Director, Postgraduate Institute of
Medical Education and Research
Chandigarh, Punjab, India

# Preface to the Tenth Edition

As we draft this preface to the Tenth edition of *Medical Emergencies in General Practice*, we are reminded of a saying of the famous Canadian physician Sir William Osler "It is astonishing with what little reading one may practice Medicine, but it is not astonishing how badly he may do so." The truth of this saying cannot be overemphasized. To be successful, a physician must have access to a powerhouse of up-to-date knowledge on which he can depend whenever confronted with a medical situation, especially an emergency. The recent COVID-19 pandemic has further highlighted the importance of deft action in the face of medical emergencies. This current edition has been revised with this ideology in mind.

The subject of *Medical Emergencies in General Practice* is not static. All sections have been updated to incorporate major medical advances since the last edition of this book was published six years ago, and a new brief section on frostbite has been added.

Readers may recall that we had thought our ninth edition might be our last, but with their continued encouragement, we are excited to release this tenth edition. We would also like to thank our new publisher Jaypee Brothers Medical Publishers (P) Ltd, New Delhi, who have facilitated nationwide distribution. We hope that this book will be of service as a helpful guide to clinical care for those in the front lines.

**SP Gupta**
**Dinesh K Gupta**

# Preface to the First Edition

*It is astonishing with how little reading a doctor can practice Medicine but it is not astonishing how badly he may do it.*
—*William Osler*

Medical science has advanced so rapidly and so dramatically in the past quarter of a century that it has become virtually impossible for any doctor to remain up-to-date even in one specialty, let alone the entire field of medicine. These advances encompass nearly all aspects of disease process but especially the physiology, biochemistry and microbiology, and have been only matched by breath-taking developments in pharmacology and therapeutics, e.g., the discovery of various antibiotics, corticosteroids, anticancer and antileukemic drugs and various antiarrhythmic measures. The availability of such powerful therapeutic agents has changed the very basis of medical care, and, in fact, the past one decade has seen the emergence of the concepts of "acute medicine" and "intensive care". As a result, the medical treatment has become far more effective, but at the same time also more intricate.

In day-to-day practice, confronted with a complex problem, the busy practitioner may find time to consult literature or his colleagues and thus deliver the goods. However, the position is entirely different in the case of a medical emergency. Here the patient and his relatives expect and the doctor has to provide immediately the very best in medical care, as far as possible. This requires the practitioner of modern medicine to possess, besides many other virtues, an up-to-date knowledge of all aspects of various emergencies, and hence scope of such a book.

Several books are already available which describe, in varying detail, management of medical emergencies. Almost all of them are, however, by Western authors and do not emphasize the medical problems encountered in tropical countries, nor take into consideration the great odds (except perhaps in big cities) against which the general practitioner has to work in this country, e.g., lack of facilities for even simple investigations such as blood urea, blood sugar and cerebrospinal fluid examination, not to speak of estimation of electrolytes and blood gases which are seldom available even in some of the teaching hospitals.

The present book has been written primarily for the generalist and aims to provide him the principles of management of common medical emergencies in as much as may be possible for him to carry out without the help of elaborate investigations and sophisticated equipment. However, the therapeutic potential of the latter has been briefly mentioned so that the reader is kept well informed and can discharge his responsibilities creditably when confronted with an emergency. If this book helps him in this regard even in a small measure, it would have served its purpose.

While I have naturally put in my best in writing this book, it is likely to have shortcomings, for which I seek the kind indulgence of my medical brethren. It is my sincere hope that readers will send their valuable suggestions which will help the book to grow in its utility, if not in weight.

**SP Gupta**
**Dinesh K Gupta**

# Acknowledgments

It is a pleasure to record my gratitude to Dr PN Chhuttani, President, National Academy of Medical Sciences of India, and Director, Postgraduate Institute Medical Education and Research, Chandigarh, Punjab, India, for graciously consenting to write a foreword for this book.

A large number of my colleagues and friends have kindly reviewed different chapters of this book. Among them, particular mention must be made of Dr MMS Ahuja, Professor and Head, Department of Medicine, All India Institute of Medical Sciences, New Delhi (assisted by Dr Bhatnagar); Dr KD Gupta, Professor, Department of Medicine and Principal, Medical College, Bikaner, Rajasthan; Dr PL Wahi, Professor, Department of Cardiology and Head, Department of Medicine, Postgraduate Institute of Medical Education and Research, Chandigarh; Dr PS Gupta, Professor and Head, Department of Medicine, Maulana Azad Medical College, New Delhi; Dr SS Jolly, Professor and Head, Department of Medicine, Medical College, Patiala Punjab; Dr NS Pathania, Professor, Department of Medicine and Principal, Medical College, Jammu; and Dr SC Srivastva, Professor, Department of Medicine, Medical College, Rohtak, Haryana. I am obliged to all of them for sparing so much of their valuable time.

I am also grateful to Dr KC Malhotra and Dr BC Bansal, Associate Professors in Department of Medicine, and Dr JS Chopra, Reader in Department of Medicine, Medical College, Rohtak, for going through certain sections of a few chapters. In the end I would like to express my thanks to Dr Sri Bhagwan, Lecturer, and Dr Rajinder Garg, Registrar in my Department, for their reading and correcting the manuscript several times.

Last but not the least, I am very grateful to the whole team of M/s Jaypee Brothers Medical Publishers (P) Ltd, New Delhi, India, who helped and guided me, Shri Jitendar P Vij (Group Chairman), Mr Ankit Vij (Managing Director), Mr MS Mani (Group President), Dr Madhu Choudhary (Director–Educational Publishing), Ms Pooja Bhandari (Production Head), Ms Sunita Katla (Executive Assistant to Group Chairman and Publishing Manager), Ms Samina Khan (Executive Assistant to Director–Educational Publishing), Dr Aditya Tayal (Team Lead—UG Publishing), Mr Rajesh Sharma (Production Coordinator), Ms Seema Dogra (Cover Visualizer), Ms Geeta Barik (Proofreader), Mr Akshay Thakur (Typesetter), Mr Radhe Shyam (Graphic Designer) and their team members, for all their support to work in this project and make it a success. Without their cooperation, we could not have completed this project.

# Contents

**Chapter 1: Cardiovascular Emergencies**   1

- Pain in Chest  *1*
- Ischemic Heart Disease  *5*
- Acute Myocardial Infarction  *10*
- Non-ST-Elevated Myocardial Infarction (NSTEMI) and Unstable Angina (UA)  *29*
- Heart Failure  *33*
- Acute Pulmonary Edema  *35*
- Cardiogenic Shock  *39*
- Pulmonary Embolism  *45*
- Hypertensive Crisis  *51*
- Hypertensive Emergency  *51*
- Cardiac Arrhythmias  *55*
- Antiarrhythmic Agents  *56*
- Tachyarrhythmias  *60*
- Bradyarrhythmias  *74*
- Stokes–Adams Syndrome  *77*
- Sudden Cardiac Death and Cardiac Arrest  *79*
- Acute Cardiac Tamponade  *84*
- Appendix  *86*

**Chapter 2: Respiratory Emergencies**   88

- Life-threatening Hemoptysis  *88*
- Foreign Body Airway Obstruction  *91*
- Acute Severe Bronchial Asthma  *93*
- Spontaneous Pneumothorax  *101*
- Acute Severe Pneumonia  *104*
- Pneumonia in Immunocompromised Patients  *112*
- Respiratory Failure  *113*
- Acute Respiratory Distress Syndrome  *118*

**Chapter 3: Gastrointestinal Emergencies**   123

- Acute Vomiting  *123*
- Acute Diarrheal Diseases  *124*
- Gastrointestinal Perforation  *128*

- Acute Gastrointestinal Bleeding   *129*
- Lower Gastrointestinal Bleeding   *135*
- Acute Hepatic Failure   *137*
- Acute Pancreatitis   *146*

## Chapter 4: Neurological Emergencies — 153

- Acute Confusional State   *153*
- The Unconscious Patient   *157*
- Cerebrovascular Catastrophes (Stroke)   *164*
- Ischemic Stroke   *167*
- Hemorrhagic Stroke   *173*
- Hypertensive Encephalopathy   *179*
- Cerebral Venous Thrombosis   *181*
- Acute Bacterial (Pyogenic) Meningitis   *182*
- Tubercular Meningitis   *188*
- Aseptic Meningitis   *191*
- Acute Viral Encephalitis   *192*
- Seizures   *194*
- Status Epilepticus   *197*
- Acute Headache   *199*
- Migraine   *201*
- Cluster Headache   *203*
- Acute Vertigo   *204*

## Chapter 5: Renal Emergencies — 207

- Clinical Fluid, Electrolyte, and Acid-base Abnormalities   *207*
- Sodium Abnormalities   *207*
- Potassium Abnormalities   *210*
- Calcium Abnormalities   *215*
- Metabolic Acidosis   *222*
- Metabolic Alkalosis   *224*
- Respiratory Acidosis   *226*
- Respiratory Alkalosis   *226*
- Acute Renal Failure   *228*

## Chapter 6: Hematological Emergencies — 241

- Classification   *241*
- Severe Anemia   *241*
- Hemostatic Disorders   *247*
- Platelet Disorders   *248*

- Henoch–Schonlein Purpura (Anaphylactoid Purpura) *254*
- Hemophilia *255*
- Disseminated Intravascular Coagulation *259*
- Neutropenia *261*

## Chapter 7: Endocrinal and Metabolic Emergencies 263

- Thyroid Gland *263*
- Thyroid Crisis ("Storm") *263*
- Thyroid-associated Ophthalmopathy *266*
- Thyrotoxic Hypokalemic Periodic Paralysis *267*
- Myxedema Coma *268*
- Acute Adrenocortical Insufficiency *270*
- Diabetic Coma *272*
- Hyperosmolar Hyperglycemic Nonketotic Coma *279*
- Lactic Acidosis *282*
- Hypoglycemia *284*
- Acute Gouty Arthritis *287*

## Chapter 8: Emergencies in Infectious and Tropical Diseases 290

- Dengue Fever *290*
- Chikungunya Fever *293*
- Ebola Virus Disease *295*
- Influenza A: Virus Infection *296*
- Leptospirosis *297*
- Enteric (Typhoid) Fever *301*
- Cholera *303*
- Mumps *305*
- Tetanus *307*
- Rabies *310*
- Malaria *314*
- Cerebral Malaria *319*
- Amebiasis *322*
- Amebic Liver Abscess *322*
- Coronavirus Disease (COVID-2019) *325*

## Chapter 9: Acute Poisoning 326

- Principles of Management *326*
- Sedative-hypnotic Toxicity *329*
- Salicylate Poisoning *330*
- Acute Opiate Poisoning *332*

- Carbon Monoxide Poisoning  *333*
- Acute Alcoholic (Ethanol) Intoxication  *335*
- Acute Withdrawal (Abstinence) Syndrome  *336*
- Methyl Alcohol (Methanol) Poisoning  *337*
- Corrosive Poisoning  *338*
- Snake Bite Poisoning  *339*
- Insecticide (Pesticide) Poisoning  *342*
- Carbamate Insecticides  *346*
- Aluminum Phosphide Poisoning  *348*
- Less Common Types of Poisoning  *351*

## Chapter 10: Iatrogenic Emergencies — 356

- Procedure-related Emergencies  *356*
- Intravenous Infusion related Emergencies  *359*
- Drug Interactions and Drug-induced Emergencies  *363*

## Chapter 11: Shock Syndrome and Critical Allergic Reactions — 376

- Shock Syndrome  *376*
- Septic Shock  *382*
- Critical Allergic Reactions  *387*

## Chapter 12: Environmental Emergencies — 391

*Acute Heat Reactions*  *391*
- Heat Edema  *391*
- Heat Syncope  *392*
- Heat Cramps  *392*
- Heat Exhaustion  *392*

*Heat Stroke and Heat Hyperpyrexia*  *393*
- Heat Hyperpyrexia  *393*
- Heat Stroke  *394*

*Hypothermia*  *398*

*Medical Emergencies in the Air*  *400*
- Adverse Effects of Altitude Hypoxia  *401*
- Adverse Effects of Pressure Changes  *402*

*Near Drowning*  *404*

*Electrical Injuries*  *406*

*High Altitude Sickness*  *407*

*Frostbite*  *409*

## Chapter 13: Miscellaneous Emergencies — 410

- Generalized Anxiety and Panic Disorders  *410*
- Syncope  *415*
- Prophylactic Immunization in Infectious Diseases  *419*
- General  *422*
- Appendix  *422*

*Index*  425

# Competency Table

| Number | COMPETENCY<br>The student should be able to: | Chapter Number | Page Number |
|---|---|---|---|
| IM2.5 | Define the various acute coronary syndromes and describe their evolution, natural history and outcomes | 1 | 5 |
| IM2.8 | Generate document and present a differential diagnosis based on the clinical presentation and prioritise based on "cannot miss", most likely diagnosis and severity | 1 | 5 |
| IM2.9 | Distinguish and differentiate between stable and unstable angina and AMI based on the clinical presentation | 1 | 10 |
| IM2.15 | Discuss and describe the medications used in patients with an acute coronary syndrome based on the clinical presentation | 1 | 16 |
| PE28.8 | Discuss the types, clinical presentation, and management of foreign body aspiration in infants and children | 2 | 91 |
| PH1.32 | Describe the mechanism/s of action, types, doses, side effects, indications and contraindications of drugs used in bronchial asthma and COPD | 2 | 93 |
| PE28.19 | Describe the etiopathogenesis, diagnosis, clinical features, management and prevention of asthma in children | 2 | 93, 98 |
| SU17.10 | Demonstrate airway maintenance. Recognize and manage tension pneumothorax, hemothorax and flail chest in simulated environment. | 2 | 101 |
| IM3.3 | Discuss and describe the pathogenesis, presentation, natural history and complications of pneumonia | 2 | 104 |
| IM3.2 | Discuss and describe the etiologies of various kinds of pneumonia and their microbiology depending on the setting and immune status of the host | 2 | 112 |
| MI3.2 | Identify the common etiologic agents of diarrhea and dysentery | 3 | 124 |
| IM15.1 | Enumerate, describe and discuss the etiology of upper and lower GI bleeding | 3 | 128 |
| IM15.10 | Enumerate the indications for endoscopy, colonoscopy and other imaging procedures in the investigation of upper GI bleeding | 3 | 129 |
| IM5.2 | Describe and discuss the etiology and pathophysiology of liver injury | 3 | 137 |
| IM5.3 | Describe and discuss the pathologic changes in various forms of liver disease | 3 | 137 |

## Competency Table

| Number | COMPETENCY<br>The student should be able to: | Chapter Number | Page Number |
|---|---|---|---|
| IM5.6 | Describe and discuss the pathophysiology, clinical evolution and complications of cirrhosis and portal hypertension including ascites, spontaneous bacterial peritonitis, hepatorenal syndrome and hepatic encephalopathy | 3 | 140 |
| IM5.16 | Describe and discuss the management of hepatitis, cirrhosis, portal hypertension, ascites spontaneous, bacterial peritonitis and hepatic encephalopathy | 3 | 140 |
| SU24.1 | Describe the clinical features, principles of investigation, prognosis and management of pancreatitis | 3 | 146 |
| IM24.3 | Describe and discuss the etiopathogenesis, clinical presentation, identification, functional changes, acute care, stabilization, management and rehabilitation of acute confusional states | 4 | 153 |
| AS7.3 | Observe and describe the management of an unconscious patient | 4,13 | 157, 415 |
| IM18.2 | Classify cerebrovascular accidents and describe the etiology, predisposing genetic and risk factors pathogenesis of hemorrhagic and non hemorrhagic stroke | 4 | 164 |
| IM18.14 | Describe the initial management of a hemorrhagic stroke | 4 | 173 |
| IM18.15 | Enumerate the indications for surgery in a hemorrhagic stroke | 4 | 173 |
| PA35.1 | Describe the etiology, types and pathogenesis, differentiating factors, CSF findings in meningitis | 4 | 182 |
| IM17.13 | Describe the pharmacology, dose, adverse reactions and regimens of drugs used in the treatment of bacterial, tubercular and viral meningitis | 4 | 182 |
| IM17.10 | Enumerate the indications for emergency care admission and immediate supportive care in patients with headache | 4 | 199 |
| IM17.3 | Classify migraine and describe the distinguishing features between classical and nonclassical forms of migraine | 4 | 201 |
| IM22.5 | Enumerate the causes and describe the clinical features and the correct approach to the diagnosis and management of the patient with hyponatremia | 5 | 207 |
| IM22.6 | Enumerate the causes and describe the clinical and laboratory features and the correct approach to the diagnosis and management of the patient with hyponatremia | 5 | 208 |
| IM22.7 | Enumerate the causes and describe the clinical and laboratory features and the correct approach to the diagnosis and management of the patient with hypokalemia | 5 | 211 |
| IM22.8 | Enumerate the causes and describe the clinical and laboratory features and the correct approach to the diagnosis and management of the patient with hyperkalemia | 5 | 212 |

# Competency Table

| Number | COMPETENCY<br>The student should be able to: | Chapter Number | Page Number |
|---|---|---|---|
| IM22.9 | Enumerate the causes and describe the clinical and laboratory features of metabolic acidosis | 5 | 222 |
| IM22.10 | Enumerate the causes of describe the clinical and laboratory features of metabolic alkalosis | 5 | 224 |
| IM22.11 | Enumerate the causes and describe the clinical and laboratory features of respiratory acidosis | 5 | 226 |
| IM22.12 | Enumerate the causes and describe the clinical and laboratory features of respiratory alkalosis | 5 | 226 |
| IM10.2 | Classify, describe and differentiate the pathophysiologic causes of acute renal failure | 5 | 228 |
| IM9.2 | Describe and discuss the morphological characteristics, etiology and prevalence of each of the causes of anemia | 6 | 241 |
| IM9.12 | Describe, develop a diagnostic plan to determine the etiology of anemia | 6 | 241 |
| PA21.3 | Differentiate platelet from clotting disorders based on the clinical and hematologic features | 6 | 247 |
| PA21.4 | Define and describe disseminated intravascular coagulation, its laboratory findings and diagnosis of disseminated intravascular coagulation | 6 | 259 |
| PA21.5 | Define and describe disseminated intravascular coagulation its laboratory findings and diagnosis of vitamin K deficiency | 6 | 259 |
| IM12.5 | Elicit document and present an appropriate history that will establish the diagnosis cause of thyroid dysfunction and its severity | 7 | 264 |
| IM12.6 | Perform and demonstrate a systematic examination based on the history that will help establish the diagnosis and severity including systemic signs of thyrotoxicosis and hypothyroidism, palpation of the pulse for rate and rhythm abnormalities, neck palpation of the thyroid and lymph nodes and cardiovascular findings | 7 | 264 |
| PA32.7 | Describe the etiology, pathogenesis, manifestations, laboratory, morphologic features, complications of la insufficiency | 7 | 270 |
| IM11.6 | Describe and discuss the pathogenesis and precipitating factors, recognition and management of diabetic emergencies | 7 | 272 |
| IM11.14 | Recognize the presentation of hypoglycemia and outline the principles on its therapy | 7 | 284 |
| PM4.1 | Describe the common patterns, clinical features, investigations, diagnosis and treatment of common causes of arthritis | 7 | 287 |

## Competency Table

| Number | COMPETENCY<br>The student should be able to: | Chapter Number | Page Number |
|---|---|---|---|
| IM4.3 | Discuss and describe the common causes, pathophysiology and manifestations of fever in various regions in India including bacterial, parasitic and viral causes (e.g., dengue, chikungunya, typhus) | 8 | 290, 293, 295, 296, 297, 301, 305 |
| IM25.1 | Describe and discuss the response and the influence of host immune status, risk factors and comorbidities on zoonotic diseases (e.g., leptospirosis, rabies) and non-febrile infectious disease (e.g., tetanus) | 8 | 298 |
| MI3.3 | Describe the enteric fever pathogens and discuss the evolution of the clinical course, the laboratory diagnosis of the diseases caused by them | 8 | 301 |
| MI3.4 | Identify the different modalities for diagnosis of enteric fever. Choose the appropriate test related to the duration of illness | 8 | 301 |
| MI3.1 | Enumerate the microbial agents causing diarrhea and dysentery. Describe the epidemiology, morphology, pathogenesis, clinical features, and diagnostic modalities of these agents | 8 | 303 |
| IM25.1 | Describe and discuss the response and the influence of host immune status, risk factors and comorbidities on zoonotic diseases (e.g., leptospirosis, rabies) and non-febrile infectious disease (e.g., tetanus) | 8 | 307, 310 |
| IM4.6 | Discuss and describe the pathophysiology and manifestations of malaria | 8 | 314 |
| IM4.23 | Prescribe drugs for malaria based on the species identified, prevalence of drug resistance and national programs | 8 | 314 |
| PH1.47 | Describe the mechanisms of action, types, doses, side effects, indications and contraindications of the drugs used in malaria, kala azar, amebiasis and intestinal helminthiasis | 9 | 322 |
| IM21.1 | Describe the initial approach to the stabilization of the patient who presents with poisoning | 9 | 326 |
| FM10.1 | Describe general principles and basic methodologies in treatment of poisoning: decontamination, supportive therapy, antidote therapy, procedures of enhanced elimination with regard to:<br>• Antipyretics: Paracetamol, salicylates<br>• Anti-infectives (common antibiotics–an overview)<br>• Neuropsychotoxicology barbiturates, benzodiazepines, phenytoin, lithium, haloperidol, neuroleptics, tricyclics<br>• Narcotic analgesics, anesthetics, and muscle relaxants<br>• Cardiovascular toxicology cardiotoxic plants—oleander, odollam, aconite, digitalis<br>• Gastro-Intestinal and Endocrinal Drugs—insulin | 9 | 329, 330, 351 |

| Number | COMPETENCY<br>The student should be able to: | Chapter Number | Page Number |
|---|---|---|---|
| FM9.6 | Describe general principles and basic methodologies in treatment of poisoning: decontamination, supportive therapy, antidote therapy, procedures of enhanced elimination with regard to ammonia, carbon monoxide, hydrogen cyanide and derivatives, methyl isocyanate, tear (riot control) gases | 9 | 333 |
| FM9.4 | Describe general principles and basic methodologies in treatment of poisoning: decontamination, supportive therapy, antidote therapy, procedures of enhanced elimination with regard to ethanol, methanol, ethylene glycol | 9 | 335 |
| PH1.21 | Describe the symptoms and management of methanol and ethanol poisonings | 9 | 335, 337 |
| IM21.3 | Enumerate the common corrosives used in your area and describe their toxicology, clinical features, prognosis and approach to therapy | 9 | 338 |
| IM20.1 | Enumerate the local poisonous snakes and describe the distinguishing marks of each | 9 | 339 |
| IM20.3 | Describe the initial approach to the stabilization of the patient who presents with snake bite | 9 | 339 |
| IM20.7 | Enumerate the indications and describe the pharmacology, dose, adverse reactions, hypersensitivity reactions of antisnake venom | 9 | 339 |
| FM9.5 | Describe general principles and basic methodologies in treatment of poisoning: decontamination, supportive therapy, antidote therapy, procedures of enhanced elimination with regard to organophosphates, carbamates, organochlorines, pyrethroids, paraquat, aluminium and zinc phosphide | 9 | 342, 346, 348 |
| FM12.1 | Describe features and management of abuse/poisoning with following camicals: tobacco, cannabis, amphetamines, cocaine, hallucinogens, designer drugs and solvent | 9 | 351 |
| PS8.1 | Enumerate and describe the magnitude and etiology of anxiety disorders | 13 | 410 |
| PS8.2 | Enumerate, elicit, describe and document clinical features in patients with anxiety disorders | 13 | 410 |
| PS9.2 | Enumerate, elicit, describe and document clinical features in patients with stress related disorders | 13 | 410 |
| PS9.4 | Describe the treatment of stress related disorders including behavioral and psychosocial therapy | | 410 |

# CHAPTER 1

# Cardiovascular Emergencies

## ■ PAIN IN CHEST

Pain in chest is one of the most frequent complaints for which medical attention is sought. Its intensity may vary in different clinical states as well as intra-individually, since pain is more of a perception, and reaction to that perception, than a sensation. Little correlation may therefore exist between the severity of chest pain and the gravity of illness. The concern is heightened by the fact that coronary artery disease (CAD) is always a possibility in such cases.

### Etiology

Because of common/overlapping neural pathways, many conditions, both cardiac and extracardiac, can result in chest pain. **Cardiac pain is mediated through upper five thoracic ganglia and spinal roots,** but ramifications from adjoining spinal roots always exist. Therefore, pain in the chest may originate from any organ/structure in thorax and upper abdomen innervated through lower cervical to D6 or D7 spinal roots.

### Evaluation of Chest Pain

In analyzing chest pain, **clinical history** holds the key to the problem. In the first place it should be determined whether the chest pain is—(1) acute, short-lived, or ongoing, (2) recurrent/episodic, or (3) persistent, sometimes for days and weeks. As in any other case of pain, clinical details are required with regard to:

- Site of pain, localized or diffuse, with radiation, if any
- Intensity and character of pain
- Precipitating and relieving factors
- Any relationship with meals/posture, and
- Any effect of local pressure, or variation with breathing, coughing, and movements of cervical spine and shoulder joints.

In general, it can be stated that *chest pain or discomfort is unlikely to be due to CAD, if*—(1) it is localized to the region of or under the left nipple, or in the skin and soft tissues, (2) it is localized to a small area (less than 2-3 cm) since anginal pain, like any visceral pain, tends to be diffuse, (3) it is chronic and persistent or recurring and momentary, (4) the chest pain is sharp, pricking, or stabbing in type, or varies with posture, breathing, and coughing, and (5) chest pain has been present for several hours but is not accompanied by appropriate electrocardiogram (ECG) changes.

## Differential Diagnosis

As many clinical details of chest pain should be inquired as possible. In fact interrogation in different form and phrase should be continued as far as time permits, until it becomes reasonably clear whether the chest pain is cardiac or non-cardiac in nature. This is the most cost-effective method of evaluating chest pain. Some typical features of important causes of chest pain are:

### Cardiac Conditions

- **Coronary artery disease:** Since *heart is embryologically a midline organ,* typical coronary pain is felt more often in the substernal region or across the chest rather than in the cardiac or left breast region. However, it may be felt only on the left side or less commonly, even on the right side of chest. It radiates classically to the left shoulder and medial side of left upper arm but may be felt in any part of the territory innervated by D1–5 and neighboring spinal segments including lower jaw, any part of left or right arm including wrist, interscapular region, and epigastrium.
  
  The **duration of anginal pain** is counted usually in minutes (and not seconds). Prolonged pain implies unstable angina (UA) or myocardial infarction (MI). The **character of pain** is usually described as choking (angina means "choking", not pain), constricting, squeezing, piercing, or burning in type. Often it is felt only as a sensation of heaviness or weight in the middle of chest or across the chest. Leading questions are often required to elicit the character and quality of pain, which may sometimes be expressed not so much by words as by gestures such as clenching the fist in front of the sternum or by placing the palm of the hand on the middle of chest across sternum. On the other hand, chest pain/discomfort, which is momentary, has a sharp stabbing or bursting character, or is described as a flying or sinking sensation, is unlikely to be angina.
  
  Anginal pain is typically **precipitated** by any activity, which increases cardiac workload and is **relieved** by rest and sublingual nitroglycerine. Such activities include hurried walking, climbing several flight of stairs, or going up an incline especially on full stomach and/or while carrying some load, e.g., a brief case. Smoking a cigarette, cold weather, strong emotions, or stressful situations are some other precipitating factors. Sometimes anginal pain is felt in the initial phase of walking but subsides with continued walking **(walk-through angina).** Anginal pain occurring at rest or increasing in frequency/duration with less and less exertion suggests UA.

- **Other cardiac (noncoronary) causes:**
  - *Pericarditis:* Most of the pericardium is insensitive to pain, and therefore, pain in pericarditis generally implies involvement of adjacent parietal pleura. This is more likely to occur in conditions associated

with pericardial inflammation (e.g., tuberculosis and rheumatic fever) rather than when pericardial involvement is localized (as in uremia or MI). ***Pericardial pain therefore often has pleural characteristics*** such as—(1) pain may be felt anywhere in areas ranging from neck and shoulder to abdomen and back, though typically it is retrosternal, (2) it aggravates with coughing, deep breathing, chest movements, and posture. Occasionally, pericardial pain recurs or persists as localized dull ache resembling MI, but is not associated with ECG changes of cardiac ischemia.
- *Pulmonary embolism (PE):* Chest pain in such cases is due either to sudden acute distension of the pulmonary artery or involvement of pleura adjacent to the area of pulmonary infarction. The former is generally retrosternal, and the latter more lateral, often with pleural characteristics. Associated features may include dyspnea, tachycardia, cough, and hemoptysis.
- *Less common cardiac causes:* These include aortic dissection, aneurysm of thoracic aorta, and severe aortic stenosis. Each of these conditions has its own clinical features. Their discussion is beyond the scope of this text.

## *Noncardiac Conditions*

- ❖ **Gastrointestinal disorders:**
  - *Esophageal disorders:* These are common causes of chest pain, which may mimic or coexist with angina pectoris.
  
    The mechanism is through either esophagitis (with or without acid reflux) or esophageal motility disorders. The differentiation from ischemic pain may be difficult as both share many common features, such as location (retrosternal), radiation, and duration of pain. To confound matters, both ischemic and esophageal pain may be relieved by sublingual nitroglycerine. However, chest pain/discomfort is more likely to be esophageal, if—(1) located in epigastrium or lower sternal region, (2) it has a burning character, often described as "heartburn", (3) the discomfort is related to meals, varies with posture (increases on lying down), and is associated with dysphagia, (4) the chest pain becomes worse after certain foods (e.g., alcohol, coffee, spices, fried food), and is relieved with milk and antacids, and (5) chest pain is intermittent, waxes, and wanes, and lasts for several hours.
    
    When doubt persist esophageal studies by endoscopy, barium meal, or pH monitoring in distal esophagus may prove useful. However, it should be recognized that both CAD and esophageal disorders are common and may coexist. Therefore, in all doubtful cases, CAD should be evaluated by appropriate studies.
  - *Other abdominal diseases:* Many other upper abdominal disorders (e.g., peptic ulcer, biliary disease, and pancreatitis) can produce moderate or severe pain in epigastrium and/or right hypochondrium, which may radiate upward into the chest and precordium. Usually however,

these disorders have their own characteristic features, which coupled with appropriate investigations make it possible to arrive at a correct diagnosis. Persistence of pain for several hours without ECG changes will further suggest that pain is noncoronary in origin.

- ❖ **Musculoskeletal disorders:**
  - *Costochondritis:* Chest pain of costochondritis is accompanied by tenderness over sternum or costochondral junctions, most often at the second and third on the left side. In some cases, there may be associated swelling of the costochondral junctions (Tietze syndrome). The pain is usually localized, sharp, may be pricking or stabbing in character, and increases with breathing, coughing, and chest wall movements. Costochondritis is sometimes a manifestation of phobic anxiety.
  - *Radiculopathy:* The pain of radiculopathy may be more difficult to differentiate from coronary pain; since it may be felt not only in the neck but also in the left upper chest, shoulder, and left arm (lower cervical and upper thoracic roots are involved as in anginal pain). Unlike angina, however, the pain is usually persistent, is related to movements of neck (and not physical exertion) and is often shooting in character. There may be accompanying sensory deficit or areas of hyperalgesia. A proper history, relevant examination of neck and shoulder regions, and suitable radiological studies usually clear the issue.
- ❖ **Psychogenic chest pain:** Pain in precordial region is not uncommon in states of anxiety and emotional instability (neurocirculatory asthenia or **Da Costa** syndrome). It is usually localized to a small area of cardiac apex but may be felt anywhere in the mammary and inframammary regions. Functional pain often presents as a dull ache on which are superimposed episodes of sharp pricking pain lasting only a few seconds, and sometimes associated with precordial tenderness. It is not related to exertion, and may be relieved spontaneously or by nonspecific measures such as rest, local pressure, or massage, and tranquilizers. Other symptoms of anxiety such as palpitation, paresthesia, sighing, and dizziness often coexist.

## Associated Symptoms

Symptoms accompanying chest pain should be inquired in detail since these can provide valuable clues in diagnosis. The most ominous is ***profuse sweating*** which points towards a catastrophic event such as acute MI (AMI), PE, or aortic dissection. *Associated dyspnea,* especially when accompanied by chest pain and perspiration will suggest either left heart failure complicating MI or pulmonary conditions such as pneumothorax, PE, or even massive pneumonia. Some cases of chest pain have accompanying ***nausea and/or vomiting or belching.*** Such symptoms ordinarily suggest upper abdominal disorders but may also occur in acute coronary syndrome (ACS). *Fever* at onset is not a feature in acute CAD and its presence will suggest an inflammatory process such as pneumonia, pleurisy, or pericarditis. On the other hand when ***multiple nonspecific symptoms*** such as hyperventilation, sighing respiration, paresthesia, dizziness, and fainting are present, the chest pain is usually psychogenic in nature.

## Diagnosis

As already stated, pain or discomfort in chest is a common presenting symptom in clinical practice, and can be due to a large number of conditions of which important ones have been discussed already. A ***good clinical history*** is the most valuable tool in making a correct diagnosis. The emphasis should be always on differentiating pain of CAD from noncoronary causes of chest pain. However, it is important to realize that the two are not mutually exclusive. The problem is compounded by the fact that CAD may present with features other than pain, such as dyspnea, fainting, fatigue, perspiration, and a feeling of "indigestion", gas, and belching (angina equivalents). However, when due to CAD, such features are episodic and short lived and have triggering and relieving factors similar to anginal pain. Proper evaluation in such cases may require detailed studies—cardiologic, radiologic, and upper gastrointestinal endoscopy. Their discussion is beyond the scope of this text.

# ISCHEMIC HEART DISEASE

Ischemic heart disease (IHD) presents either as stable angina pectoris (due to chronic CAD) or as ACS. The latter encompasses all acute phases of (IHD), i.e., UA, non-ST-Elevated MI ***(NSTEMI),*** and ST-Elevated MI ***(STEMI).*** Introduced during last decade of the previous century, the term "ACS" is now commonly employed to cover all cases of IHD presenting with acute chest pain, at rest or on minimal exertion.

## Acute Coronary Syndrome

The term "Acute Coronary Syndrome" encompasses all acute phases of coronary heart disease (CHD), which usually present with acute chest pain at rest or on minimal exertion.

### *Pathogenesis*

As already stated, most of such cases have a common presentation with acute chest pain of presumed coronary origin. Pathologically also there is a common mechanism in most of such cases in that inflammatory and certain other processes render ***some atheromatous plaques vulnerable to rupture,*** and thus unstable **(Fig. 1.1)**. This understanding forms the basis of management of ACS. Clinical consequences of such changes in plaque morphology (compounded by platelet aggregation and chemical mediator-induced vasoconstriction) can vary from UA through non-Q-wave MI to Q-wave type AMI, and sudden ischemic death. All these states in fact present a continuum of the disease process characterized by ***an abrupt reduction in coronary flow.*** This is in contrast to patients with stable CAD in whom angina usually

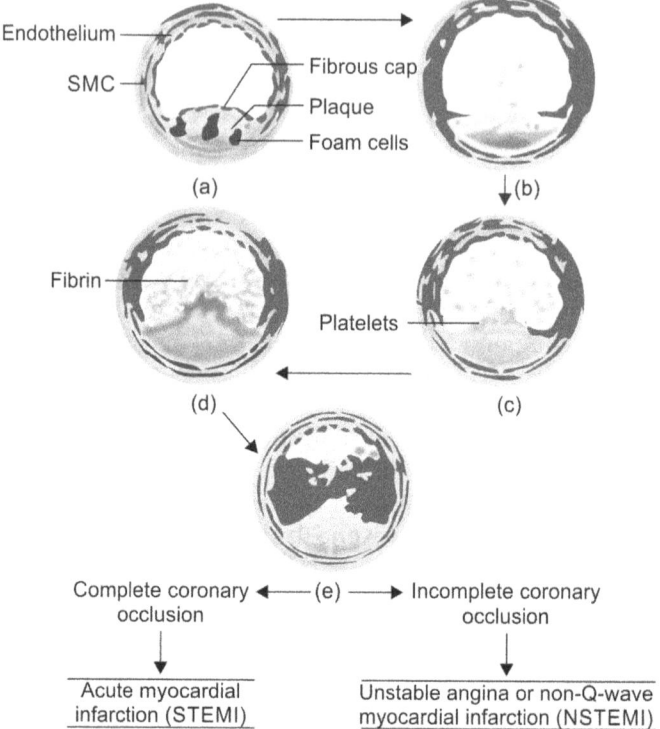

**Fig. 1.1:** Pathogenesis of acute coronary syndrome. (a) Vulnerable plaque with large eccentric lipid-rich pool with foam cell infiltration, and thin fibrous cap; (b) plaque rupture; (c) platelet activation, adhesion, and aggregation; (d) conversion of fibrinogen to fibrin; and (e) thrombus formation.
(SMC: smooth muscle cells)

results from increase in myocardial oxygen demand (e.g., on exertion) that exceeds the ability of the stenosed coronary arteries to increase its delivery. The atheromatous disease including plaques is generally stable in such cases so that acute reductions in coronary blood flow, and thereby, acute ischemic events do not occur.

### Pathophysiology

In most of the acute ischemic episodes, formation of an **intraluminal thrombus** at the site of plaque disruption is central to the initiation of pathology, and it is the subsequent behavior of this thrombus and associated local factors that determine the pattern of ACS. Three broad patterns are recognized. Their differential features are given at **Table 1.1 and Flowchart 1.1**.

- ❖ **ST-segment Elevated MI (STEMI):** Such cases usually present with persistent ST-segment elevation, and result from an intraluminal thrombus, which is **completely occlusive,** fixed, and persistent. Consequently, there is abrupt cessation of myocardial perfusion resulting in necrosis of the involved myocardium. Most of these cases develop Q-waves in the ECG

## Chapter 1: Cardiovascular Emergencies

**Table 1.1:** Diagnosis of acute coronary syndrome.

| Parameter | ST-elevated MI | Non-ST-elevated MI | Unstable angina |
|---|---|---|---|
| ECG<br><br>S-T segment<br>T-waves | Elevated (Persistent)<br><br>Inverted ↑ | Depressed<br><br>Inverted ↑ | Depressed or slightly elevated (transitory)<br>Poor/inverted ↑ |
| Cardiac enzymes<br>CPK (MB)<br>-Troponins | Present | Present | Normal or slightly absent |

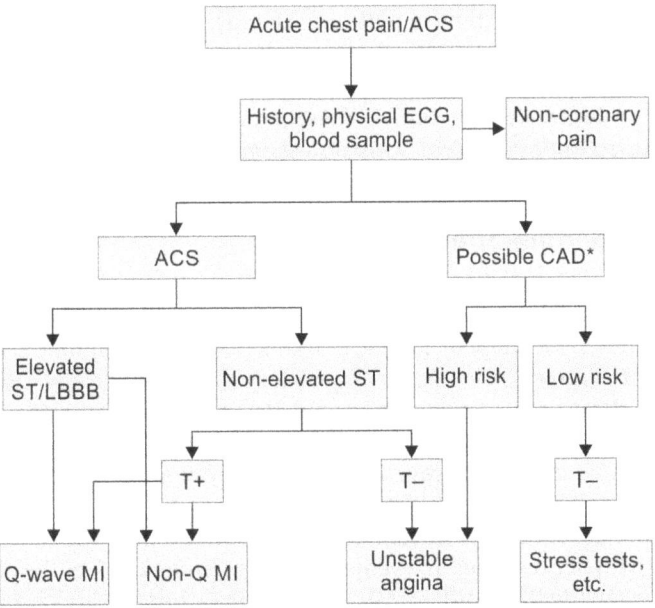

**Flowchart 1.1:** Diagnostic evaluation of acute chest pain and acute coronary syndrome (ACS).

(CAD: coronary artery disease; T: troponins)

during the next 12–24 hours, and hence these cases are also termed as **"Q-wave MI"**. A small proportion may, however, develop only non-Q wave MI.

❖ **Non-ST-segment Elevated MI:** Such cases present without ST elevation, and are usually due to **sub-occlusive intraluminal thrombus.** A few cases may develop complete occlusion but such patients have either good distal collaterals, or the occlusion is soon followed by spontaneous reperfusion and resolution of vasospasm. These factors limit the duration of myocardial ischemia and prevent extensive necrosis. **ECG changes** generally comprise ST-segment depression of at least 1 mm and T-wave inversion >0.1 mV in two consecutive leads. Serum cardiac markers are usually detectable since variable degree of myocardial necrosis does occur in such cases.

- **Unstable angina:** This is a heterogeneous group in which alterations in coronary perfusion may result from one or more of the following mechanisms:
  - Plaque rupture or erosion leading to *superimposed thrombus, which is usually sub-occlusive. This is sometimes intermittent,* so that there may be single or recurrent episodes of angina. This is believed to be the most common cause of UA. The thrombus often undergoes spontaneous lysis.
  - There may be only dynamic obstruction due to coronary spasm.
  - In a few cases, UA may result not so much from intraluminal events and coronary vasospasm, but from a transient increase in myocardial oxygen demand as in tachyarrhythmias, sudden increase in blood pressure, or unaccustomed exercise especially on a full stomach.

  In view of such a diverse pathophysiology, the clinical picture is often variable, which accounts for a variety of terminology used earlier to describe UA, e.g., *intermediate syndrome, acute coronary insufficiency, crescendo angina, preinfarction angina.* All these patterns of myocardial ischemia are now grouped under the term **"Unstable Angina".** If the thrombus progresses to complete occlusion it may end up in AMI.

### *Evaluation and Risk Stratification*

As soon as a patient with ACS is identified, a quick history should be taken, relevant physical examination conducted, an ECG recorded, and blood samples drawn for study of cardiac markers (especially troponins) and other traditional coronary risk factors. The history should especially include—(a) nature of chest pain/anginal symptoms, (b) previous history of CAD, heart failure, diabetes or hypertension, (c) earlier admission (s) for ACS, (d) previous medication, and (e) prior revascularization procedures, if any. As soon as possible an echocardiogram should also be done.

On the basis of such information, it should be possible to risk stratify patients with acute ischemic events into those *at high risk* of developing an adverse event (death, non-fatal MI, or recurrent ischemia), and those who are at a *relatively low risk* for such complications. Such an approach is helpful in designing therapy in ACS. However, it should be remembered that a normal ECG at the start doses not rule out MI.

- **High-risk group:** These cases have following features:
  - Elderly people (>65 years)
  - Past history of CAD or prior admission (s) for ACS
  - Recurrent chest pain (more than two angina episodes in 24 hours) especially when associated with ST-T changes
  - Positive troponins
  - Hemodynamic instability
  - Tachycardia/ventricular arrhythmias
  - Low left ventricular ejection fraction (LVEF <40%) or history of heart failure
  - Previous coronary interventions (within 6-12 months) or bypass surgery

- Diabetes mellitus, and
- Multiple (three or more) coronary risk factors.

❖ **Low-risk group:** This group comprises patients of ACS comparatively younger in age (<50 years), without significant risk factors, who have no recurrent chest pain and in whom ECG changes are minimal or absent. Cardiac enzymes will be normal in such cases.

❖ **Intermediate-risk group:** Such patients initially have characteristics in between high and low-risk groups. Most important risk markers in such cases will be—(1) age over 70 years, (2) presence of diabetes mellitus, peripheral arterial or cerebrovascular disease, and (3) ECG changes of old CAD. Such cases should be admitted to ICU for 24–48 hours and observed for development of high-risk features.

## *Management Plan*

Central to the management of ACS are the ECG **abnormalities** at the time of presentation, and detection of blood **markers of myocardial necrosis.** Based on these parameters, a rational approach to diagnosis and management of ACS can be planned (**Flowchart 1.2**).

Details about modality of treatment are provided in subsequent sections on "AMI" and "UA". It must however, be emphasized that all cases of ACS should receive both **anti-ischemic treatment** *(nitrates and beta blockers)* as well as **antithrombotic therapy** *[aspirin, clopidogrel, and low-molecular weight heparin (LMWH)].* In addition, identifiable risk factors must be controlled aggressively, especially serum lipids. **Statins and beta-blockers** also help in long-term plaque stabilization.

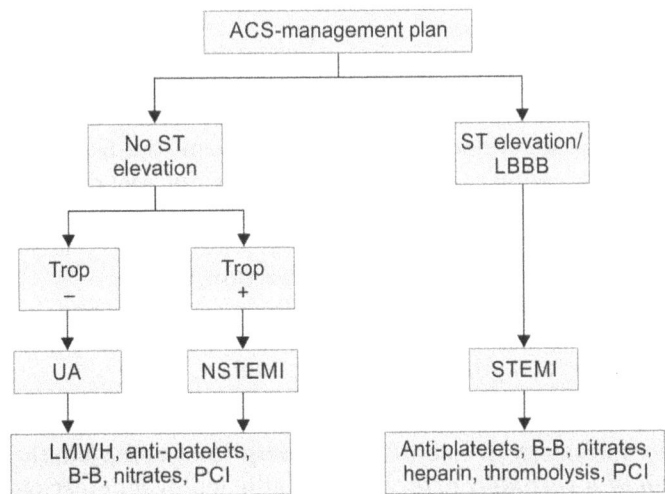

**Flowchart 1.2:** Acute coronary syndrome with principles of management.

(B-B: beta-blockers; LMWH: low molecular weight heparin; NSTEMI: non-ST-elevated MI; PCI: percutaneous interventions; STEMI: ST elevated MI; UA: unstable angina)

Early coronary angiography followed by appropriate revascularization procedure should be considered in all high-risk patients (vide supra). In low-risk patients a conservative approach can be adopted coupled with a close watch on the patient for any rest pain and/or fresh ECG changes.

## Summary

Coronary heart disease has become a very serious health hazard in our country, and indications are that its prevalence will continue to show a steep rise in the years to come. With increased understanding of pathogenesis of ACS, newer therapeutic options have emerged, which have been largely standardized. Since most of such patients initially contact a primary care doctor or a physician rather than a cardiologist, it is essential that the latest concepts of ACS, outlined in this section, are well understood by the primary care providers, so that they are able to deliver appropriate and timely treatment to these critically ill patients.

# ACUTE MYOCARDIAL INFARCTION

Acute myocardial infarction is one of the most common medical emergencies encountered in clinical practice, and unfortunately its prevalence is continuously increasing. More ominous is the fact that AMI is being increasingly encountered at comparatively younger age, and both among the poor as well as in women. Moreover, despite all the advances during the past quarter century, it still carries a high-early mortality (10–20%), and approximately half of these fatalities occur within the first few hours of the event, chiefly due to ventricular fibrillation (VF).

## Etiology

Myocardial infarction is most often a manifestation of ***underlying coronary atherosclerosis,*** and results from an occluding ***coronary thrombus***. Infrequently, prolonged vasospasm or sudden hypotension with consequent inadequate myocardial blood flow may be the precipitating factors. Rare causes include embolic coronary occlusion, vasculitis, aortic root dissection, and in young people, cocaine abuse.

Depending upon ECG findings, such cases are currently classified as:
- **ST-segment elevated myocardial infarction**, and
- **Non-ST-elevated myocardial infarction.**

### ST-Segment Elevated Myocardial Infarction

*Pathogenesis*

The basic pathology in STEMI is an ***abrupt and complete thrombotic occlusion of a coronary artery*** already afflicted by atherosclerosis, with consequent sudden decrease in coronary blood flow. Slower occlusions do not usually result in STEMI because of supportive collateral network, which develops over a period of time. The thrombus invariably develops at the site of plaque disruption, which results in platelet activation and aggregation. As a result thromboxane A2 is released and coagulation cascade is activated. Consequently, prothrombin is converted to thrombin, which then converts fibrinogen to fibrin.

The exact cause of atheromatous plaque disruption (fissuring, ulceration, and rupture) is not known. Plaques with thin fibrous cap and rich-lipid core containing fat laden macrophages are more vulnerable. *Triggers* of plaque disruption include sudden unaccustomed exertion, acute emotional stress (often associated with anger), hypertension, and cigarette smoking.

*Precipitating factors*

Besides triggers of plaque disruption (vide supra), MI may be precipitated by an intercurrent illness (especially chest infection), ischemic stroke, episode of hypotension, anesthesia, surgery, etc. In many cases, however, no such history is available, and symptoms (of MI) appear while the subject is at rest or engaged in routine activities.

*Clinical features*

Although an attack of MI may develop suddenly, quite often nearly one out of every three cases has some form of **prodromal symptoms** arising from transient episodes of cardiac ischemia. These may comprise sudden appearance of transitory chest discomfort resembling angina pectoris, accelerating angina (increase in duration and/or frequency of pre-existing angina), or rest angina. Other prodromal features may take the form of an episode of syncope, sudden fatigue, or unusual "indigestion/gas". Unfortunately, because of their diversity, such prodromal symptoms are often overlooked, sometimes with tragic consequences.

*The most common presenting symptom of MI is acute chest pain occurring at rest,* usually in the early morning hours. The pain is often severe and prolonged, lasting more than 30 minutes and sometimes for several hours. The pain may begin with the subject at rest or during exertion, but even in the latter situation (unlike angina pectoris) it does not subside with cessation of physical activity. The pain may be described as a load on the chest, or as squeezing, crushing, or less often stabbing or burning in type. Typically, this is located in the retrosternal region, and may radiate to one or both shoulder or arms, to the neck, in the interscapular region or the epigastrium (see also section on "Pain in Chest"). In fact coronary pain may be felt anywhere between the occiput and umbilicus. A frequent location is epigastrium where it is often mistaken for "acidity" or "gas".

The intensity of pain varies a great deal, and although a severe, excruciating, and prolonged pain usually denotes an extensive infarction, it is important to remember that there may be *little correlation between the intensity of chest pain and the gravity of the underlying pathology.* In fact extensive MI may be associated with only mild chest pain or, on occasions, be entirely painless. This is especially true in elderly patients, in long-standing diabetics, or in the presence of heart failure.

Features of **sympathetic over-activity** often accompany other symptoms of MI, and include anxiety, restlessness, tachycardia, profuse perspiration, peripheral vasoconstriction, and/or cyanosis. In a smaller group of patients with inferior MI, **vagotonia** may predominate with resulting bradycardia, pallor, and even syncope. Vomiting is not infrequent. Other associated or even presenting features of AMI include dyspnea, shock, dysrhythmia, syncope, severe change in mental status, or a stroke. Sudden death, of course, is a constant fear.

**Physical examination** may not be of much diagnostic help, but is important in assessing the severity of cardiac dysfunction. The heart rate may vary from marked bradycardia (usually in inferior MI) to tachycardia resulting from increased sympathetic activity. Likewise, blood pressure may remain unaltered or be even raised though more often it drops by a variable degree. Occasionally, arrhythmias or features of heart failure may dominate the clinical picture.

Auscultation of the heart is usually unimpressive. A soft first sound reflects decreased left ventricular (LV) contractility. An atrial gallop (S4) is common, but ventricular gallop (S3) is uncommon and indicates significant LV dysfunction.

An evanescent and localized pericardial rub may be audible, usually in cases with transmural infarction. However, such signs are likely to be missed by an unaccustomed ear.

Systolic murmurs are often heard and are due to mitral regurgitation resulting from papillary muscle dysfunction/rupture. A comparatively uncommon cause (of systolic murmur) is rupture of ventricular septum in cases with transmural septal infarction. The murmur in such cases is generally loud and holosystolic. Special attention should be paid to **auscultation of the lungs.** Inspiratory rales, with or without rhonchi, may be heard at the lung bases (pulmonary congestion), and indicate LV dysfunction, which worsens in proportion to the progression of pulmonary congestion up the lung fields. Presence of right ventricular failure (secondary to LV failure or right ventricular infarction) is indicated by high-jugular venous pressure and tender hepatomegaly.

## Diagnosis

Acute chest pain can occur in a large number of conditions besides IHD (see section on "Pain in Chest"). A careful history and physical examination are of great help, but the diagnosis of MI essentially rests on findings of ECG and biological markers of cardiac necrosis.

### *Electrocardiogram*

This is the most important and commonly employed tool for the diagnosis and localization of AMI, as well as to (fairly) prognosticate such cases. Abnormalities often appear in the ECG soon after the onset of STEMI, and are generally well developed within a few hours. Sometimes, however, the changes of AMI may not be obvious for 24–48 hours after the onset of symptoms.

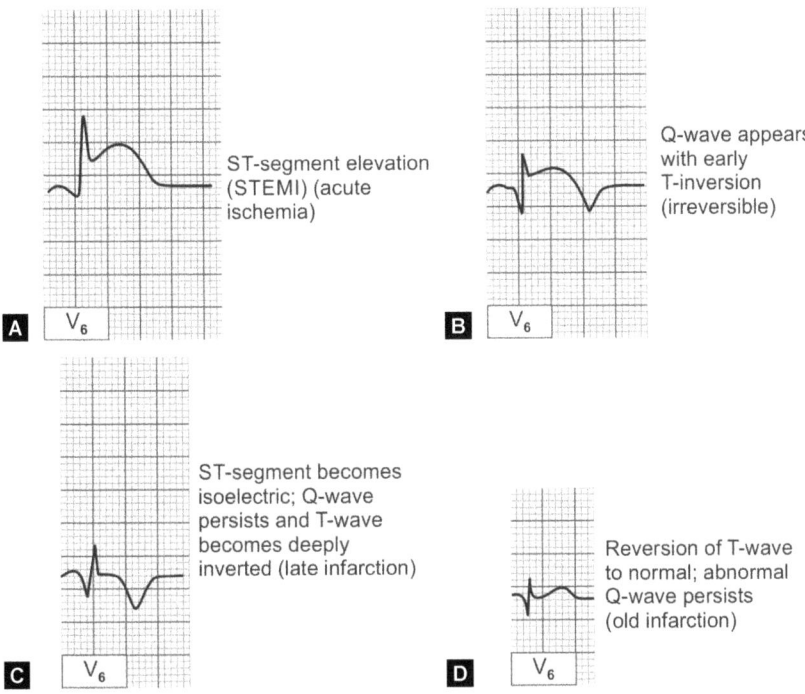

**Figs. 1.2A to D:** ECG patterns (V6) in evolving myocardial infarction. (A) Within minutes to hours; (B) Several hours to days; (C) Days to weeks; (D) Months to years.

- ❖ **Diagnostic evaluation:** The classical finding in initial phases of STEMI is *ST-elevation* in the leads overlying/reflecting the involved area. However, sometimes in the very early stages of ischemia, tall t-waves *(hyperacute T-waves)* appear over the ischemic zone. Within a period of hours to days, elevation of ST-segments is followed by evolving T-wave inversions **(Figs. 1.2 and 1.3)**. Marked ST-elevation in multiple leads generally indicates severe myocardial injury. *Q-waves are not specific for STEMI, since presence of abnormal Q-waves only indicates significant myocardial necrosis, and may be seen in both STEMI and NSTEMI.*
  If the cardiac damage does not extend to epicardial surface, ST-segments are depressed with inverted T-waves **(Fig. 1.4)**. Earlier called *"subendocardial infarction",* such cases are now termed NSTEMI. This differentiation of AMI into STEMI and NSTEMI has important therapeutic implications as will be discussed later.
- ❖ **Localization of MI:** An ECG also provides valuable information regarding the location of AMI, and thereby in identifying the infarct-related artery **(Table 1.2)**.
- ❖ **Prognostic value of ECG in MI:** An ECG may also be helpful in the assessment of prognosis especially as to the risk of death and recurrence of acute ischemic events. **Highest risk** is indicated by the presence of marked ST-segment elevation, significant conduction defects (e.g., left bundle branch block) and LV hypertrophy. On the other extreme, patients

**Chapter 1:** Cardiovascular Emergencies

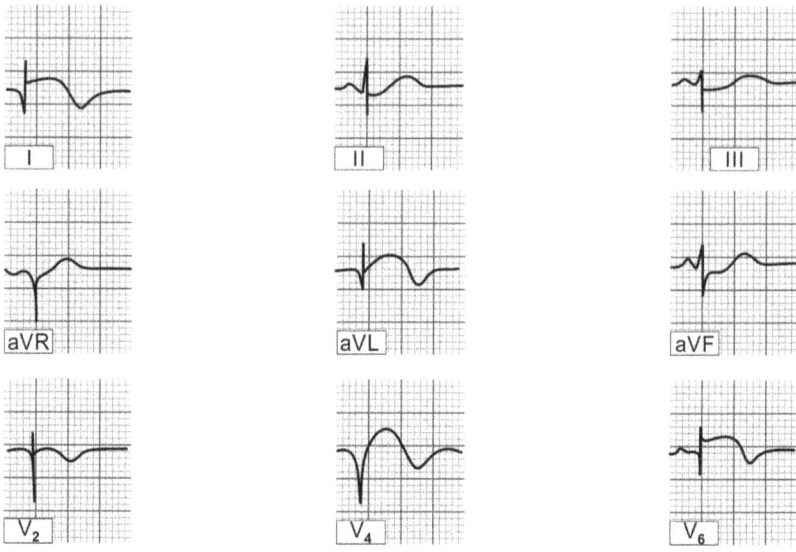

**Fig. 1.3:** ST-elevated myocardial infarction (STEMI).

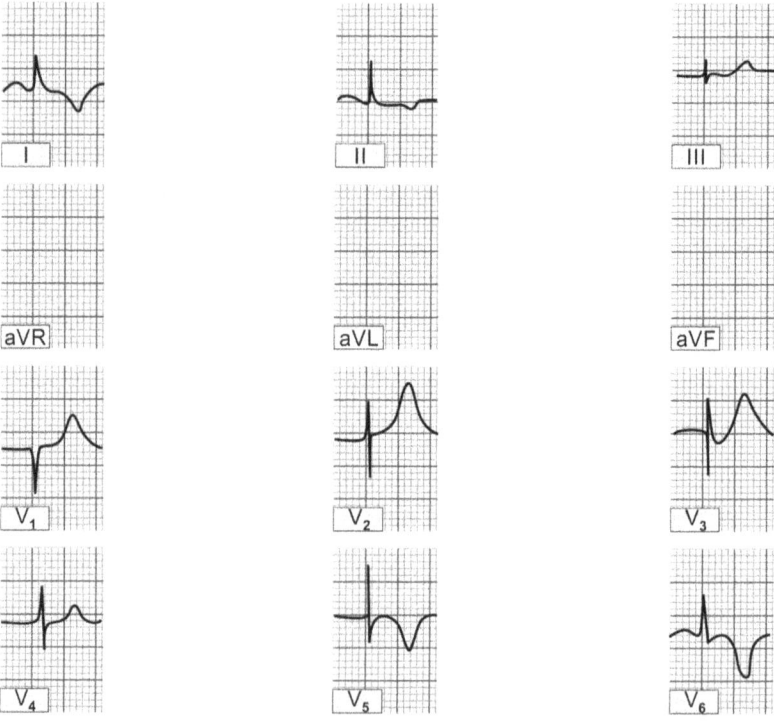

**Fig. 1.4:** Non-ST-elevated myocardial infarction (NSTEMI).

**Table 1.2:** Electrocardiographic localization of myocardial infarction.

| ECG changes* | Area of infarct | Probable artery involved |
|---|---|---|
| Leads II, III, a VF | Inferior | Right coronary artery |
| V1–V3 | Anteroseptal | Left anterior descending |
| V2–V4 | Anterior | Left anterior descending |
| I, aVL, V4-6 | Lateral | Left circumflex |
| V1-V2 | Posterior† | Posterior descending |

*ST-elevation, T-wave inversion, or new Q-waves
†Tall R-waves with ST-depression; T-wave is inverted initially but becomes upright over a period of time

with isolated T-wave inversions or near normal ECGs are **at least risk**. In the **intermediate risk** category will be most of the patients in whom ECG changes comprise only modest ST-segment alteration with T-wave inversions. Presence of such changes in three or more ECG leads and/or ST-segment alteration >0.2 mV add to the gravity of the risk.

## Serum Enzymes

Certain biochemical cardiac markers provide useful information in the diagnosis of myocardial necrosis:

- ❖ **Creatine phosphokinase (CPK):** The enzyme CPK comprises several isoenzymes. Results are more specific (for myocardial injury) when its MB isoenzyme *(CPK-MB)* is studied. The enzyme level begins to rise within 6–8 hours of onset of MI, peaks at 18–24 hours, and returns to normal in 3–4 days. An early peaking occurs in patients who receive thrombolytic therapy. An elevated total CPK with an MB-fraction >5% is diagnostic. *Peak CPK activity usually correlates with the extent of muscle necrosis.*
- ❖ **Cardiac-specific troponins:** Study of troponins *(troponin-I and troponin-T)* is a very sensitive and specific test to detect myocardial necrosis in cases of MI. Troponins are normally not detectable in the blood of healthy persons, and therefore these are the preferred biochemical markers of MI. Furthermore, the test results are rapidly available. Cardiac troponins can be detected within 3–6 hours of a severe ischemic episode and remain elevated for 7–10 days after MI.

   Troponin assays with varying sensitivities are now available. "Sensitive" or "contemporary" assays have been used for last several years, but recently "high-sensitivity" troponins have been introduced for measurement of both Troponin I and T. The Fourth Universal Definition of Myocardial Infarction recommends use of these assays. Since multiple companies manufacture these assays, they have different reference ranges. A troponin level must be above the 99th percentile of the upper reference limit to be abnormal.

   Troponin elevations usually begin in two to three hours after the onset of acute MI, and ideally, a rise or fall of the troponin value should be observed.

### Echocardiogram

Since abnormalities in regional wall motion occur soon after myocardial ischemia/necrosis, echocardiography is extremely useful for *early detection and assessment of MI*. It can be especially useful when the history is compatible with AMI but the ECG is non-diagnostic. Furthermore, since echocardiography provides a *very good estimate of LV functions*, it is valuable both in planning the treatment and in establishing prognosis after AMI. Its sensitivity is highest for cases with Q-wave infarction and least for patients with unstable angina who are free from pain at the time of the study. It may also detect right ventricular infarction (often missed in 12-lead ECG), papillary muscle dysfunction, ventricular septal rupture, pericardial effusion, and LV thrombus.

### Management

Recent advances in our knowledge of the pathogenesis of AMI are well-reflected in the newer concepts of its treatment. Accordingly, the **current therapeutic approach is aimed at:** (1) establishing *early reperfusion in cases with STEM* who are suspected to have complete arterial occlusion (according to ECG findings), (2) *control of platelet aggregation* at the site of plaque disruption, and (3) *increasing stability of the atheromatous plaque.* Management is best considered under two heads—**prehospital and hospital management.**

#### Prehospital Care

- **Aspirin therapy:** Since *platelet aggregation* at the site of intimal disruption plays an important role in the early stages of thrombus formation, this should be inhibited as early as possible. The drug most commonly used is *aspirin,* which has a rapid antithrombotic effect due to *inhibition of enzyme cyclooxygenase and blocking production of thromboxane A2 in the platelets (Flowchart 1.3).* The action occurs almost instantly after administration of aspirin and continues for 4–6 days (after a single dose) till a new generation of platelets enters circulation. The best way is to ask the patient to chew half to one tablet (162–325 mg) of aspirin since buccal absorption of the drug allows a faster absorption. Ideally, aspirin should be administered within 6 hours of onset of symptoms.
- **Nitrates:** Every patient of proven or even suspected AMI should receive sublingual nitrate in the form of *isosorbide dinitrate* (5 mg). This may be repeated once or twice as required, at 5-minute intervals. Persistence of symptoms beyond 15 minutes, or return of chest pain after initial favorable response, especially if associated with other features of on-going ischemia (in ECG) is an indication for intravenous nitroglycerine and/or coronary intervention. *Nitrates help to diminish or abolish chest pain by relieving coronary spasm, improving collateral flow, and decreasing myocardial oxygen demand (by lowering preload).* **Therapy with nitrates is contraindicated** in patients who have low systolic pressure (<100 mm Hg), have associated right ventricular

**Flowchart 1.3:** Aspirin therapy.

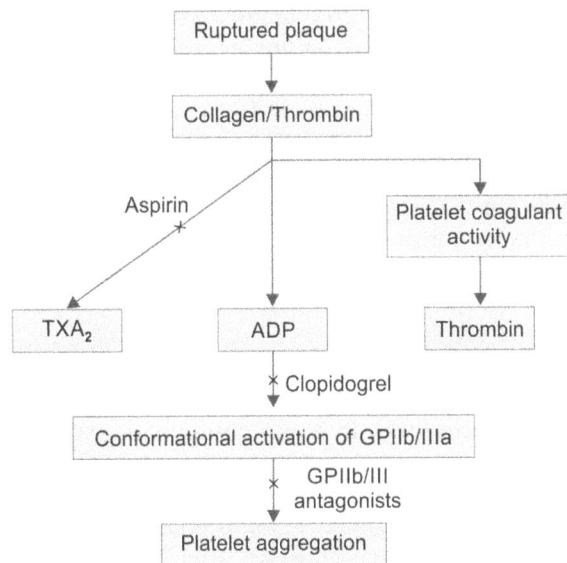

infarction, or who have taken sildenafil (for erectile dysfunction) within past 24 hours. **Long-acting nitrates should not be used in the very initial stages of AMI.**

*Home versus hospital care*

With the benefits of fibrinolytic therapy fully established, every patient of STEMI should be hospitalized. Even when thrombolysis is not possible, hospitalization is advisable if the patient belongs to high-risk group (*see* section on "Acute Coronary Syndrome").

*Patients with following features deserve immediate admission in ICU:*
- Cardiac pain is severe or recurrent
- Infarction is extensive, is associated with STEMI, and involves anterior wall
- Features of heart failure exist
- Significant arrhythmia is present
- Patient has had an earlier MI or has an associated disease of significance such as uncontrolled hypertension or diabetes mellitus.

In other situations, the patient may be allowed to stay at home especially, if first 24 hours of illness have elapsed, there is no complication of MI, and adequate medical supervision is available.

## Treatment in the Hospital

On the arrival at the hospital every patient with a possible diagnosis of AMI should have an immediate ECG, a blood sample drawn for serum enzyme studies, and a quick history and physical examination to determine the time frame of onset of symptoms, status of vital signs, any arrhythmia, evidence of left/right ventricular dysfunction, or any other complication of MI. At this stage contraindications to fibrinolysis and/or anticoagulation should also be evaluated. The information thus obtained will guide the precise nature of treatment required in a given case. *Following specific measures are, however, common to all cases of fresh MI.*

- **Antiplatelet agents:** A number of drugs are known to inhibit platelet activation and aggregation **(Flowchart 1.3)**:
    - *Aspirin:* This is a powerful antiplatelet agent but its action is limited to **inhibition of the enzyme cyclooxygenase.** Aspirin does not affect the alternative pathways of platelet activation and aggregation, which include thrombin, adenosine diphosphate (ADP), collagen, and epinephrine. Furthermore some cases may be aspirin-resistant or respond to it only partially.
    - *Clopidogrel:* It is a thienopyridine derivative, which selectively and irreversibly inhibits ADP-induced platelet activation **(blocks platelet adenosine receptors).** In combination with aspirin, it provides a significantly greater protection in cardiovascular death or stroke in all cases of ACS including STEMI.
    
        Clopidogrel is now routinely administered (along with aspirin) in all cases of AMI in a once daily dose of 75 mg. The antiplatelet effect starts within 1 hour. A loading dose of 300-600 mg reduces the time to achieve maximum platelet inhibition.
    - *Platelet GpIIb/IIIa receptor antagonists:* Platelet activation and agglutination is a complex process involving many chemical agents and pathways. In the end (at the receptor level) however, all these act through Gp IIb/IIIa receptors, which are abundant on the platelet surface.
    
        GpIIb/IIIa receptor-antagonists act by occupying the receptors, preventing fibrinogen binding, and thereby inhibiting platelet aggregation. These are highly specific anti-platelet agents (abciximab, eptifibatide, and tirofiban), but are expensive, have a short half-life, and can be used only intravenously. Currently, these drugs are used in cases of ACS either as an adjunct to percutaneous coronary intervention (PCI) or in high risk cases, in combination with heparin.
- **Analgesics:** Since the pain of AMI is due to continuing ischemia of living, jeopardized myocardium rather than to the effects of completed myocardial necrosis, complete bed rest, and use of NG sublingually should be the initial measures to relieve chest pain. If chest pain persists or is severe, it should be controlled with morphine sulfate or buprenorphine **(Norphine).** The usual dose of morphine is 10-15 mg IM (or 2.5 mg IV, if pain is severe), and of norphine 0.2-0.3 mg IM or IV. Repeated injections may be required in cases of intractable pain but the total dose in 24 hours should not exceed 60 mg morphine or 1.2 mg norphine. Respiratory depression may occur with such large doses and should be treated with naloxone (0.1-0.2 mg IV) or nalorphine (5-10 mg IV).

    Both these drugs (especially morphine) may produce troublesome vomiting, and should therefore be combined preferably with promethazine **(Phenergan)** in a dose of 12.5-25 mg. It is also useful to remember that *morphine may produce hypotension* (due to venous pooling) *and bradycardia* (due to enhanced vagal tone), and therefore, should be avoided, if any of these complications is present or anticipated, especially in inferior myocardial infarction. Narcotic analgesics, in general, should be withheld, if the patient is confused or delirious (usually due to cerebral anoxia) or has features of shock.

- **Oxygen therapy:** Some degree of hypoxemia is invariable in all but the mildest cases of AMI, and is due to ventilation-perfusion abnormalities secondary to overt or subtle LV failure. Oxygen should therefore be administered to all cases of AMI for first 24–48 hours by nasal prongs at a rate of 3–4 L/min. Patients with heart failure and other MI complications may need longer and more aggressive oxygen therapy.
- **Intravenous nitroglycerine:** In patients with ACS including AMI, nitroglycerine (NG) infusion is indicated for *relief of persistent pain,* or as a vasodilator when there is *associated LV failure.* In the absence of ischemic pain or heart failure its role is suspect especially if the patient has been fibrinolyzed successfully. NG infusion is likely to be most beneficial in patients with large Q-wave type MI especially of the anterior wall, and in those with recurrent chest pain. It has been found to increase myocardial perfusion and diminish the risk of mechanical complications of MI. However, to achieve maximum benefit NG infusion should be started soon after the onset of MI, if the hemodynamic status is stable.

  Nitroglycerine is infused initially at a rate of 5 µg/min and then increased in a stepwise manner, in increments of 5 µg/min at a time, up to 20 µg/min or even up to 50 µg/min. Throughout the infusion a careful watch should be keep on the blood pressure so as not to reduce mean arterial pressure (diastolic pressure + 1/3 pulse pressure) below 90 mm Hg since greater reductions may decrease collateral blood flow, and actual increase infarct size.

  NG infusion should be continued for at least 24 hours, but usually not beyond 48 hours as *prolonged infusion carries the risk of inducing tolerance to nitrates, methemoglobinemia, and alcohol intoxication* (commercially available NG solution for IV use is prepared with ethanol as a diluent). When discontinuing NG infusion, *it should be tapered gradually* by titrating down 5 µg/min every 10 minutes since abrupt discontinuation of infusion can result in sudden increase in blood volume due to release of blood that was sequestrated in the venous capacitance bed.

  **Intravenous nitroglycerine is contraindicated** in the presence of hypotension, hypovolemia, raised intracranial pressure, constrictive pericarditis or pericardial tamponade, and should be used cautiously in patients with inferior myocardial infarction associated with right ventricular infarction.
- **Antiarrhythmics:** Some or the other type of arrhythmia occurs in almost all cases of AMI, if closely monitored. Patients who manifest ventricular premature beats (VPBs) more than 6/min, especially if multiform, or in

whom VPBs occur in couplets or in short runs of ventricular tachycardia (VT), should be considered for antiarrhythmic therapy during the acute course of the disease (3-5 days, or even longer in some cases). The standard treatment in such cases is **IV lidocaine** administered initially as 50-100 mg bolus followed by infusion at the rate of 1-4 mg/min. If ventricular ectopy is not satisfactorily controlled or there are contraindications to the use of lidocaine (such as hypotension), **amiodarone** becomes the drug of choice (for further details *see* section on "Cardiac Arrhythmias").

It may be added that beta-blockers, which are generally used in the initial treatment of all patients with AMI (vide infra), also have potent antiarrhythmic effect in such a setting.

❖ **Antithrombotic therapy:** The standard antithrombin agent used in clinical practice is ***heparin,*** which plays a key role in the management of patients of MI. This is because partial or complete coronary thrombotic occlusion is the underlying cause in most of these patients. The mechanism of action of heparin is complex. For the purpose of this text, it may be stated that heparin activates antithrombin, which then inactivates thrombin, the enzyme central to formation of fibrin. Given IV along with fibrinolytic agents that have a short half-life (UK, tPA), unfractionated heparin facilitates thrombolysis, and helps to establish and maintain patency of infarct-related artery (IRA). Standard heparin is used and administered IV in a dose of 12-15 units/kg/hour (maximum 1,000 units/hour over 24 hours), and monitored by ***partial thromboplastin time (PTT),*** which should be maintained between 1.5 and 2 times the control values. A loading dose is not required when the patient has been already fibrinolyzed. The infusion should be continued for 48-72 hours.

In cases in whom fibrinolysis cannot be offered for any reason or when it is not advisable (non-Q-wave MI), heparin is nearly always administered (unless contraindicated) along with aspirin and Clopidogrel, to arrest progression and recurrence of MI. Two schedules are available for heparinization in such cases:

1. *Intravenous heparin:* Standard (unfractionated) heparin is used IV; an initial bolus of 60 units/kg (maximum 5,000 units) is followed by infusion, which may be continued according to the reperfusion strategies.
2. *Subcutaneous heparin:* Low molecular weight heparin is more often used since (compared to standard heparin) it has better bioavailability, quicker onset of action, longer half-life, and a more predictable anticoagulant effect, thus obviating need for frequent PTT estimation. Any of the available LMWHs may be used in recommended dosage, and administered for 5-7 days.

ote

All intramuscular injections should be avoided in patients receiving fibrinolytic therapy or IV heparin.

❖ **Fibrinolytic therapy:** Since, most of the cases of STEMI are due to complete thrombotic occlusion of the IRA, fibrinolytic therapy has a very rational basis. Best results are obtained when therapy is instituted within the first hour *(the golden hour)* of onset of symptoms. When appropriately instituted fibrinolytic therapy reduces infarct size, limits LV dysfunction, and reduces the incidence of serious complications, such as cardiogenic shock, septal rupture, and serious ventricular arrhythmias. These benefits however, have been found to be limited to cases of AMI associated with complete occlusion of the coronary artery. Such cases are recognized on ECG by ST-segment elevation of >0.1mV in two inferior or lateral leads or two contiguous precordial leads, or by new onset of left bundle branch block.

*Choice of fibrinolytic agent*

There are two broad groups of fibrinolytic agents: (a) Exogenous agents produced by beta-hemolytic streptococci [such as **Streptokinase** (SK)], and (b) Endogenous agents that are derived from human sources—**Urokinase (UK)** and **Alteplase** (recombinant tissue Plasminogen Activator; t-PA).

All fibrinolytic drugs activate plasminogen to its active form, plasmin (Flowchart 1.4), which specifically degrades fibrin to degradation products, and results in clot lysis. It is to be noted that *none of these drugs is "thrombus-selective",* and that all fibrinolytic agents produce almost equal degree of fibrin dissolution both in the thrombus and in hemostatic plugs; hence in the therapeutic doses employed their bleeding complications are almost similar.

*Streptokinase (SK)*

This was the first plasminogen activator introduced in clinical practice, and continues to be the most widely used, at any rate in India, primarily because of cost factors. It has a comparatively long half-life (30 minutes). The usual dose is 1.5 million units administered as infusion over 1 hour (of which 250,000

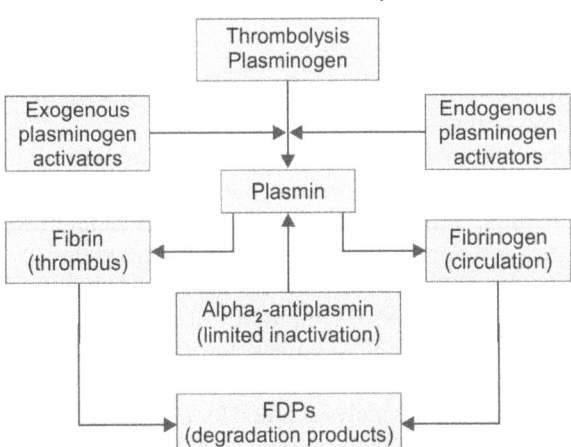

**Flowchart 1.4:** Fibrinolysis.

is given as bolus). Just before starting SK therapy, 100 mg hydrocortisone and 25 mg pheniramine are administered IV to minimize the risk of allergic reactions, which may include rash, fever, nausea, hypotension, serum sickness like syndrome, and rarely anaphylactoid reaction.

*Urokinase*

This has a short half-life (16 minutes) with fibrinolytic properties almost similar to SK. The recommended dose is 2 million units, and since, it is free from allergic side effects, it is given IV as a bolus, usually over 5 minutes.

*Tissue plasminogen activator (t-PA; Alteplase)*

A variety of protocols have been used for t-PA therapy. Currently favored regimen comprises administration of a 15 mg bolus followed by 50 mg IV over 30 minutes, and then by 35 mg over the next 60 minutes. It is non-antigenic and probably achieves a more rapid and complete patency rate in the IRA than either SK or UK. It is especially preferable in the subgroup of patients presenting within 3 hours of onset of symptoms since, in such patients, the speed of reperfusion is of great importance. Since, t-PA has a shorter half-life than SK, concomitant use of heparin is mandatory.

*Reperfusion*

The success of fibrinolytic therapy is judged by reperfusion occurring within 1 hour of start of infusion. **Successful reperfusion is usually indicated** by the following criteria:
- ❖ Reduction in chest pain
- ❖ Early peaking of (CPK) and CPK-MB level (8–15 hours instead of 18–24 hours)
- ❖ Rapid evolution of ST segment shift on ECG
- ❖ Certain reperfusion arrhythmias may occur immediately upon successful reperfusion, and can persist up to 12–24 hours. Typically, these are ventricular in type, the most characteristic being accelerated idioventricular rhythm.

*Selection of patients for fibrinolytic therapy*
- ❖ Fibrinolytic therapy is indicated **only in patients with STEM** (cases with ST-elevation or new-onset LBBB).
- ❖ Greatest benefit is seen in patients with large anterior infarcts. However, fibrinolytic therapy is also useful in patients with inferior MI presenting with ST-segment elevation especially when associated with posterior/lateral extension or reciprocal precordial ST-depression.
- ❖ Though the "therapeutic window" for fibrinolysis has been enlarged up to 12 hours after the onset of symptoms (especially in cases with on-going chest pain and persistent ST-segment elevation), best results are observed when carried out within 6 hours (the sooner, the better).
- ❖ The upper limit of age usually accepted for fibrinolytic therapy is 75 years. It may, however, be beneficial in patients who are even 80 years of age or

more, if they are otherwise in good health, are seen soon after onset of symptoms, and have continuing ischemic pain.
- ❖ Diabetes mellitus, hypotension, sinus tachycardia, or features of heart failure at the time of presentation are additional factors, which favor institution of fibrinolytic therapy.

*Prehospital fibrinolysis*

As the advantages of fibrinolysis in AMI are being appreciated by a wider section of the medical fraternity and even by the public at large, there is increasing desire to offer early fibrinolysis in domiciliary practice and in remote areas when removal to a hospital is likely to be delayed.

The practicability, safety, and advantages of such prehospital fibrinolysis are now well-established and it is being increasingly offered to patients in mobile intensive coronary care units and in emergency rooms. The precondition is that the diagnosis of AMI should be established beyond doubt, and the therapy preferably restricted to cases likely to derive maximal benefit with minimal risk, i.e., cases of anterior MI associated with STEMI, and without hypertension especially if they are younger than 75 years and have associated diabetes mellitus.

The problem is a little more complex in the rural and semi-urban areas of India where the CAD is becoming increasingly common. There is a great need and scope of prehospital fibrinolysis in such cases. However, given the poor health delivery system, lack of education, poverty, and the fear of consumer protection laws, practice of prehospital fibrinolysis in *mofussil* areas at present may be fraught with several problems.

*Contraindications to fibrinolysis*
- ❖ **Absolute contraindications**
    - Active internal bleeding
    - Suspected aortic dissection
    - Recent head trauma or known intracranial neoplasm
    - Diabetic hemorrhagic retinopathy or other hemorrhagic ophthalmic condition
    - Pregnancy
    - Blood pressure more than 200/120 mm Hg
    - Hemorrhagic stroke within past 1 year
- ❖ **Relative contraindications**
    - Recent head trauma or surgery more than 2 weeks ago
    - Prolonged or traumatic cardiopulmonary resuscitation (CPR)
    - History of chronic severe hypertension with or without drug therapy
    - Active peptic ulcer
    - Ischemic cerebral stroke within past 6 months
    - Known bleeding diathesis or current use of anticoagulants
    - Significant liver dysfunction
    - Dental extraction within 14 days
    - Active menstruation or lactation

- Previous allergic reaction to SK between 5 days to 12 months (SK antibodies develop in such cases); urokinase or t-PA may be used.

*Complications of fibrinolytic therapy*

Fibrinolytic therapy is generally safe, if administered carefully in properly selected cases. However, following complications may be encountered:

- ❖ **Systemic bleeding:** While minor bleeding is not uncommon (up to 20% cases), major hemorrhage is rare. The most serious complication is intracranial bleeding (0.5–1.0% of patients), the rate being slightly higher with t-PA than with SK. The risk is more marked in elderly patients (>70 years) and those with hypertension. It is, however, important to remember that following fibrinolysis, a defibrinated state may persist for several hours, and therefore, all needle punctures should be avoided for 24 hours, and blood drawn from an indwelling venous catheter for laboratory testing.
- ❖ **Allergic reactions:** Though uncommon, allergic reactions may follow use of SK, which should be avoided if already administered within 1 year. Allergic features may comprise rash, fever, serum sickness-like syndrome, and most importantly, hypotension.
- ❖ **Reperfusion arrhythmias:** Transient arrhythmias occasionally occur during fibrinolytic therapy (vide supra). These are usually short lived and in fact have been regarded as indicators of successful reperfusion. In view of their innocuous nature, no prophylactic antiarrhythmic therapy is necessary.

*Other pharmacological measures*

The process of thrombus formation in the coronary arteries is a complex one involving platelets, coagulation system, and blood-flow conditions. Adjunctive therapy is designed to inhibit this ongoing occlusive cascade and stabilize the atheromatous plaque. Such measures are recommended in all cases of AMI, whether fibrinolyzed or not. In this context, the role of antiplatelet agents and heparin has already been discussed.

- ❖ **Beta-blockers:** Intravenous beta-adrenoreceptor blockers (followed by oral agents) given early in the course of AMI reduce heart rate, blood pressure and cardiac index, and thus help to limit the infarct size, relieve chest pain, and decrease the risk of ventricular arrhythmias. The effects are especially favorable in patients of AMI with hypertension and sinus tachycardia, recurrent or persistent chest pain, and tachyarrhythmias. Such patients invariably have large infarcts or compromised LV functions, and these are the very cases likely to suffer the side effects of treatment, notably heart failure. Therefore IV beta-blockers should be employed only in patients admitted in ICU, and ***after echocardiographic evaluation of LV functions.*** Contraindications to beta-blockade include hypotension (systolic pressure <90 mm Hg), bradycardia (heart rate <60/min), incipient or overt heart failure, heart block, and history of bronchial asthma.

  The treatment schedule comprises administration of metoprolol IV slowly in a dose of 3–5 mg. If the heart rate continues to be above 70 beats/min, and systolic pressure >110 mm Hg, another 3–5 mg metoprolol may be given once or twice (up to a maximum of three doses) at intervals of 10-15 minutes. Thereafter, if the patient is hemodynamically stable, metoprolol is continued orally in a dose of 25–50 mg twice daily. In case of uncertainty regarding the safety of beta-blockade, an ultra-short acting beta-blocking agent *(esmolol)* with a half-life of only 9 minutes may be used to determine whether the patient can tolerate beta-blockade.

❖ **Angiotensin-converting enzyme (ACE) inhibitors:** Unless hemodynamically unstable (systolic pressure <100 mm Hg), these drugs should be prescribed to all cases of STEMI within 24 hours. ACE inhibitors reduce mortality rate in the acute phase (complimentary to anti-platelets and beta-blockers) and lower the risk of subsequent heart failure when administered on long-term basis (by reduction in the process of ventricular remodeling). The beneficial cardiac effects are a "class effect" of ACE inhibitors (or receptor blockers), and there is no conclusive evidence to favor any particular agent. However, when blood pressure is already on the lower side, treatment with short-acting Captopril may be preferable, at any rate initially.

❖ **Calcium channel blockers (CCB):** As a class, *CCB have not been found be useful in cases of STEMI, and hence their routine use is not recommended.* However, in patients in whom beta-blockers are contraindicated, diltiazem may be used for relief of ongoing ischemia especially in NSTEMI, or for control of tachycardia. *Long-acting nifedipine should not be used in the early stages of AMI as it may result in unpredictable drop in blood pressure.* Pharmacological profile of three commonly used CCBs is given at **Table 1.3**.

A new CCB **"Cilnidipine"** is now available which is especially useful in the treatment of hypertension. Since, there is *little venodilatation, pedal edema is not a problem* (a common side effect of amlodipine). It is also *cardioprotective* (no increase in heart rate or cardiac contraction) and *renoprotective* (increases renal blood flow along with decrease in rennin secretion).

❖ **Other agents:**
- *Nitrates:* Both sublingual and IV nitrates are useful (vide supra) in relieving pain in the initial stages of STEMI (and also in UA/NSTEMI). IV nitroglycerine can be helpful in relieving on-going ischemic pain, and possibly in reducing infarct size. This is especially beneficial in

**Table 1.3:** Pharmacological profile of common calcium channel blockers.

| Name of drug | Arterial vasodilatation | Coronary vasodilatation | Myocardial depression | Decreased AV node conduction |
|---|---|---|---|---|
| Nifedipine | +++ | +++ | 0 | 0 |
| Diltiazem | ++ | ++ | ± | ± |
| Verapamil | + | + | + | ++ |

cases with large anterior infarcts associated heart failure, persistent ischemia or hypertension, and in patients of AMI in whom fibrinolysis is not possible. ***Long-acting nitrates should be avoided in the very early stages of AMI*** especially inferior MI associated with right ventricular infarction. Long term use of nitrates after MI, though often advised, is without proven benefits except in cases with complicating angina or heart failure.

- *Statins:* Lipid-lowering therapy reduces the incidence of acute ischemic events in patients of ACS by various mechanisms, including increase in plaque stability. The most commonly used drugs are HMG-CoA reductase inhibitors (**statins**). Any one of the available statins should, therefore, be administered to all cases of ACS within 24–48 hours), especially those found to be hyperlipidemic. ***The treatment should be started during the acute phase and statins*** continued on a long-term basis in appropriate dosage, the aim being to keep level of low-density lipoprotein (LDL) below 80 mg%.
- *Other measures:* Suitable drugs should be prescribed, for any associated disease, such as **diabetes mellitus** *(avoid glitazones)* and **hypertension** (ACE inhibitors are anyway routinely prescribed in STEMI, unless contraindicated).

Additionally, ***measures to control coronary risk factors (especially smoking) and improve life style*** should be encouraged with a view to prevent further episodes of coronary disease.

*Acute percutaneous coronary intervention (PCI)*

Most of the cases of can be stabilized during the acute phase by conservative treatment and fibrinolysis (if instituted within the first few hours of onset of MI)

**Symptoms:** Nevertheless, ***primary PCI*** (performed without preceding fibrinolysis) is being ***increasingly offered*** to such patients especially when cardiogenic shock has supervened/threatened, fibrinolysis is contraindicated or has failed, or there is substantial delay in instituting it (fibrinolysis).

The role of PCI in patients of ACS without ST-elevation (**NSTEMI or UA**) depends upon the risk profile of the patient. However, urgent or semi-urgent coronary angiography with suitable reperfusion procedure should be considered on a priority basis in high-risk patients who are troponin positive, have recurrent or persistent ischemic pain, depressed LV functions, and associated diabetes mellitus.

*Major complications of myocardial infarction (STEMI)*

Nearly half of all patients developing STEMI have no significant complication. In others, most of the serious complications occur within the first 5 days, and may be either electrical or mechanical in nature. The former comprise various types of arrhythmias, which can be immediately detected and treated in a well-equipped and staffed ICU (*see* section on "Cardiac Arrhythmias"). It is the control of mechanical complications of MI which is more challenging. There are two main mechanical complications:

1. **Pump failure:** This may take the form of acute pulmonary edema or cardiogenic shock. Both these conditions are discussed in subsequent sections of this Chapter.
2. **Rupture of a part of the myocardium involving:** *(1) Papillary muscle or interventricular septum* leading respectively to acute mitral regurgitation and ventricular septal defect; and *(2) Ventricular-free wall* with resultant tamponade. Such complications usually occur between 2 and 7 days following infarction, but may occur within the first 24 hours. The clinical course is invariably catastrophic, and the prognosis is grave especially in those with free wall rupture.

### *General Measures*

These are of no less importance in the overall management of AMI and should be diligently observed.

- **Bed rest:** Strict bed rest continues to be the sheet-anchor of treatment of AMI. Therefore, as soon as a diagnosis of AMI is made or even suspected, the patient should be put to bed. Depending upon the severity and extent of MI, the period of rest varies from 5 to 7 days. Ambulation is encouraged early, so that in an uncomplicated case the patient is allowed to sit in the chair on the 3 or 4 days, and move around in the room and use adjoining toilet by 4 or 5 days. If these activities are well tolerated, physical activity should be gradually increased, and if there is no untoward incident the patient may be discharged from the hospital in about a week provided good domiciliary medical care is available.

  *Longer period of bed rest* may be required in high-risk cases with the following features: (1) Age over 80 years, (2) Extensive transmural anterior MI, (3) Previous myocardial infarction, and (4) Associated diabetes mellitus, heart failure, shock, recurrent chest pain, or arrhythmias.

- **Antiarrhythmics:** One or the other type of arrhythmia occurs in almost all cases of AMI if closely monitored. Patients who manifest multiple ventricular premature beats (VPBs) >6/min especially if multiform, or in whom VPBs occur in couplets or in short runs, should be considered for antiarrhythmic therapy with lidocaine or amiodarone (for further details *see* section on "Cardiac Arrhythmias").

- **Tranquilizers and sedatives:** Patients with AMI should be kept calm and well sedated with alprazolam or diazepam for first 48–72 hours to allay the anxiety that is so common in such a setting. An additional dose of nitrazepam 5–10 mg may be required at night to ensure good sleep.

- **Diet:** A liquid or semisolid diet should be advised for first 2–3 days to avoid vomiting. This should be followed by a 1,200–1,500 calories soft, easily digestible food, low in salt, and divided into multiple small feeds for another 2–3 days. Finally, in the absence of complications, a more or less normal diet, low in cholesterol, can be permitted after about a week. However, strong tea or coffee should be avoided for several weeks because

of the risk of arrhythmias. Smoking is particularly dangerous as it may lead to sudden death, and should be totally prohibited.
- **Care of the bowel and bladder:** Mild laxative should be given from day-1 to avoid constipation and straining. If constipation does occur, it may be relieved by a low glycerin enema. Some patients find it difficult to pass stool while lying in bed. In such cases, it is preferable to let them use a bedside chair commode (after 2–3 days of MI) rather than strain on the bed pan.

*Bladder*

Urinary retention occasionally occurs in men in the immediate postinfarction period, and some may be unable to pass urine in lying-down position; they should be permitted to sit up with support or even to put their legs across the bed, if that helps them in passing urine. If urinary retention persists, bladder should be catheterized with aseptic technique.

## Summary

With the general acceptance of the concept of "vulnerable plaque" in the pathogenesis of acute coronary syndrome, management strategies in AMI have been largely standardized. The key points can be summarized as follows:
- Rupture of the atheromatous plaque with consequent acute coronary thrombosis is generally accepted as the cause of AMI. Patients with STEMI usually have complete intraluminal obstruction.
- Platelet aggregation and clogging of the artery should be inhibited by immediate administration of **anti-platelet drugs** *(aspirin, Clopidogrel),* **and heparin.**
- Timely *fibrinolysis* in patients of AMI with elevated ST-segment (STEMI) or fresh onset LBBB improves both short- and long-term survival. The challenge is to diagnose such cases and institute fibrinolytic therapy in the shortest possible time (hospital door to drug <30 minutes).
- Myocardial oxygen consumption should be decreased in the immediate postinfarction phase by complete bed rest and by limiting heart rate with beta-blockers. Analgesics to relieve pain and tranquilizers to allay anxiety are also helpful.
- Anti-ischemic treatment with **nitrates and beta-blockers** should be instituted early (unless contraindicated) to improve myocardial oxygen supply and limit heart rate. *Supplemental oxygen* for first 24–48 hours is generally beneficial.
- Treatment with ACE **inhibitors** should be instituted within 24–48 hours (as soon as the patient is hemodynamically stable) to reduce infarct size and minimize risk of ventricular dysfunction.
- Lipid-lowering drugs **(statins)** should be introduced in the therapeutic schedule at the earliest. *The five drugs in bold print (except perhaps nitrates) should be continued for at least 1 year after AMI, while low dose aspirin and an appropriate dose of a statin continued indefinitely.* Ideally, LDL cholesterol should be maintained ≤ 80 mg%.

❖ Urgent coronary angiography and a suitable reperfusion procedure should be considered in all cases of STEMI especially in patients in whom fibrinolysis either fails or is contraindicated. In other cases of acute coronary syndrome, coronary angiography and optimal intervention should be considered on priority.

# NON-ST-ELEVATED MYOCARDIAL INFARCTION (NSTEMI) AND UNSTABLE ANGINA (UA)

## Definition

Along with STEMI, NSTEMI, and unstable angina (UA) constitute a pathophysiological continuum in ACS (though not necessarily a clinical continuum). In all three conditions disruption of atheromatous plaque is the initial pathology leading to platelet aggregation and thrombosis at the site of plaque rupture/erosion. The pathological difference between the various disease states is that in patients with NSTEMI and UA, the thrombus is only partial and sub-occlusive whereas in STEMI, it is completely occlusive. Further differentiation between NSTEMI and UA is possible by study of cardiac biomarkers indicative of myocardial necrosis; these are elevated in patients with NSTEMI and are within normal limits in UA.

## Pathophysiology

Both NSTEMI and UA are the result of a rapidly developing mismatch between the oxygen supply and/or increase in myocardial oxygen demand on the background of coronary obstruction, usually due to atherosclerosis. A *non-occlusive thrombus* develops at the site of plaque disruption, with the result that what was a subcritical coronary atherosclerotic lesion (usually 50% or less) becomes critical, resulting in sudden acute myocardial ischemia. Such a thrombus in UA forms intermittently, remains sub-occlusive, and often undergoes spontaneous lysis. Since, the speed and pattern of such pathological changes are often variable, UA was known in the past by a variety of names, such as "Intermediate Syndrome", "Crescendo Angina", "Acute Coronary Insufficiency", "Preinfarction Angina", etc. Currently however, all these patterns of myocardial ischemia are grouped under "Unstable Angina". If the thrombus proceeds to complete obstruction, it may end up as AMI.

## Clinical Features

Unstable angina has been classified according to its severity as follows:

**Class I:** This comprises two types of cases: **(1) Crescendo angina** characterized by a recent increase in the frequency, severity, or duration of anginal pain in patients of stable AP. Accordingly, angina occurs with lesser and lesser exertion, lasts longer than usual, and becomes increasingly resistant to sublingual nitrates; **(2) New-onset** severe and frequent angina (within 2 months of presentation), but without rest angina.

**Class II:** This is marked by onset of one or more episodes of **rest angina** during the past 4 weeks but not within preceding 24 hours (subacute cases).

**Class III:** In this category, the patient has one or more episodes of **new onset acute angina within past 48 hours,** occurring at rest or on minimal exertion. This is often the first manifestation of CHD in such patients.

The pain of UA is identical to that of effort-induced angina (*see* section on "Pain in Chest") but is usually more severe, lasts longer (even up to 30 minutes), may be nocturnal, and radiate to a new site. It is incompletely relieved by sublingual nitrates, and may be accompanied by symptoms, such as nausea, vomiting, dyspnea, perspiration, hypotension, and other features of LV dysfunction.

## Diagnosis

The diagnosis of UA is based on the clinical patterns of ischemic pain described above coupled with transient ST-segment depression and/or inversion of T-waves, especially if ECG is recorded during chest pain. It is important to remember that patients with NSTEMI present in a similar manner, and the distinction between the two can be made only later when the results of cardiac serum markers (CPK-MB or troponins) become available. Since significant myocardial necrosis does not develop in cases of UA, cardiac enzyme CPK-MB is usually within normal limits or only marginally increased, and troponins cannot be detected **(Table 1.1 and Fig. 1.2).** New-onset Q-waves do not occur in UA but may develop in a minority of cases of NSTEMI.

## Management

The immediate objective of management in UA and NSTEMI is to control both the acute symptoms as well as prevent worsening of ischemia and progression to STEMI. The condition is potentially dangerous, and the consequences of misdiagnosis may be serious. Ideally therefore, every patient suspected of UA should be hospitalized and observed for 24 hours before excluding the diagnosis. However, since this may not be practical, some risk stratification is desirable. **Admission in an ICU is mandatory in high-risk group,** which comprises patients with:

- Age >70 years
- Recent, prolonged or recurrent chest pain
- Definite ECG changes indicative of ischemia in multiple leads
- Associated disease of significance, such as previous MI, diabetes mellitus, or significant hypertension
- Aggravating angina when already on aspirin and other anti-ischemic drugs.

### General Measures

All patients with UA and NSTEMI should be advised bed rest or permitted very limited activity for 3–5 days. The *period of bed rest* may be prolonged in cases with ongoing pain. Some degree of *anxiety* is always present, and should be controlled with benzodiazepine. Blood pressure should be maintained near lower level of normal, and the heart rate lowered to 60–70/min with beta-blockers (unless contraindicated). All hospitalized patients should receive supplemental oxygen. Any *associated disease* which may temporarily increase myocardial oxygen demand (such as infection, hypertension, thyrotoxicosis, concurrent pulmonary or gastrointestinal illness, anemia, tachyarrhythmia, or severe bradycardia), should be promptly diagnosed and appropriately treated. For risk factor modification, *see* section on STEMI.

## Specific Measures

- **Antiplatelets** *(aspirin and Clopidogrel),* and **anti-ischemic drugs** *(nitrates and beta-blockers)* **should** be **administered as** early as **possible** in all cases **suspected** of NSTEMI or UA (for **details** *see* section on **STEMI).**
- **Anticoagulation:** Since intravascular thrombosis plays a *prominent role in* the pathogenesis of UA and NSTEMI and their progression to MI, heparinization (usually LMWH) is recommended in all such patients of UA. When given along with aspirin and **Clopidogrel,** heparin reduces risk of MI and sudden death (for details *see* section on Acute Myocardial Infarction).
- **Nitrates:** As in cases with STEMI, nitrates are administered sublingually at the start of chest pain in all patients of UA/NSTEMI. By promoting coronary blood flow, nitrates not only relieve anginal pain, and prevent recurrence of acute ischemic events, but also improve LV functions. If the pain is prolonged and the patient can be closely monitored, nitroglycerine (NG) infusion may be considered (*see* section on STEMI) and administered for 24-48 hours, according to intervention strategy planned. If intervention is not possible or is denied by the patient or his relatives, oral nitrates should be substituted. However, it should be noted that long-term use of nitrates, though often prescribed, is likely to be beneficial only in cases with recurring anginal pain. Their continued use is not known to alter mortality or the rate of MI in patients with UA.
- **Beta-adrenergic blocking agents:** Unless contraindications exist, beta-blockers should be combined with nitrates in all cases of UA, adjusting the dose so as to maintain the heart rate between 60 and 70 beats/min. The combination (of nitrates and beta-blocker) reduces the frequency of recurring ischemic episodes. Even if the patient is already taking nitrates and calcium antagonists, beta-blockers should be added. However, such patients should be carefully monitored since a *combination of beta-blockers and calcium antagonists (especially verapamil or diltiazem) may precipitate heart failure and undue bradycardia.*
- **Calcium channel blockers:** These drugs have not been found to improve the outcome in such patients and should not be used unless beta-blockers are contraindicated, when cilnidipine may be added, especially if hypertension coexists.

**Chapter 1:** Cardiovascular Emergencies

> **Box 1.1: Criteria for high-risk cases of NSTEMI/UA.**
> - Persistent angina at rest or on minimal activity
> - New ECG changes - ST depression or T-wave inversion
> - Elevated cardiac biomarkers
> - Associated features of heart failure
> - Significant hypokinesia on echocardiography; EF <40%
> - Fall in blood pressure
> - Past history of myocardial infarction or coronary interventions

- **Fibrinolytic therapy:** Since coronary thrombus is usually sub-occlusive in patients with UA and NSTEMI, and often undergoes rapid spontaneous lysis, *fibrinolytic therapy is not recommended in such cases (including high-risk cases).*
- **Percutaneous coronary intervention (PCI):** Patients with UA and NSTEMI have an unpredictable course, and therefore early coronary angiography (CAG) with appropriate reperfusion procedure is desirable, especially in high-risk cases **(Box 1.1)**.

**Elective PCI:** Limited medical facilities generally available (especially in *mofussil* areas) coupled with economic constraints in most of the patients in India and other developing countries restrict the scope of routine coronary angiography in these cases. Furthermore, a great majority of such patients often stabilize and become pain-free with medical therapy. These patients should however, undergo non-invasive testing a few days after they have been stabilized. Such an approach will identify high-risk subset of patients who should undergo CAG (followed by PCI or coronary bypass grafting) without much delay. However, **all through this period, treatment with antiplatelet drugs, nitrates, and beta-blockers must continue.** If beta-blockers are contraindicated, the new CCB *(cilnidipine)* should be prescribed.

### Subsequent Measures

After the acute phase of disease is controlled with medical therapy, with or without coronary intervention, **long-term management must be stressed.** This should include life-style modifications, control of comorbidities (especially diabetes and hypertension), and appropriate medication which comprises *five classes of drugs: (1) Antiplatelets* (aspirin should be continued life-long, and Clopidogrel for about one year), *(2) Statins* (improve dyslipidemia and help plaque stabilization), *(3) ACE inhibitors* (help plaque stabilization), *(4) Beta-blockers* (as anti-ischemic agent), and *(5) Nitrates* which are employed in acute phase to relieve chest pain, and on long-term basis to improve exercise tolerance in patients with recurring angina.

## Summary

NSTEMI and UA represent a clinical syndrome characterized by *acute myocardial ischemia due to subocclusive coronary thrombus.* The

cardiac ischemia is more marked in the former and, unlike UA, is associated with myocardial necrosis and elevated serum enzymes. Key points in the management of such cases are:
- Admission to an ICU should be considered for all cases especially those in high-risk group.
- **All cases should receive antiplatelet drugs (aspirin and Clopidogrel), nitrates, and (unless contraindicated) beta-blockers.** When beta-blockers are contraindicated, cilnidipine (the new **CCB**) should be prescribed, especially if hypertension coexists.
- IV nitroglycerine for first 12-24 hours is beneficial in such cases, especially if there is on-going pain.
- All cases should be heparinized by subcutaneous LMWH for first 3-5 days.
- Fibrinolysis is not beneficial in such cases and may actually be harmful.
- Any exacerbating factor should be identified and treated (hypertension, arrhythmia, heart failure, acute infection, thyrotoxicosis, severe anemia, etc.).
- Early CAG is desirable in all but the mildest cases; it should be performed on priority in high-risk cases, and combined (as required) with appropriate intervention.

# HEART FAILURE

Heart failure (HF) is a clinical state in which an abnormality in cardiac function or structure impairs the ability of the heart to pump blood commensurate with the metabolic needs of the tissues. It is the result of damage to heart muscle by another primary cause most commonly hypertension and CAD. Depending on the cause, heart failure may occur gradually over many years or it may occur quickly if a significant part of heart muscle is damaged at once—as after massive MI.

## Terminology

In order to properly understand the syndrome of HF, it is necessary to be familiar with certain terms:
- **Ejection Fraction (EF):** This is a manifestation of the amount of blood pumped out of LV with each beat. In a normal person, the EF equals about 55% or more. In patients with systolic failure the EF will be 20-40% or even less.
- **Ventricular remodeling:** When heart failure develops, the LV undergoes certain changes such as: (a) inside of the ventricle gets bigger, (b) its walls become thicker, and (c) the heart changes shape and becomes more round rather than pear shaped. These changes worsen the heart's ability to pump blood, stress the heart and may cause mitral valve to leak.
- **Systolic heart failure (systolic dysfunction):** This implies that LV does not contract with enough force, so there is not enough oxygen-rich blood pumped throughout the body. An EF <40% indicates systolic HF.

❖ **Diastolic heart failure** (diastolic dysfunction with preserved LV systolic function). In this state heart contracts normally (a normal EF) but the ventricle does not relax or fill properly or is stiff, and less blood enters the heart during normal filling. The two types (systolic and diastolic) HF are differentiated by echocardiography.

## Types of Heart Failure

❖ **Left-sided heart failure/left heart failure (LHF):** This type occurs whenever left ventricular functions are compromised and EF decreases to 20–40% or even less. LHF may be predominantly systolic or mostly diastolic HF (vide supra), and these two types need to be differentiated because drug treatment is different for the two types.
❖ **Right-sided heart failure/right heart failure (RHF):** Most often this occurs secondary to left sided HF. When the left ventricle fails, increased fluid pressure is transferred back through the lungs, ultimately damaging the right ventricle.
Another important cause of RHF is disorders of the lungs, the most common being chronic obstructive pulmonary disease (corpulmonale)
❖ **Congestive heart failure (CHF):** This is a type of HF in which blood returning to the heart through the veins backs up, causing congestion in the body's tissues (mostly dependent parts). The classical clinical triad in such cases comprises increased jugular venous pressure (JVP), enlarged tender liver and pedal and leg edema. Fluid may also collect in the alveoli resulting in shortness of breath especially in supine position. In advanced state this can result in pulmonary edema, which is described in the next section.

## Management

Heart failure being generally a chronic condition, only essentials of management are described. While controlling the underlying cardiac/lung disease and treating (any) precipitating factor(s) are obviously a priority, some general measures are also important. These include restricted physical activities according to severity of HF, low salt diet, abstinence from alcohol and smoking and appropriate treatment of comorbidities, such as diabetes mellitus, hypertension, hyperlipidemia, etc.

### *Specific Measures*

The most effective drugs in both systolic and diastolic HF are diuretics, ACE inhibitors/receptor blockers, spironolactone and beta-blockers especially in cases associated with tachycardia. In systolic HF additional measures, which may be considered include nitrates/vasodilators and (in selected cases) digitalis therapy especially in patients with fast atrial fibrillation/flutter.

## Advanced Chronic Heart Failure

Advanced or resistant HF represents a stage in HF when patients do not improve despite optimal therapy that includes diuretics, ACE inhibitors, and beta-blockers, and when indicated cardiac resynchronization therapy. Such patients have all or most of the following features: (1) Severe symptoms with dyspnea/fatigue at rest or on minimal exertion, (2) LVEF less than 30%, (3) Elevated B-type natriuretic peptides, and (4) One or more hospitalizations for HF in the past 6 months.

**Newer methods:** (1) Cardiac transplantation introduced in 1967 is an accepted procedure in the treatment of advanced HF, and can prolong life by about 5 years. However, its scope is greatly limited by the number of "donor hearts" available, (2) Introducing embryogenic stem cells, and "gene therapy" are new modalities still in experimental stages.

## ACUTE PULMONARY EDEMA

### Etiology

Acute pulmonary edema is a grave medical emergency, which may complicate a variety of clinical conditions. It can be broadly classified into two types, **cardiogenic and noncardiogenic (Table 1.4)**. The description that follows pertains to cardiogenic pulmonary edema.

*Acute pulmonary edema of cardiogenic origin represents acute LHF of the severest type.* It may develop suddenly in patients with known cardiac disease, acute or chronic, or may result from acute intensification of pre-existing LHF. Any disease on the left side of the circulation, distal to the pulmonary capillaries, can result in acute LHF, e.g., rheumatic, ischemic and hypertensive heart disease, cardiomyopathies, acute myocarditis, and diseases of the pulmonary veins.

The *precipitating factors* include acute ischemic myocardial injury, tachyarrhythmias, acute infections especially respiratory, undue physical exertion, and increase in blood volume and venous return as in pregnancy or following large rapid IV infusions (especially on the background of cardiac disease—valvular or myocardial).

### Pathogenesis

Acute (cardiogenic) pulmonary edema/acute LHF usually occurs whenever there is imbalance between the opposing hemodynamic forces of pulmonary capillary pressure (normally 8–12 mm Hg) and plasma oncotic pressure (normally about 25 mm Hg). In LHF, the pulmonary capillary pressure is increased, and pulmonary edema usually occurs whenever there is an acute, critical elevation of pulmonary capillary pressure beyond the plasma oncotic pressure. Consequently, fluid transfer from the capillaries into the interstitial tissues is increased. Initially, this excessive fluid in the interstitium is removed

Table 1.4: Classifications of pulmonary edema.

| Cardiogenic | Noncardiogenic |
|---|---|
| **Secondary to LV failure**<br>• Coronary artery disease<br>• Hypertension<br>• Aortic valve disease<br>• Myocarditis<br>• Cardiomyopathies | **Altered permeability of alveolar-capillary membrane**<br>All types and causes of "acute respiratory distress syndrome" (see Chapter 2) |
| **Increased pulmonary capillary pressure (without LV failure)**<br>• Mitral stenosis<br>• Diseases of pulmonary veins<br>• Rapid large IV infusions | **Insufficiency of pulmonary lymphatics**<br>• Lymphangitis carcinomatosis<br>• Fibrosing alveolitis |
|  | **Miscellaneous**<br>• High-altitude pulmonary edema<br>• Neurogenic pulmonary edema (CNS trauma, subarachnoid hemorrhage)<br>• Eclampsia<br>• Heroin overdose<br>• Pulmonary embolism<br>• Postanesthetic<br>• Narcotic intoxication<br>• Cardioversion<br>• Cardiopulmonary bypass |

by the lymphatic flow. However, when the capacity of the lymphatics is exceeded, the fluid starts collecting in the interstitial tissues, tracks into the interstitial space around the alveoli, and disrupts the tight junctions of the alveolar membrane. Finally, the fluid pours into the alveoli and drains into the bronchi. It is this sudden flooding of the lungs, which is responsible for most of the symptoms in such cases.

### Clinical Features

In a well-developed attack of LHF, the history and appearance of the patient are characteristic. Most of the attacks come during sleep, unless there are particular precipitating factors as mentioned above. The patient is suddenly awakened from his sleep by cough and a feeling of suffocation; he has to sit up and soon becomes extremely breathless. The secretions in the respiratory passage mix with the air and form froth which, to some extent, obstructs air-flow through bronchi. There may also be reflex bronchial constriction with diffuse wheeze **(cardiac asthma)**.

Persistent cough develops and is associated with frothy sputum which may be blood tinged. The patient appears to be fighting for life and extreme anxiety grips him resulting in profuse perspiration, cold clammy skin, and marked tachycardia. Cyanosis often develops and is due both to hypoxemia and intense peripheral vasoconstriction resulting from sympathetic over-activity. *Auscultation of the lungs* reveals rales and rhonchi that appear at first over the lung bases but then extend upward as the condition worsens. Cardiac auscultation may be difficult because of respiratory "noises", but an S3 gallop and accentuated pulmonary closure sound are often present. In addition, evidence of underlying cardiac pathology may be discovered.

The attack may be cut short by treatment or, rarely, may subside spontaneously. If severe and untreated, it often progresses into frank right ventricular failure and/or cardiogenic shock.

## Diagnosis

In the presence of typical clinical features described above the diagnosis of acute LHF is usually easy. Evidence of an underlying cardiac pathology will provide additional support. An ECG is of great value, if MI is suspected. This may not however, be immediately available and if the history is not carefully elicited or is atypical, the presence of appreciable wheezing may lead to an erroneous diagnosis of bronchial asthma. Old patients may have associated emphysema and may present genuine problem in differential diagnosis. In such cases, furosemide 40-60 mg may be given IV as a therapeutic test. This will induce a brisk diuresis and provide appreciable relief in dyspnea, if it is of cardiac origin. Narcotics should be withheld if there is the slightest doubt of the patient having primary respiratory failure or bronchial asthma.

**Investigative work up** should include complete blood count, and estimation of blood sugar, urea, creatinine, electrolytes, and preferably also blood gases. A **CXR** will show blurring of vascular outlines, vascular redistribution in the lungs, and a characteristic butterfly pattern of alveolar edema. A more specific investigation is **echocardiography** which provides quick and valuable information regarding the nature and extent of LV dysfunction, any valvular lesion, or pericardial disease.

## Management

As soon as a diagnosis of cardiogenic pulmonary edema is made, prompt and effective measures should be instituted to: (1) Lower the venous return and thereby decrease pulmonary congestion; (2) Improve myocardial function; and (3) Clear the air passages. A more definite aim would be to correct underlying abnormalities.

### Specific Measures

- **Posture:** The patient should be made to sit in a chair, or else a cardiac bed provided, if available. Lowering the legs reduces the venous return (preload) thereby relieving pulmonary congestion. Use of rotating tourniquets is outmoded.
- **Narcotics:** Morphine sulfate is an extremely valuable drug in such cases. Besides allaying anxiety, restlessness and distress of acute dyspnea, it

diminishes central sympathetic outflow, and results in venous dilatation thereby decreasing preload and relieving pulmonary congestion. Morphine should be given IV in a dose of 3-5 mg slowly over a 3-minute period, and may be repeated after 15-30 minutes, if necessary. If morphine is not available, norphine (0.3-0.6 mg IV) or pethidine (75-100 mg IM) may be given initially and repeated in smaller doses after 4-6 hours, if required. However, narcotic drugs should be avoided in patients with chronic obstructive pulmonary disease. Naloxone should be readily available in case respiratory depression supervenes.

- ❖ **Diuretics:** Coupled with morphine/norphine, rapidly acting *loop diuretics are the mainstay of treatment in acute LHF* 40-60 mg furosemide should be injected IV slowly over 2-3 minutes and repeated every 4-6 hours as required. Besides inducing diuresis, these agents produce venodilatation which often occurs even before the onset of diuresis. After the acute attack is over, maintenance therapy should be continued with oral diuretics. Serum electrolytes must be carefully monitored while patient is receiving IV furosemide.
- ❖ **Nitrates:** By reducing both blood pressure and LV filling pressure, nitrates have a beneficial effect in acute LHF especially in cases of pulmonary edema due to MI or hypertension. *Sublingual NG or isosorbide dinitrate should be given as an emergency measure followed by NG infusion* starting at 5 mcg/min and titrating the dose upward in increments of 5 mcg/min every 5-7 minutes until pulmonary edema is relieved or systolic pressure drops to 100 mm Hg (for more details, *see* section on "Acute Myocardial Infarction"). After the acute phase is over, IV NG should be withdrawn gradually and ACE inhibitors added to the regimen.
- ❖ **Bronchodilators:** Intravenous aminophylline can be very useful when given in a dose of 5 mg/kg slowly over 7-10 minutes (provided the systolic pressure is not less than 100 mm Hg), especially when bronchospasm is prominent. Depending upon the clinical response, it may be repeated in a dose of 250 mg once or twice at 6-8 hours intervals. Besides relieving bronchospasm, aminophylline reduces pulmonary congestion by its positive inotropic action, and mild venodilator and diuretic effect. *Treatment with inhaled beta-adrenergic agonists may also be helpful in relieving bronchospasm.*
- ❖ **Other measures:** All cases of severe acute LHF/pulmonary edema should receive oxygen at high flow rates through binasal prongs. If significant hypoxia exists ($PaO_2$ <60 mm Hg), noninvasive pressure support ventilation should be tried. However, if severe respiratory distress **persists,** endotracheal **intubation** and assisted ventilation may become necessary.

The etiologic and precipitating factors, as mentioned earlier, should be carefully sought in every case of cardiogenic pulmonary edema, and appropriately treated. Dramatic relief may follow their successful treatment, e.g., control of arrhythmias.

## General Measures

As soon as acute cardiorespiratory problem has been somewhat controlled, care should be taken to provide adequate fluids *orally*. Urine output should be properly recorded. Patient should be nursed in the semi-recumbent position, a light diet provided for first few days, and fluid and electrolyte balance carefully maintained.

After the patient comes out of the acute attack he should be carefully watched, dosage of oral diuretics and vasodilators (ACE inhibitors) adjusted, and moderate salt restriction continued. Physical activities should be restricted for 2-3 weeks to consolidate recovery.

## Complications
- Acute renal failure
- Cardiogenic shock

## Summary

Acute pulmonary edema may have an acute onset (as in acute MI), or result from gradual deterioration in LV functions. Marked respiratory distress develops along with tachycardia, cyanosis, and diffuse pulmonary rales and rhonchi. The most useful investigations include ECG and echocardiogram. Salient points in the management of acute pulmonary edema are as follows:
- Morphine and furosemide given intravenously are the frontline drugs in such cases.
- Nitroglycerine infusion and IV aminophylline are also very effective, and should be employed keeping a close watch on blood pressure.
- Supportive measures are important and include proper posturing of the patient, and supplemental 100% oxygen.
- Dopamine and dobutamine are the most appropriate inotropic agents, if hypotension develops.

# CARDIOGENIC SHOCK

## Definition and Etiology

Cardiogenic shock (CS) is a life-threatening emergency—***the result of severe LV failure.*** It is a clinical syndrome characterized by acute, severe and prolonged hypotension (systolic pressure <85 mm Hg) with evidence of hypoperfusion of skin, kidneys, and brain. It results from sudden failure of heart as an effective pump, and is encountered mostly in patients with acute MI (usually ST-elevated *type).* Less often, acute severe primary myocardial failure may be seen in cases with cardiomyopathy, myocarditis, or cardiac tamponade.

It needs to be emphasized that, in cases of acute MI cardiogenic shock should not be diagnosed on the basis of hypotension alone since this may be the result of intravascular hypovolemia and reduction in LV preload due to factors, such as vomiting, diaphoresis, lack of oral intake, and certain medications (e.g., nitrates, narcotics, beta-blockers, or CCBs).

Such cases are not uncommon (up to 20%), and can be differentiated from true CS by measuring central venous pressure (a reading <12cm water is highly suggestive of hypovolemia). Hypotension usually resolves in these patients following administration of IV fluids, and prognosis is relatively better than when CS is entirely due to myocardial damage.

## Pathogenesis

The frequency of CS in AMI is directly related to the extent of myocardial necrosis. Typically, it manifests when at least 40% of the LV myocardium is damaged. Cardiogenic shock is relatively uncommon with inferior MI unless there is associated right ventricular infarction.

Cardiogenic shock may be the presenting feature in a case of AMI, but more often it manifests a few hours after the onset of infarction since ischemic injury is progressive over time and its full impact on hemodynamic alterations may evolve over several hours. Occasionally, it is ushered in by other serious complications of acute infarction, such as tachy-or-bradyarrhythmias, pulmonary embolism, A-V blocks, acute papillary muscle dysfunction or rupture of interventricular septum.

## Pathophysiology

The basic disturbance in cases of CS is *decreased* **cardiac output** (cardiac index being <2.2 L/m$^2$/min, often 1.6 L/m$^2$/min) **coupled with elevated pulmonary capillary pressure** >18 mm Hg *(often about 25 mm Hg).* The blood volume is essentially normal, and it is this feature which distinguishes cardiogenic shock from majority of other cases of shock (*see* Chapter 11).

Acute MI results in both systolic and diastolic dysfunction with consequent decrease in stroke volume, on the one hand, and elevation of LV end-diastolic pressure (with associated pulmonary congestion, on the other). Systemic blood pressure drops resulting in coronary hypoperfusion, and coupled with hypoxia (on account of pulmonary congestion) leads to increasing ischemia and progressive myocardial dysfunction. A vicious circle, thus, develops which is only worsened by lactic acidosis and a systemic inflammatory response which may accompany large infarcts and shock.

## Clinical Features

Many patients with CS have continuing chest pain, and appear, restless, sometimes ***confused and even drowsy due to cerebral under-perfusion.*** Compensatory peripheral vasoconstriction due to sympathetic over-activity results *in diaphoresis, cold clammy skin, and peripheral cyanosis.* Systolic pressure falls progressively, is usually below 85 mm Hg (or lower by 60 mm Hg than former levels in hypertensive subjects), ***and pulse is weak and rapid,*** usually between 100 and 120 beats/min. ***Tachypnea and Cheyne-Stokes respiration*** may be present along with elevated jugular venous pressure; rales are often audible. In the final phase oliguria usually sets in with urine output <20–30 mL/hour.

## Diagnosis

Given the background of AMI or some other type of severe cardiac disease, a diagnosis of cardiogenic shock is not difficult if the patient has **signs of marked hypoperfusion** coupled with ***features of peripheral vasoconstriction and pulmonary congestion.*** Clinical features of systemic venous congestion may or may not be present. Cardiogenic shock in MI is usually associated with advanced age, ST-elevated MI, history of previous MI, and often diabetes mellitus **(high-risk group** *see* section on "Acute Coronary Syndrome").

## Investigations

An ***ECG and echocardiogram*** are the basic investigations in CS. The latter will determine its etiology, and also assess the extent of myocardial damage. In cases due to acute MI ***cardiac markers including troponins are always elevated.*** Hepatic transaminases may be markedly increased and reflect hepatic hypoperfusion. Investigations may also reveal elevated white cell count, altered renal functions and electrolytes, hypoxemia, and metabolic acidosis.

## Management

Once fully developed treatment of cardiogenic shock is difficult and complex, and often unrewarding. The disease carries an in-hospital mortality of 50–80% depending upon the quality of medical care available. Prognosis is better when facilities exist for continuous hemodynamic monitoring [measurement of pulmonary capillary wedge pressure (PCWP) and online arterial pressure/blood gas analysis], and intra-aortic balloon counter pulsation (IABC).
**Two main objectives of management should be:**
1. To maintain adequate cardiac output and perfusion pressure by continuous recording of systolic pressure (which should be maintained ≥ 90 mm Hg), and an hourly record of urine output through an indwelling catheter.
2. To preserve the integrity of jeopardized myocardium, and limit infarct size as best as possible.

### *Specific Measures*

The patient should be hospitalized immediately in a suitable facility (vide supra), if not already admitted. It is important that therapeutic measures are instituted even while a clinical and laboratory assessment of the patient is under way. Chest pain (if present) should be relieved as it may be responsible for some vasodepressor reflex activity. However, narcotics should be avoided as far as possible because of risk of fall in blood pressure.

**Overall management comprises:**
- Raising blood pressure with vasopressors
- Treating coexisting hypovolemia, if any, by infusion of crystalloids to maintain PCWP about 20 mm Hg or CVP ~ 15 cm $H_2O$.
- Correcting associated acidosis, hypoxemia, and any other identifiable contributory factor (vide supra).

1. **Vasopressors:** Intravenous vasoactive drugs are the mainstay to improve blood pressure and cardiac output. Commonly used inotropic/vasopressor agents and their hemodynamic profile are given in **Table 1.5**.

   All vasopressors activate both alpha-and beta receptors in varying degree, and no ideal vasopressor agent is available so far. Most favorable results are likely to be achieved with agents that provide maximal inotropism and effective vasoconstriction while inducing minimal tachycardia (chronotropic effect). *Dobutamine has positive inotropic action but very little peripheral vasoconstrictive effect* (alpha-effect). *Dopamine, on the other hand, has both chronotropic and inotropic effects (beta-receptor stimulation), and also vasoconstrictor effect* (alpha-receptor stimulation) at higher doses (>10 µg/kg/min). Further, this alpha-effect is dose-dependent, and becomes progressively more intense with increasing doses of the drug (up to a maximum of 30 µg/kg/min).

   As a practical rule, vasopressor therapy in CS is initiated with dopamine at a dose of 5-10 µg/kg/mm. The dose is then titrated if required, upward every 5-7 minutes to achieve reasonable systolic pressure (~90 mm Hg). However, at doses higher than 20-25 µg/kg/min, its hemodynamic profile comes to resemble that of norepinephrine with predominant chronotropic (tachycardia) and marked vasoconstrictive (alpha-adrenergic) effect. Accordingly systemic vascular **resistance (afterload) greatly increases**

**Table 1.5:** Common inotropic drugs—pharmacodynamic profile.

| Drug | Receptor (s) activated* | Inotropic | Chronotropic | Vasoconstrictor |
|---|---|---|---|---|
| Norepinephrine | α**β**$_1$ | +++ | +++ | ++++ |
| Dopamine | **α**β$_1$ | +++ | ++ | (+) to (++)† |
| Dobutamine | αβ$_1$**β**$_2$ | +++ | + | (0) to (+)† |
| Epinephrine | **α**β$_1$β$_1$ | +++ | +++ | ++ |
| Isoproterenol | β$_1$**β**$_2$ | ++++ | ++++ | - |
| Methoxamine | **A** | 0 | 0 | ++++ |
| Amrinone | 0 | +++ | 0 | - |

Chief property: α-agonist: vasoconstriction; β$_1$-agonist: chronotropic and inotropic; β$_2$-agonist: vasodilatation and bronchodilation.
*Bold letters indicate predominant adrenergic receptor activity
†Adrenergic effect varies with drug concentration

and this coupled with tachycardia, is likely to aggravate myocardial ischemia. **Such large doses** of **dopamine** are **therefore** best avoided in CS associated with MI.

If dopamine in moderate doses (up to 20 µg/kg/min) is unable to increase blood pressure to satisfactory level, dobutamine should be added to achieve additional inotropic action (in doses of 2.5–10 µg/kg/min). In fact *dopamine and dobutamine have a complimentary* role in a manner that is most beneficial in such patients.

*Norepinephrine* has powerful (alpha) vasoconstrictor action (increases afterload) and also possesses beta-agonist activity that increases contractility and heart rate. Since both vasoconstriction and tachycardia are associated with increased myocardial oxygen consumption, norepinephrine should be reserved for patients in desperate situations. It is usually started in a dose of 4 µg/min and can be increased gradually up to 15 µg/min, beyond which it is unlikely to be further beneficial.

**ote**

See Appendix at the end of this chapter for details of weight adjusted doses of common drugs administered as bolus/infusion in cardiovascular emergencies.

2. **Correction of hypovolemia:** An important contributory factor in the pathogenesis of shock following MI can be hypovolemia (in 15–20% of cases). Though the need for IV fluid therapy may to some extent, be judged from details of history (excessive fluid loss or poor intake), it is best assessed by measuring PCWP, or more simply (though less satisfactorily) by central venous pressure (CVP). PCWP <15 mm Hg or CVP <12 cm water is highly suggestive of hypovolemia.

    Since patients of cardiogenic shock with significant hypovolemia have a better prognosis, these cases should be actively identified and treated with successive boluses of 100 ml normal saline given rapidly (20–40 mL/min) until PCWP reaches 15–18 mm Hg or CVP 12–15 cm water. If the blood pressure improves and signs of pulmonary congestion do not appear or worsen, 500 mL of normal saline should be infused rapidly in 30–60 minutes keeping a close watch on PWP/CVP and clinical signs of fluid overload. This should result in considerable hemodynamic improvement. The speed of fluid administration is important since it is only by such *rapid infusions* that one can be certain of acute expansion of vascular compartment, and thereby augmentation of venous return. Thereafter, IV fluids should be continued at a slower rate monitored by serial records of BP, pulse rate, urine output, and PWP/CVP.

3. **Intra-aortic balloon counterpulsation (IABC):** If the vasopressors and other symptomatic measures fail to rapidly improve blood pressure and cardiac output, IABC should be instituted. It decreases left ventricular work and oxygen demand by reducing afterload while simultaneously improving

coronary perfusion by increasing aortic diastolic pressure. IABC improves hemodynamic status in most of the patients *though this improvement may be temporary.*
4. **Revascularization:** Since cardiogenic shock usually occurs in patients with large anterior ST- elevated infarcts early reperfusion therapy significantly decreases the risk of complications including cardiogenic shock. What is important to rapidly establish blood flow in the infarct-related artery. If fibrinolytic therapy fails to improve circulatory status, early angiography and some revascularization procedure should be planned keeping in view the overall condition of the patient. Even primary angiography (before fibrinolysis) and revascularization is being increasingly considered in such cases, but the choice has to be individualized.
5. **Other measures:** Any precipitating or aggravating factor should be promptly identified and managed. This could be an inappropriate medication, acute infection, blood gas or electrolyte disturbance, and brady-tachy-arrhythmias.

### *General Measures*

The patient should be kept in ***supine position*** with legs slightly elevated to improve venous return. However, this position may be impracticable in the presence of significant LHF; such patients should be placed in a semi-recumbent position. All patients should be given supplemental oxygen through binasal prongs at fast rates (6–8 L/min), or by intratracheal intubation, if pulmonary edema coexists. Two IV lines should be established, and a Foley's catheter inserted to record urine output every 2 hours. Restlessness and agitation, if marked, should be controlled with benzodiazepines. Heavy sedation should be avoided.

### Summary

Cardiogenic shock in a case of AMI implies a large infarct often involving both endocardium and epicardium (STEMI). Management of such cases is complex, and results are often nongratifying. Important steps in management are as follows:

- After taking care of airways and breathing, at least minimal hemodynamic monitoring in the form of CVP recording should be promptly established. A low CVP (<8–10 cm of water) implies some degree of hypovolemia. This should be quickly corrected, and CVP maintained near 12–15 cm of water.
- Vasopressors are invariably required to maintain adequate tissue perfusion; dopamine should be used first, and its dose gradually titrated to achieve desired results, failing which dobutamine should be added.
- Patients with inadequate response to these measures should be considered for IABC and, in selected cases, even for emergency percutaneous intervention.

❖ Reversible factors such as severe acidosis (pH<7.0), hypokalemia, acute infections, **tachy-brady-arrhythmias, and profound hyperglycemia should be quickly identified and suitably treated.**
❖ Proper positioning of the patient, supplemental oxygen and other general measures must be taken care of.

# PULMONARY EMBOLISM

Pulmonary embolism also referred as pulmonary thromboembolism (PTE) implies blockage of a major artery of the lung or one of its branches. Most commonly the block is by a blood clot that breaks loose and travels to the lungs through the bloodstream *(embolism).* Most common site of origin of such emboli is deep venous thrombosis (DVT) in the deep veins of the legs or pelvis. Less frequently some foreign material like air (from central venous catheters), fat (after blunt trauma and long bone fractures), tumor fragments, and septic emboli (acute infective endocarditis) may embolize to the pulmonary circulation.

## Risk Factors

Major *predisposing factors for DVT include* venous stasis, injury to blood vessels, and hypercoagulability **(Virchow's triad).** Venous stasis increases with the duration of immobility (especially postoperatively), in advanced stages of pregnancy, chronic heart failure, prolonged travel and sitting as in an airplane, and in obesity. Blood vessels may be damaged by fracture/surgery on lower limbs, trauma, or prior episodes of venous thrombosis. Hypercoagulability may occur in several conditions such as malignancy, extensive surgery, in sepsis, nephrotic syndrome, after medication (oral contraceptive pills), in postpartum period, or can be inherited. Contributory factors include smoking, advanced age, and obesity.

## Clinical Features

Clinical presentation of PE depends largely on two factors—*size of the embolus, and pre-existing cardiopulmonary status.* Accordingly, the clinical features can be extremely varied ranging from breathlessness through hypotension and shock to sudden death. No single sign or symptom, or even their combination, is specific for PE. The most prominent symptoms are:
❖ Sudden onset of chest pain with pleuritic features
❖ Unexplained dyspnea in a patient predisposed to DVT
❖ Cough, usually dry but may be tinged with blood
❖ Other symptoms may include sudden shortness of breath, worsening of underlying heart failure, or sudden unexplained supraventricular tachycardia.

**Physical examination** is unreliable for the diagnosis or exclusion of both DVT and PE. The signs of DVT are related to venous obstruction and inflammation.

Unfortunately neither of the two may be present even in cases found to have DVT on Doppler studies. The most important feature suggestive of DVT is the presence of asymmetric leg swelling, which may or may not be painful. Pain is a symptom more of superficial thrombophlebitis which may be associated with local erythema and a palpable tender **(cord-like)** vein. Homans' sign is a **nonspecific indicator of** calf inflammation, and is rather uncommon in DVT.

The *fate of the embolus reaching the lungs* depends upon the size of the **embolus,** previous episodes of pulmonary embolization, and any coexistent cardiorespiratory disease. Broadly speaking, clinical presentation of acute PE can be classified into three categories depending upon size of the embolus:

- **Massive PE:** Such cases have 50-80% (or even more) obstruction in pulmonary blood flow with consequent abrupt increase in pulmonary artery pressure and right ventricular dysfunction. If death does not occur immediately, a distinctive clinical picture develops dominated by sudden dyspnea or chest pain or both. The chest pain may be angina-like, and is often mistaken for myocardial infarction. Other features include syncope, hypotension, tachypnea and cyanosis. Acute right ventricular strain may develop indicated by engorged neck veins, tender hepatomegaly, gallop rhythm, and accentuated pulmonary closure sound **(acute cor pulmonale).**

- **Moderate or submassive PE:** This is associated with involvement of significant portion (~50%) of pulmonary arterial tree. Such cases often have *right ventricular hypokinesia on electrocardiography but systemic blood pressure is normal* The presenting symptoms are unexplained dyspnea, tachycardia, and chest pain. Cases with pre-existing cardiac disease may also develop HF and various atrial arrhythmias. Examination of the lungs is unremarkable. Cyanosis may or may not be present but arterial hypoxemia is common (due to increase in physiological dead space).

- **Small PE:** These are cases of low-risk PE and have *neither arterial hypotension nor right ventricular dysfunction.* Some of these cases develop **pulmonary infarction** though it is uncommon because of dual blood supply from pulmonary as well as bronchial artery. Symptoms of pulmonary infarction usually develop 3-7 days after embolism, and comprise pleuritic chest pain, cough, mild fever, and hemoptysis. A pleural or pleuropericardial friction rub is often heard, and signs of consolidation and/or pleural effusion may appear.

### Diagnosis and Investigations

Like amoebic abscess of liver, PE often masquerades and mimics a host of disease such as myocardial infarction, cardiac tamponade, congestive heart failure, pericarditis, pneumonia, pneumothorax, asthma, and chronic obstructive pulmonary disease. A high index of suspicion is therefore, required to guide diagnostic work up. Evidence of proximal (above the knee) DVT on

Doppler ultrasound is highly suggestive. Simultaneous venous ultrasonography may reveal inability to fully compress the common femoral or popliteal veins (positive predictive value of **97%**).

**The initial investigations always include CXR and ECG.** The former is **required to exclude other common lung diseases. In their absence, it is** often reported normal but a careful study may reveal relative oligemia (increased lung translucency) in the area of embolism, and an abrupt cut-off of pulmonary vessels. After 24–48 hours, nonspecific radiological signs may manifest such as **elevation** of diaphragm on affected side, small wedge-shaped pleural-based infiltrate, atelectasis, and pleural effusion (often hemorrhagic).

**Electrocardiogram** is also normal or shows only nonspecific T-wave abnormalities in majority of patients. With large/massive PE pattern of acute right heart strain (**Fig. 1.5**) may be seen: (1) prominent S-wave in lead I; (2) significant Q-wave with inverted T-wave in lead III, which may be mistaken for inferior myocardial infarction; (3) inverted T waves in **V1** to **V3/V4**; (4) prominent spiky P waves; and (5) occasionally, incomplete or complete right bundle branch block. These abnormalities are often transitory, unlike acute MI.

**Echocardiography:** Right ventricular dysfunction, when present, is indicative of significant obstruction of pulmonary artery so that right ventricle is unable to match the pressure. Additionally, it reliably excludes other acute illnesses that may mimic PE (e.g., acute MI, pericardial tamponade, and aortic dissection).

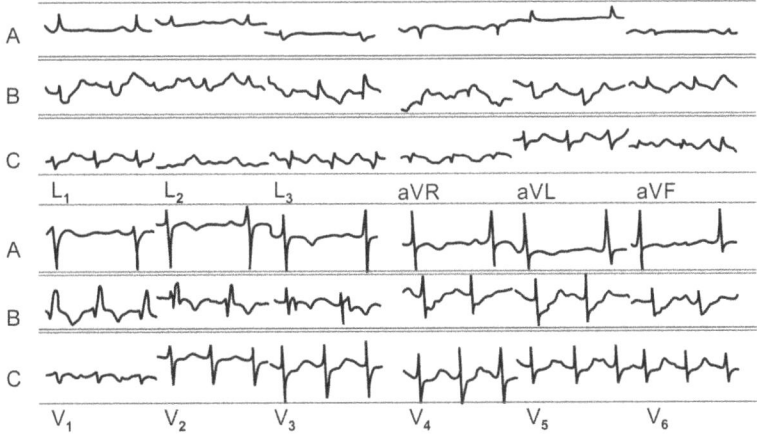

**Fig. 1.5:** ECG changes in massive pulmonary embolism: (A) Basal-65 years male, chronic smoker, admitted with extensive anterior wall ischemia; QRS duration 92 ms, P-axis 14, T-axis 57; (B) Two hours after chest pain and breathlessness-note prominent P in L2 and L3, appearance of deep Q and inverted T in L3 and a VF with right bundle branch block; QRS duration 124 ms, P-axis 79, R-axis 111, T-axis 13; (C) 24 hours later Q3 T3 persists but intraventricular conduction has improved (QRS 84 ms) and P and R-axis have decreased to 71 and 86, respectively.

## Special Diagnostic Tests

- **D-dimer estimation:** Plasma D-dimer is a degradation product of fibrin, and can be estimated by quantitative enzyme-linked immunosorbent assay (ELISA). Its study is based on the principle that endogenous fibrinolysis is an ongoing process in most of the cases of PE. Such fibrinolysis (insufficient by itself to prevent PE) results in breakdown of some of the fibrin clot into D-dimer which is *highly sensitive for PE, but lacks specificity.* Its absence indicates that there is less chance of PE, but even when elevated it may be nonspecific since many conditions which may be associated with PE can cause an elevation of this test (e.g., cancer, recent surgery, infection, any systemic illness, and pregnancy).
- **Ventilation/perfusion (V/Q) scanning:** In this test a radioactive substance is used to show how well oxygen and blood are flowing to the lungs. In PE there is a mismatch between areas that are ventilated but not perfused. Such scans however, are complex to interpret and have low specificity since many other lung diseases (e.g., tuberculosis, carcinoma, sarcoidosis, and emphysema) can also result in scan defects. It is most valuable when negative (rules out diagnosis of PE), or a "high-probability" scan. However, this test is now seldom used because of greater availability of CT technology.
- **CT chest and CT pulmonary angiography** are now the recommended first line diagnostic imaging tests in all suspected cases of massive/sub-massive PE, and have largely replaced pulmonary angiography (an invasive process) long considered the gold standard for diagnosis of PE.

## Management

**Once PE occurs the outcome is uncertain since it** often **recurs,** and moreover, the very first episode of PE (if massive) may be fatal. The patient should therefore, be immediately hospitalized, if not already in the hospital.

Several approaches are available for management of patients with PE *according to risk stratification* based on clinical findings, laboratory evaluation, echocardiographic changes, and perfusion lung scan. **On the basis of such a work up two types of cases of PE can be recognized:**

- Patients with acute PE, but with normal blood pressure and without any evidence of RV dysfunction. Such cases have a stable course and can be treated with anticoagulation alone.
- Patients with echocardiographic evidence of right ventricular enlargement and hypokinesia. These are at increased risk of adverse events and early mortality, and are strong candidates for fibrinolytic therapy.
- **Anticoagulation:** In most cases of PE anticoagulant therapy is the mainstay of treatment. Three drugs are available: (1) unfractionated heparin, (2) low molecular weight heparin, and (3) fondaparinux.

Details of **heparin and LMWH** therapy have been provided in the section on AMI. Heparin retards additional thrombus formation by preventing further fibrin deposition, and thus allows endogenous fibrinolytic system to dissolve the clot. To that extent **it provides only secondary prevention in PE.** Nevertheless, it constitutes the frontline treatment of PTE.

Heparin should be started at the earliest in all moderate to high-risk patients of PE, sometimes even while awaiting the results of various investigations, if there are no contraindications. Heparin should be continued for 5-7 days, and oral anticoagulants introduced on day-1 or day-2 of heparin therapy, adjusting its dosage to achieve prothrombin time to 1.5-2.5 times the control [international normalized ratio (INR) 2.0-3.0]. An overlap of 4-5 days should be allowed with heparin therapy.

*Fondaparinux:* This is a synthetic polysaccharide derived from the antithrombin binding region of heparin. Like LMWH this is also administered subcutaneously but once a day only. The choice between fondaparinux and LMWH should be based on cost factor, availability, and familiarity of use.

There is no consensus as to the ***duration of anticoagulant therapy*** in patients of PE or proximal DVT (merit of heparin therapy in cases of DVT below the knee is uncertain). It will depend upon potential reversibility of risk factors, likely risk of bleeding, patient's age and his preference for continued therapy. Most of the authorities recommend continuing anticoagulation for 3-6 months after the first episode, if the risk factor is transitory, 12 months in idiopathic PTE, and 12 months to indefinitely if the disease is recurrent or the risk factors are nonreversible.

- **Fibrinolytic therapy:** In patients with acute large PTE who are hemodynamically *unstable and/or have RHF,* fibrinolysis is the treatment of choice. Any of the three conventional drugs may be used (streptokinase, urokinase, and rt-PA) since all of them increase plasmin levels, and thereby rapidly dissolve the obstructing intrapulmonary arterial thrombus (primary treatment). Additionally, fibrinolysis results in lysis of the residual clots in the pelvic or deep leg veins thus reducing the chances of recurrence. Fibrinolysis should be initiated as early as possible after the diagnosis has been confirmed, though the "therapeutic window" in such cases is much longer (even up to 10-14 days after the onset of symptoms) than in cases of acute MI. The dosage schedule for fibrinolytic agents is given in **Table 1.6**.
- **Interventional therapy:** Catheter-based methods are currently being studied to extract pulmonary embolus or to induce its mechanical fragmentation in cases where heparinization and pharmacological thrombolysis has failed. Surgical procedures in PE include caval interruption and embolectomy with cardiopulmonary bypass. Their discussion is beyond the scope of this text.
- **Treatment of DVT:** When DVT involves proximal vessels, heparin infusion is recommended for 7-10 days followed by oral anticoagulation. The treatment of patients with calf vein thrombosis is controversial.

| Table 1.6: Dosage schedule of fibrinolysis in acute PTE. | |
|---|---|
| **Lytic agent** | **Dosage regimen** |
| Streptokinase | 250,000–500,000 units IV as loading dose over 15 min, followed by 100,000 units/hr for 24 hours |
| Urokinase | 4,400 units/kg as loading dose over 10 min, followed by 4,400 units/kg/hr for 24 hours |
| Alteplase (t-PA) | 100 mg infusion over 2 hours |

Symptomatic patients should be hospitalized and anticoagulated with either IV unfractionated heparin or by LMWH. On the other hand, in asymptomatic patients, anticoagulant therapy can be safely withheld until serial ultrasonography reveals proximal propagation of thrombus.

❖ **Other measures:** Pleuritic pain when present should be relieved with conventional analgesics or NSAIDs. Hypoxia is invariably present in all but the mildest cases of PE, and therefore, oxygen should be administered at fast rates in acute stage of the disease in all cases. Broad-spectrum antibiotics are also generally required both to prevent secondary infection of pulmonary infarct as well as for any thrombophlebitis in the legs. Some cases have severe bronchospasm due to serotonin. They will need salbutamol nebulization and/or aminophylline infusion in appropriate dosage (*see* section on "Acute Severe Asthma"). When features of acute right heart failure or shock supervene, these should be appropriately managed as described in earlier sections of this Chapter.

## *Prophylaxis*

Though prevention of disease is always the best treatment, in a condition like PE it may be the only practical measure since the very first episode of PE may prove fatal. Since PE is really a complication of DVT, prevention of the latter will constitute the most effective management of PE **(DVT and PE are two manifestations of the same disease).**

It is to be noted that virtually all surgical procedures which necessitate confinement to bed increase the risk of DVT, the risk being maximum for orthopedic surgery in the region of the pelvis. This risk increases in patients who are older than 40, are obese, have carcinoma, a past history of DVT or PE, or when surgery is likely to last longer than one hour. The increased risk persists for about a month after hospital discharge. Likewise, patients with medical disease necessitating prolonged bed rest (e.g., low output HF, complicated MI) are at high risk of developing DVT.

In most of such cases LMWH is used, the first dose being given 2 hours preoperatively, and then treatment continued for seven days postoperatively or till the patient becomes ambulatory. Other preventive measures include leg physiotherapy, deep breathing exercises, use of compression stockings, and intermittent pneumatic compression.

## Summary

- DVT or pulmonary embolism is likely to occur in patients who have venous stasis, some abnormality of blood vessels, or hypercoagulability *(Virchow's triad)*. Risk of PE is especially high when DVT involves vessels above the knee.
- Most common causes include surgery, orthopedic injuries around pelvis, malignancy, and prolonged recumbence in cases of heart failure.
- The classic presentation of PE is sudden onset of dyspnea with tachypnea in a predisposed patient. Diagnostic suspicion is strengthened, if echocardiogram and V/Q scan reveal typical findings.
- Heparin anticoagulation is the cornerstone of treatment, and should be started in full doses, at the earliest, in all patients with a strong suspicion of PE, even before diagnostic evaluation is complete (provided it is not contraindicated).
- Fibrinolysis should be seriously considered in cases of established PE with RV dysfunction who are hemodynamically unstable and are at high risk of death.

# HYPERTENSIVE CRISIS

Hypertensive crisis (HC) is an all encompassing term for hypertensive emergency and hypertensive urgency, which may occur whenever blood pressure (BP) becomes very high. In the former the BP is so high that organ damage is imminent, and BP must be reduced immediately to prevent (further) organ damage.

In *hypertensive urgency,* BP rises rapidly (180/120 or higher), but there is no damage to the body's vital organs. In these cases BP can be brought down safely within a few hours (12–24 hours) with *oral therapy,* and hospitalization is not necessary. Almost all oral antihypertensive drugs are effective, but a combination regimen should be preferred, the goal being a reduction in BP by about 20–25%. An initial relief in BP may be obtained quickly by chewing 25 mg **Captopril** (as in cases with hypertensive emergency). Given these characteristics, hypertensive urgency is not really a medical emergency, and some authorities consider the term has little meaning, minimal utility, and should be dropped. Further discussion is confined to hypertensive emergency.

# HYPERTENSIVE EMERGENCY

## Etiology and Pathophysiology

Formerly called *"malignant hypertension"* the etiology of hypertensive emergency is not well understood. Fluctuations in (normal) BP are common throughout the day (in reaction to emotional or physical stress), as well as over the course of a long period of time. Usually in the range of 30–40 mm Hg, wider swings (60–80 mm Hg) can occur in hypertensive subjects and affect the reactivity of the blood vessels, especially if hypertension is not well controlled. Often such patients are "asymptomatic until a crisis" occurs *(hypertension is a "Silent Killer")*. It is to be remembered that hypertensive emergency is not uncommon sometime or the other in the course of hypertensive patients, if the blood pressure is not frequently monitored.

Many factors can be contributory in hypertensive crises. One main cause is the discontinuation of antihypertensive medication. Other common causes are concurrent use of drugs such as NSAIDs, nasal decongestants (especially pseudoephedrine), migraine medications (which relieve headache but also constrict blood vessels throughout the body), and cocaine, and amphetamines.

*An abrupt rise in systemic vascular resistance* and failure of normal autoregulation are typical initial components of the disease process. This leads to dilatation of arterioles resulting in leakage of fluid into the tissues. Additionally, endothelial injury occurs with fibrin deposition and consequent fibrinoid necrosis of small arteries which is responsible for target organ damage. These changes can be largely reversed by effective antihypertensive treatment instituted in time.

## Clinical Features

Hypertensive emergencies occur **most commonly** in middle-aged patients, and men are at greater risk **than women**. Major organs affected are cardiovascular system, central nervous system, and renal vasculature. Within the brain, features of raised intracranial tension appear such as headache, vomiting, altered mental status, hypertensive encephalopathy, and subarachnoid or intracerebral hemorrhage. Funduscopy often reveals papilledema, and retinal hemorrhage/exudates *(hypertensive retinopathy)*.

*Cardiovascular manifestations* can include chest pain, dyspnea, LV failure and pulmonary edema, acute coronary syndrome, and arrhythmias. Damage to the *kidneys* may be asymptomatic though often small vasculature (glomerular) is affected with increased intraglomerular pressure resulting in proteinuria, hematuria, and even renal failure. Some patients may have pre-existing renal pathology and develop worsening renal functions with challenging diagnostic and therapeutic issues.

Less common features of hypertensive emergency include *severe epistaxis, eclampsia, and aortic dissection.*

## Diagnosis

Hypertensive emergency is diagnosed on the basis of very high BP (diastolic pressure >120 mm Hg) coupled with evidence of target-organ damage. The latter can be detected by routine investigations such as urinalysis, serum BUN and creatinine, chest X-ray, and ECG. An ECG is in fact essential to determine left ventricular hypertrophy or acute ischemia. Echocardiogram can be optional. Funduscopy would have been covered in physical examination and reveals changes of retinopathy (papilledema, soft exudates, and hemorrhages). Patients with neurologic findings will require CT head to diagnose intracranial bleeding, edema, or infarction. Additionally, complete blood count, blood sugar, and serum electrolyte levels may provide useful information for management of the patient.

## Management

The treatment of hypertensive emergencies is based on a rapid and controlled reduction in BP (but not too abruptly). The aim should be to reduce the diastolic BP by about 20-25%, or to between 100 and 110 mm Hg within minutes to 1 or 2 hours, and then to a level of 160/100 mm Hg during the next 3-6 hours. It is to be remembered that individuals with a history of chronic hypertension may not tolerate a "normal" BP, and that excessive reduction in BP can precipitate coronary, cerebral, or renal ischemia.

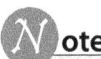ote

> The American Heart Association 2017 report on the classification of blood pressure is given in the appendix at the end of this Chapter.

### Initial Therapy

Immediate reduction in BP is best achieved in such cases by IV medication (vide infra). However, as a first aid measure 25 mg captopril may be chewed and swallowed. Sublingual nifedipine is not recommended since this can result in precipitous fall in BP.

### Subsequent Therapy

Patient should be admitted in an intensive care unit since intravenous medications (which are fast-acting and easily titrable) are generally used. The preferred agents are sodium nitroprusside, nitroglycerine, labetalol, cilnidipine (class IV CCB), fenoldopam, and nicardipine. The choice will depend upon the type of hypertensive emergency, and availability and experience with the drug. Their dosage and other pharmacological properties are given in **Table 1.7**.

Though all these drugs are effective in most of the hypertensive emergencies, yet some drugs are preferred in certain conditions **(Table 1.8)**.

### Maintenance Therapy

Once the BP has been brought under control, treatment should be continued with oral antihypertensive agents, preferably by combining drugs with different class effects in a manner best suited for the clinical state being treated. A small dose of a diuretic should however, be added to all such regimens.

**Table 1.7:** Intravenous drugs for hypertensive emergencies.

| Name of drug | Dose | Onset of action | Duration of action | Special indications |
|---|---|---|---|---|
| Sod. nitroprusside IV infusion | 0.3–0.5 µg/kg/min | Immediate usual dose 3–5 µg/kg/min (not to exceed 8 µg/kg/min) | 1–2 min | Most HE; caution with raised ICP or azotemia |
| Nicardipine | 5–15 mg/hr IV | 5–10 min | 15–30 min may be >4hrs | Most HE except acute HF; caution coronary ischemia |
| Nitroglycerine | 5–100 mg/min IV infusion | 2–5 min | 5–10 min | Coronary ischemia |
| Labetalol | 20–80 mg IV bolus | 5–10 min every 10 min, or 0.5–2.0 mg infusion | 3–6 hrs | Most HE except acute heart failure; avoid in cases with associated bronchial asthma |
| Fenoldopam* | 0.1–0.3 µg/kg/min | <5 min | 30 min | Most HE; caution glaucoma |

*Fenoldopam is a peripheral dopamine-1 receptor agonist that causes a dose-dependent reduction in BP without any major side effects.

[HE: hypertensive emergencies; HF: heart failure; hr: hour; ICP: intracranial pressure; min: minute(s)]

**Table 1.8:** Target-organ specific treatment of common hypertensive emergencies.

| Hypertensive emergencies | Treatment |
|---|---|
| Acute ischemic stroke | Intravenous therapy preferred if BP >200/120<br>**Goal of therapy:** 10–15% reduction in BP<br>**Preferred drug:** IV labetalol or nicardipine<br>**Second choice:** IV nitroprusside |
| Acute intracerebral hemorrhage | Intravenous infusion for aggressive reduction in **BP** if systolic pressure >200 mm Hg<br>**Preferred drug:** Nicardipine |
| Acute pulmonary edema | Intravenous therapy is mandatory<br>**Goal of therapy:** Symptomatic relief<br>**Drugs of choice:** Nitroglycerine and lasix<br>**Second choice:** Nitroprusside |
| Myocardial infarction/unstable angina | **Drugs of choice:** Nitroglycerine, IV beta-blockers |
| Pre-eclampsia/eclampsia | **Goal of therapy:** BP to 140/90 mm Hg<br>**Preferred drugs:** Labetalol, nicardipine |

## Summary

The most common cause of HC, presenting either as an "emergency" or "urgency" is interruption of previously effective antihypertensive medication.

Not infrequently however, it is the first manifestation of undiagnosed hypertension ("silent killer"). The diastolic pressure is markedly elevated (often >120 mm Hg), but the correlation between blood pressure level and end-organ damage is poor. The management of such patients can be summarized as follows:

- Every case of severe hypertension (diastolic pressure >120 mm Hg) should have a quick evaluation of cardiovascular, neurological, and renal systems.
- As initial treatment, **captopril** 25 mg may be given to be chewed and swallowed.
- Hypertensive emergencies require parenteral therapy. The drugs most commonly used are IV nitroprusside, labetalol, and nitroglycerine. The aim should be to achieve a target BP (diastolic pressure ~ 110 mm Hg within minutes to 1-2 hours. Excessive/precipitous lowering of BP should be avoided since it can result in cardiac, cerebral, or renal ischemia.
- In cases of hypertensive urgency, oral medication (preferably more than one drug) alone should suffice to lower BP to safe levels over 12-24 hours.
- Maintenance therapy with appropriate drugs should then be continued, and adequate follow-up ensured.

## CARDIAC ARRHYTHMIAS

Brady-or-tachy-dysrhythmia may be encountered in the course of any type of heart disease—ischemic, rheumatic, thyrotoxic, cor pulmonale, constrictive pericarditis, acute myocarditis, and cardiomyopathy. Other important causes include digitalis overdose, and acid-base or electrolyte imbalance. Sometimes the exact etiology remains unknown.

Clinical spectrum of cardiac arrhythmias may vary from nonconsequential to life-threatening state. Arrhythmias are detrimental when symptomatic or associated with hypotension (leading to reduced tissue perfusion) and/or marked tachycardia (increased myocardial oxygen demand).

### Management

Management of each patient with cardiac arrhythmia needs to be individualized depending upon the type of rhythm disturbance, probable cause, and whether it is symptomatic or not. Several measures are available for treatment of cardiac arrhythmias but invariably pharmacological therapy is employed initially, and usually proves satisfactory. The various antiarrhythmic drugs available have complex and diverse modes of action, and hence defy a simple

**Table 1.9:** Site of action of antiarrhythmic drugs.

| SA node and/or atrium | AV node | Ventricle |
|---|---|---|
| Beta-blockers | Verapamil | Lidocaine |
| • Verapamil | Beta-blockers | Disopyramide |
| • Disopyramide | Quinidine | |
| Procainamide | Mexiletine | |
| Quinidine | Phenytoin | |
| Amiodarone | Amiodarone | |

classification. Nevertheless, it is desirable to have some knowledge of their site of action within the heart and their electrophysiological properties. These are given in **Tables 1.9 and 1.10**, respectively.

**The aims of treatment are:**
- Control arrhythmia
- Eliminate the cause of arrhythmia/treat underlying disease, and
- Prevent recurrence of the arrhythmia.

### General Guidelines to Antiarrhythmic Therapy
- A correct interpretation of a given arrhythmia is essential.
- Any cardiac arrhythmia of acute onset should be controlled as fast as possible to prevent various untoward sequels such as angina pectoris, heart failure, fainting, dizziness, convulsions, cerebral ischemia, and even death.
- The possible cause of a given arrhythmia should be determined, and then eliminated/controlled.
- **Not** all drugs in the same group have identical effects, e.g., amiodarone, **sotalol,** and bretylium (class III drugs) are quite different; on the other hand some drugs in different classes have overlapping actions, e.g., class IA and IC drugs.
- Some drugs have important drug interaction, e.g., serum digoxin level increases when quinidine is administered simultaneously, so that features of digitalis toxicity appear more frequently.
- Refractory arrhythmias often require a combination of antiarrhythmic drugs and DC shock/artificial pacemaker.
- *In general practice it is better to get familiar with a few antiarrhythmic agents, and use only these drugs as far as possible.*

## ANTIARRHYTHMIC AGENTS

Most of the currently available antiarrhythmic drugs are listed in **Table 1.10**. Only a few of these, however, are ordinarily used in general practice, and these are briefly described here.

| Table 1.10: Classification of antiarrhythmic drugs on electrophysiological basis. ||
|---|---|
| Class | Drugs |
| Class I | Drugs which block influx of Na$^+$ into myocardial cells. Three subclasses are defined according to effects on Purkinje fiber action potential: |
| I a | Slow the rate of rise of the action potential (moderate depression of phase 0 upstroke) and prolong its duration, thus slowing conduction and increasing refractoriness:<br>• Quinidine<br>• Procainamide<br>• Disopyramide |
| I b | Shorten action potential duration, but do not effect conduction or refractoriness (minimal depression of phase 0 upstroke):<br>• Lidocaine<br>• Phenytoin<br>• Tocainide, mexiletine |
| I c | These drugs result in maximal depression of phase 0 upstroke, thus slowing conduction and increasing refractoriness, more so than Class Ia drugs:<br>• Flecainide<br>• Encainide |
| Class II | These drugs block beta-adrenergic receptors (decrease automaticity and prolong conduction):<br>• Propranolol<br>• Metoprolol<br>• Atenolol, etc. |
| Class III | Block K$^+$ channels in repolarization (outward flux of K$^+$), prolong repolarization with widening of QRS and QT intervals:<br>• Amiodarone<br>• Sotalol<br>• Bretylium |
| Class IV | Block slow-calcium channels (decrease automaticity and atrioventricular conduction):<br>• Verapamil<br>• Diltiazem |

**Note:** (i) This classification is based on in vitro electrophysiological studies, and in clinical practice their usage remains largely empirical, (ii) All these drugs can exacerbate arrhythmias (proarrhythmic effect), and many depress LV function.

## Lidocaine

Lidocaine is the drug of choice in the treatment of acute onset ventricular arrhythmias especially when associated with MI, cardiac surgery, anesthesia, or cardiac catheterization. Lidocaine depresses automaticity in the ventricles but has little or no effect at AV node and atria. It is therefore, of not much use in the treatment of supraventricular tachycardia (SVT).

## Dosage

To achieve therapeutic blood levels rapidly, lidocaine therapy should be initiated with IV bolus injection of 1 mg/kg (not exceeding 100 mg) at a rate of approximately 25 mg/min. Additional bolus injections of 0.5 mg/kg can be given every 8-10 minutes, if necessary, up to a total of 4 mg/kg. In most cases the arrhythmia is quickly controlled. Thereafter, the drug is continued as IV infusion at a rate of 1.5-3.0 mg/min (in a 60 kg patient) for 24-48 hours and then weaned off. If there is risk of recurrence of arrhythmia, one of the oral antiarrhythmics should be started 6 hours before lidocaine infusion is to be discontinued.

Half-life of lidocaine varies according to the state of myocardium and the hemodynamics. It is about 1-2 hours in normal subjects, more than 4 hours in patients with noncomplicating MI, more than 20 hours in patients of MI complicated by cardiac failure, and even **longer** in the **presence** of cardiogenic shock. **Maintenance** dose of lidocaine should therefore, be appropriately reduced when cardiac output is diminished.

The drug should be used cautiously in patients over 70 years of age. Prolonged administration of lidocaine also reduces its clearance. It is eliminated almost exclusively by the liver. The drug has a wide margin of safety but when used in large doses (over 4 mg/min) or for a prolonged period (over 48 hours) it may result in certain adverse reactions. These are mostly confined to central nervous system and include nausea, drowsiness, dizziness, confusion, slurred speech, numbness of lips and tongue, muscle twitching, respiratory distress or arrest, double vision, and tremor. Occasionally, cardiovascular toxic symptoms are encountered such as bradycardia, hypotension, and sinus arrest.

## Beta-adrenergic Blocking Agents

Beta-blockers comprise several drugs with important pharmacological differences. However, so far as their antiarrhythmic action is concerned, there is nothing much to choose between them (Sotalol, a beta-blocker with unique antiarrhythmic action, is an exception). The description that follows applies to metoprolol, which is a cardioselective beta-blocker. The antiarrhythmic action of these *drugs* is attributed largely to their beta-blocking effect, which prevents arrhythmias arising from activation of autonomic nervous system. A weak quinidine-like or direct membrane **stabilizing** action also possibly exists. ***Chief indications of beta-blockers are:***

- ❖ Catecholamine induced arrhythmias (e.g., arrhythmias precipitated by exertion or emotional stress)
- ❖ Arrhythmias associated with thyrotoxicosis, pheochromocytoma, and anesthetics
- ❖ Tachyarrhythmias associated with WPW syndrome (drug of choice)
- ❖ Digitalis-induced arrhythmias such as atrial tachycardia, premature ventricular beats, and VT without any associated AV block (in the presence of such blocks lidocaine is preferred).

## Chapter 1: Cardiovascular Emergencies

- Atrial fibrillation or flutter (to reduce ventricular rate which responds inadequately to digitalis), and
- As an adjunct to other antiarrhythmic therapy, e.g., in atrial fibrillation, ventricular tachyarrhythmias.

*Beta-blockers are contraindicated* in the presence of bradyarrhythmia, heart failure, bronchial asthma and chronic obstructive pulmonary disease. Its role in the control of VPBs or VT in patients of MI is limited.

In **acute situations,** *metoprolol should be given IV slowly,* in the intensive care unit, and after echocardiography has excluded severe myocardial dysfunction. The treatment is initiated with a dose of 2.5-5 mg; this may be repeated once or twice every 5-10 minutes until desired effect is achieved. If doubt exists about the safety of beta-blockade, a short-acting beta-blocker (esmolol) may be tried initially. In less urgent situations, metoprolol can be given orally, 25-50 mg twice daily. Higher doses can be given under close supervision. Untoward cardiovascular effects include hypotension, **bradycardia** and heart **failure.**

### Amiodarone

**Amiodarone was introduced initially as a vasodilator to treat** angina pectoris, but was later found to possess powerful antiarrhythmic properties. It is a near ideal antiarrhythmic drug, and combines, to some extent, electrophysiologic properties of all four classes of antiarrhythmic agents.

*Hemodynamically,* amiodarone is a peripheral and coronary vasodilator, and also induces alpha-and-beta-antagonism. When administered IV it decreases heart rate and systemic vascular resistance, possibly with some increase in cardiac output. Amiodarone does not significantly reduce LVEF, yet because of its antiadrenergic properties it should be used cautiously (especially intravenously) in patients with cardiac impairment. The drug has wide-ranging indications comprising *all types of tachyarrhythmias (supraventricular, ventricular, and those associated with WPW syndrome), VPBs, and nonsustained VT.*

The drug has a large volume of distribution (chiefly liver, adipose tissue, myocardium, kidneys and thyroid). It therefore has a delayed onset of action (2-3 days), and requires a large loading dose. It also has a long half-life (almost 7-8 weeks) and consequently, the duration of antiarrhythmic action as also adverse effects are relatively long even when the drug is discontinued.

It has important interactions with a number of other drugs **(Table 1.11)**. When concomitant therapy with amiodarone is warranted, these drugs must be used cautiously, and their dosage reduced appropriately (up to one-third to one-half).

### Calcium Channel Blockers (CCB)

The two drugs in this group have antiarrhythmic effect—verapamil and diltiazem. Their *principal action is at the AV node whereby the drugs prolong*

**Table 1.11:** Interactions of amiodarone with other drugs.

| Drug | Result of interaction |
|---|---|
| **Pharmacokinetic interactions** | |
| Digoxin | Increased digoxin concentration |
| Flecainide | Increased flecainide concentration |
| Procainamide | Increased procainamide concentration |
| Quinidine | Increased quinidine concentration |
| Warfarin | Increased warfarin concentration |
| **Pharmacodynamic interactions** | |
| Diltiazem | Sinus arrest and hypotension |
| Propranolol | Bradycardia, sinus arrest |
| Quinidine | Torsades de pointes ventricular tachycardia |

*refractory period as well as conduction time* (more with verapamil). Heart rate decreases due to a direct effect on the sinoatrial (SA) node. In effect, however, the sinus rate may show only little change since their peripheral vasodilator effect results in reflex sympathetic stimulation.

Significant bradycardia occurs only when verapamil is given to a patient who is also receiving a beta-blocker. This is a dangerous drug combination and should be avoided. QRS duration is not much altered. Currently, only diltiazem is used for termination of paroxysmal SVTs.

Occasionally, these are also used to reduce the ventricular rate in atrial fibrillation or flutter. The drugs have little effect, if any, on VPBs or VT. These are contraindicated in the presence of hypotension, compromised LV functions, AV block, brady-tachy-arrhythmias, WPW syndrome, and any tachyarrhythmia associated with wide QRS complexes.

### *Dosage*

For termination of acute attack of SVT diltiazem is preferred and given IV in a dose of 0.25 mg/kg as bolus over 2 minutes, followed by a similar dose after 15–30 minutes, if necessary. Oral dose has a wide range (90–360 mg), and should be adjusted according to the patient's response.

### Types of Cardiac Arrhythmias

Cardiac arrhythmias can be classified as **tachyarrhythmias** (supraventricular or ventricular) and **bradyarrhythmias** (including AV blocks). The former are defined as fast rhythms with rates greater than 100 beats per minute (bpm), and the latter as slow heart rates (less than 60 bpm).

## TACHYARRHYTHMIAS

All tachyarrhythmias, both supraventricular (SV) and ventricular, have heart rates >100 bpm. The rhythm can be regular or irregular, P-waves may or may not

**Flowchart 1.5:** An approach to diagnosis of tachycardia.

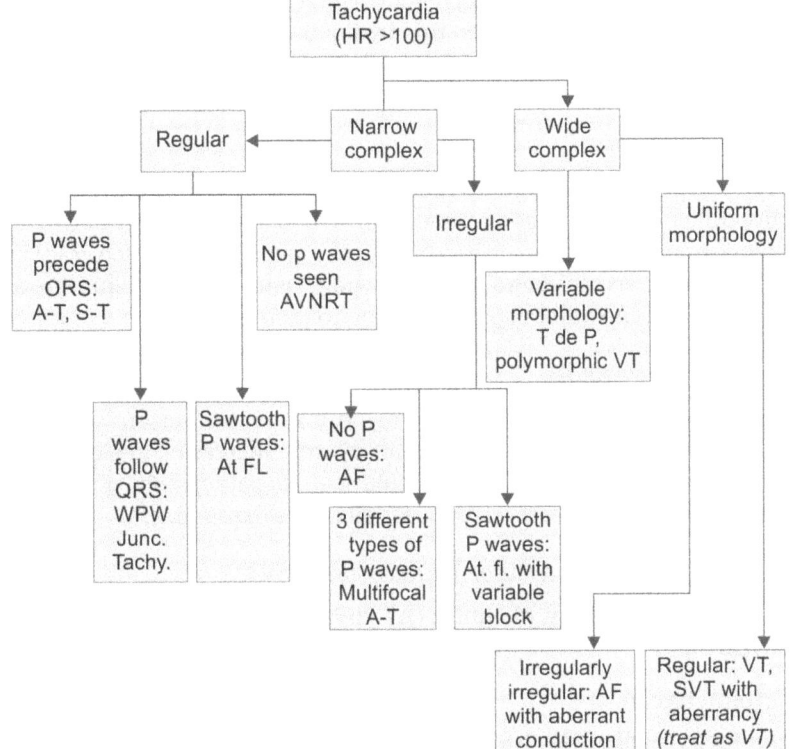

(AF: atrial fibrillation; At.Fl.: atrial flutter; A-T: atrial tachycardia; AVNRT: A-V nodal re-entry tachycardia; S-T: sinus tachycardia; SVT: supraventricular tachycardia; TdeP: torsades de pointes; VT: ventricular tachycardia; WPW: Wolff–Parkinson–White syndrome)

be visible, and QRS complexes may be narrow or wide. A schematic approach to diagnosis of tachycardia is given in **Flowchart 1.5**.

## Supraventricular Tachyarrhythmias

Supraventricular tachyarrhythmias generally have narrow QRS complex (<100 msec) except when associated with aberrant conduction or pre-existing bundle branch block. *The therapeutic approach varies according to QRS-width, i.e., whether SV tachycardia is of "narrow-complex" or "wide-complex" type.*

### Sinus Tachycardia

Tachycardia (heart rate ≥100 bpm) arising from SA node is termed as sinus tachycardia. It is usually physiological, and aims at increasing cardiac output in response to metabolic demands (e.g., exercise, fever, thyrotoxicosis). It may also result as a physiological response in states of hypovolemia, or may be due to heightened sympathetic activity as in anxiety, pain, and hypotension.

When inappropriate to the clinical state of the patient, sinus tachycardia should be regarded primarily as a potential indicator of an underlying disorder. In fact, **in susceptible patients, this by itself may precipitate myocardial ischemia since it: (i) increases myocardial oxygen demand, and (ii) impairs** cardiac perfusion by reducing diastolic phase of the cardiac cycle.

*Treatment*

The causative factor should be identified and treated appropriately. Sinus tachycardia per se requires treatment only when associated with myocardial ischemia or patient is aware of it/complains of palpitation. In such cases beta-blockers may be administered provided hypotension and heart failure are ruled out, and there is no other contraindication to their use.

### Atrial Premature Beats

Atrial premature beats occur frequently in normal people, and are never a sufficient basis for the diagnosis of heart disease. Increasing the heart rate by any means usually abolishes such ectopic beats. In patients who may be aware of such premature beats, reassurance is all that is required.

### Paroxysmal Supraventricular Tachycardia (PSVT)

This may be in the form of either: **(A) Atrial tachycardia, or (B) Re-entry tachycardia.**

*Atrial tachycardias*

**Atrial tachycardia (Fig. 1.6):** This is usually a **non-reentrant** type of SVT, which arises from *enhanced automaticity of an ectopic focus in the atria*

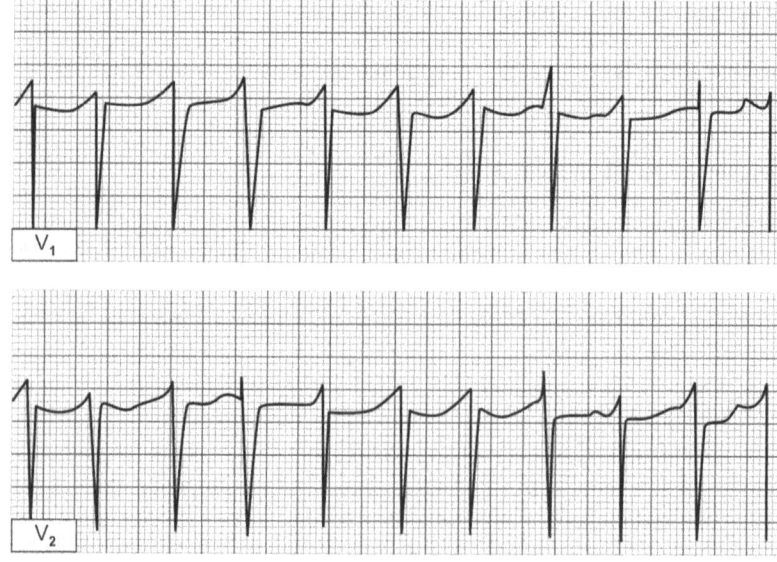

**Fig. 1.6:** Atrial tachycardia.

generally associated with some pulmonary or cardiac disease. Occasionally, it is due to digitalis intoxication (often accompanied by hypokalemia) and then is associated with variable atrioventricular block (*paroxysmal atrial tachycardia with block*). In a classical case, during tachycardia ECG will reveal P-waves preceding QRS-complex, with morphology different from that seen during sinus rhythm.

*Treatment*
This is on the same lines as that of PSVT due to re-entry.

*Multifocal atrial tachycardia (MAT)*

This is characterized by presence of P-waves of three or more different morphology arising from multiple ectopic foci within the atria, which have achieved enhanced automaticity. **RR interval is markedly irregular,** rate is usually between 100 and 140/min, and AV block is unusual. It is generally seen in elderly patients with chronic lung disease and hypoxemia, but may also occur in CAD, metabolic crisis, sepsis, and toxicity with digitalis or theophylline. Distinction from atrial fibrillation may sometimes be difficult.

*Treatment*
The most effective treatment of MAT is to reverse the underlying pathology. For temporary slowing or controlling MAT, verapamil may be used. It acts by decreasing the frequency of atrial beats. Beta-blockers can also be useful, if not contraindicated. Cardioversion or digitalis is not beneficial in such cases. On the whole, this particular arrhythmia is very difficult to manage.

*Re-entry tachycardia*

Most cases of PSVT (approximately 90%) have a re-entry mechanism, and usually occur in patients without any organic heart disease. The re-entry circuit involves a **dual pathway, and may be located either in the AV node or in the form of an accessory pathway between the atria and the ventricles.** Of the two, the former is much more common and is termed as AV **nodal re-entrant tachycardia (AVNRT).** In such cases **SVT is** nearly always precipitated by a critically placed atrial premature beat. P-waves are either not visible in the ECG or are seen as upright P-waves at the end of the QRS complex in $V_x$ or $V_2$ (Fig. 1.7).

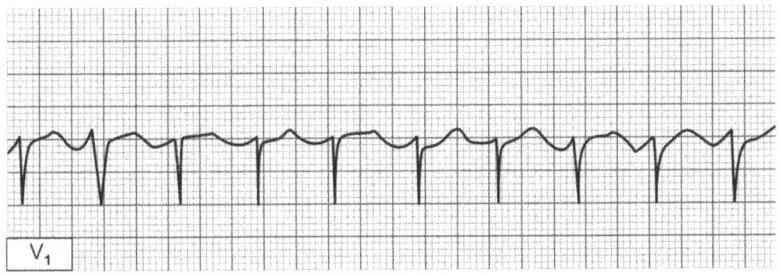

**Fig. 1.7:** AV nodal re-entrant tachycardia (AVNRT).

Less commonly *re-entry tachycardia is due to accessory (bypass) pathways with different refractory pathways.* This is referred to as *(orthodromic)* AV **re-entrant tachycardia *(AVRT).*** Such cases have (retrograde) *inverted P-waves, which follow QRS.*

## Clinical Features

Paroxysmal supraventricular tachycardia manifests as repeated attacks of tachycardia with heart rate usually between 150 and 200/min. Each attack starts abruptly, lasts for several minutes or hours (less commonly even for days), usually ends spontaneously, and is often accompanied/followed by profuse diuresis. The general condition of the patient remains remarkably well during the attack except when the episode is much prolonged or there is associated organic heart disease. In such cases PSVT may precipitate heart failure, hypotension, or coronary pain.

## Diagnosis

The diagnosis may be suspected from typical history but becomes clear if the patient is seen during the attack. The cardiac rate is invariably over 150/min (usually around 200/min), and the rhythm is quite regular.

## Electrocardiogram

Whenever possible an ECG should be recorded during an episode of PSVT. It will not only confirm the diagnosis but also help to define the exact nature of tachycardia. ***Study of ECG should start by:***

- **Making a note of the P-wave**—its presence or absence, and its relationship to the QRS-complex. P-waves that precede the QRS complex indicate sinus or atrial tachycardia **(Fig. 1.6)**. P-waves are either not visible (buried in QRS) or follow QRS complex in AVNRT **(Fig. 1.7)**, WPW syndrome, and junctional tachycardia.
- **QRS-width should be studied next**—whether it is narrow (<0.12 seconds) or wide (>0.12 seconds). Wide QRS-complex may be seen in patients with SVT who have either pre-existing bundle branch block (recognition possible only, if an earlier ECG is available) or have aberrant intraventricular conduction. The distinction between the latter and VT can be very difficult.

***Features favoring VT include:*** (1) QRS complex more than 0.14 seconds, (2) AV dissociation, (3) presence of fusion or captured beats, (4) left axis deviation with right bundle branch block morphology, and (5) concordant QRS pattern (all positive or all negative deflections) in all precordial leads. In addition, presence of structural or some other type of serious heart disease is a strong predictor of VT. On the other hand, younger age of the patient (<35 years), and a history of similar episodes for >3 years is suggestive of SVT

***Supraventricular origin is favored by:*** (1) a triphasic QRS-complex especially if the initial component of QRS is negative in V1 and V6, (2) ventricular rate

\>170/min, (3) QRS duration >0.12 sec but not longer than 0.14 sec, and (4) presence of WPW syndrome.

## Treatment

- **Mechanical maneuvers:** Since about 90% cases of SVT have a re-entry mechanism, mostly in the AV-node, the initial treatment should be mechanical maneuvers that increase vagal tone, and interrupt the conduction at some point in the re-entry circuit. These include Valsalva maneuver, carotid sinus massage and coughing, lowering the head between the knees, and tickling the pharynx to induce vomiting (ocular pressure is not recommended). *Carotid sinus massage is done (after excluding carotid bruit)* by applying firm but gentle pressure and massage first on the right (non-dominant) carotid sinus for 10–20 seconds and, if unsuccessful, on the left carotid sinus. It is desirable that continuous ECG monitoring is available during carotid massage otherwise at least continuous cardiac auscultation should be done during the procedure.

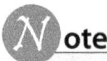ote

Carotid pressure should never be applied on both sides at the same time.

- **Drug therapy:** If mechanical measures mentioned above do not terminate the attack, two rapidly acting IV agents are available that will control the arrhythmia in more than 90% of episodes.
    - *Adenosine:* This is the ***drug of first choice.*** It binds to cardiac alpha-1 receptors in the SA and AV node, has a negative chronotropic effect on SA node, and depresses conduction and increases refractoriness in the AV node. The drug is administered IV initially as 6 mg bolus over 1–2 seconds followed by a saline flush. If no response is obtained after 1–2 minutes, a 12 mg bolus should be given in a similar manner. Methylxanthines and dipyridamole interfere with the action of the drug. Adenosine is quite safe and well-tolerated, though often associated with dose-related symptoms of dyspnea, flushing, and chest discomfort or pain. All these effects are however, short-lived, lasting an average of 5–20 seconds. The drug should be used cautiously in patients with bronchial asthma.
    - *Calcium channel blockers:* **Diltiazem** is also quite effective in such cases but should be avoided when supraventricular origin of the tachycardia is in doubt, and if the systolic pressure is <100 mm Hg. Diltiazem is used IV [0.25–0.35 mg/kg (over 2–3 minutes)] followed by a second bolus, if necessary.
- **Cardioversion:** If adenosine and diltiazem fail to control PSVT, and the patient is hemodynamically unstable or has angina or AMI, **synchronized** cardioversion should be done without delay. This is almost universally

successful. However, it should be avoided, if the patient is already digitalized.

If facilities for cardioversion are not available, an alternative is a short acting beta-blocker (esmolol) used in a dose of 500 µg/kg IV over 1–2 minutes followed by an infusion of 25–200 µg/min.

### Prevention

* **Drugs:** In patients with frequently recurring tachycardia, or when attacks of tachycardia are poorly tolerated hemodynamically (regardless of the frequency of the attacks), *long-term control* should be maintained by verapamil, beta-blockers, or amiodarone. All these drugs act by slowing conduction through AV node.

ote

> Diltiazem should never be administered IV for control of PSVT, *if accessory pathways are suspected* since by shortening refractory period of the accessory pathways, it can facilitate conduction down the bypass tract resulting in a more rapid ventricular response.

* **Radiofrequency ablation:** This is the treatment of choice in patients with recurring symptomatic re-entrant SVT whether it is due to a dual pathway within the AV node or to an accessory pathway. It is especially indicated, if the patient is irregular with his medication or is unable to tolerate antiarrhythmic medication.

## Special Types of SV Tachycardia

### *Wolff-Parkinson-White Syndrome*

It is a special type of supraventricular tachycardia due to accessory pathway in which the *bypass tracts are composed of muscle strands placed around AV rings.* Unlike AVRT, the antegrade conduction is through the bypass tract and therefore avoids conduction delay of the AV node. *During sinus rhythm the ECG will therefore reveal a short P-R interval* (<0.12 seconds) and an early delta-wave (indicative of early ventricular excitation) at the onset of wide-slurred QRS complex **(Fig. 1.8)**. During PSVT in WPW, there is usually antegrade-conduction of impulse over normal AV node, and retrograde through the bypass tract, and therefore *during tachycardia the ECG reveals the same pattern as PSVT due to AVRT.*

### *Treatment*

Patients with WPW or other pre-excitation syndromes with normal sinus rhythm require no treatment. Episodes of PSVT requiring immediate control should receive DC cardioversion. In less urgent situations IV lidocaine (3–5 mg/kg administered over 20 minutes) may be tried to slow the ventricular rate. Beta-blockers are usually not beneficial. Recurrence of SVT in such patients

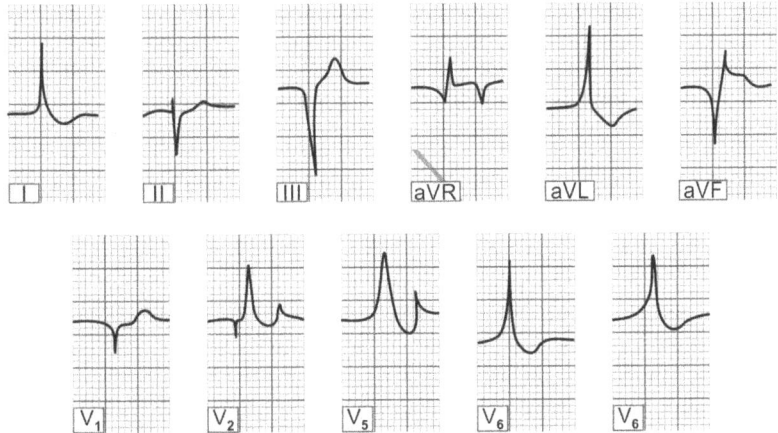

**Fig. 1.8:** Wolff-Parkinson-White syndrome (WPW).

**Table 1.12:** Treatment of common cardiac arrhythmias.

| Arrhythmia | Treatment of choice | Alternatives | Comments |
|---|---|---|---|
| Supraventricular ectopic beats | No medication or mild sedation | Verapamil, digoxin, propranolol | Treat only if symptomatic; digoxin if associated with heart failure |
| Paroxysmal SV tachycardia (PSVT) | Vagal stimulation adenosine | Diltiazem, propranolol, cardioversion | Cardiovert if drugs fail or hypotension/angina develop |
| PSVT with block (digitalis induced) | KCl, lidocaine, | Propranolol, Digibind | Stop digitalis and diuretics |
| Multifocal atrial tachycardia | Amiodarone | Propranolol, verapamil/diltiazem | Treat basic disorder; correct hypoxemia/acidosis |
| Atrial flutter/fibrillation | Cardioversion, amiodarone, digoxin | Rate control in stable patients with digoxin, calcium channel or betablockers | Unstable patients cardioversion or amiodarone, digoxin, if heart failure is present |
| Ventricular premature beats | Lidocaine | Amiodarone | IV infusion in urgent situations, otherwise oral medication |
| Ventricular tachycardia | Cardioversion, lidocaine | Amiodarone, propranolol/sotalol | Unstable patients cardioversion; stable-amiodarone, lidocaine |
| Ventricular fibrillation | Thumpversion DC shock | Lidocaine | If DC shock: unsuccessful, cardiopulmonary resuscitation |

may be prevented by catheter ablation of the bypass tract, or by amiodarone or Class IA antiarrhythmic drugs administered orally **(Table 1.12)**.

### SVT with Aberrant Conduction (Wide-complex Tachycardia)

Despite various ECG criteria (vide supra), it may not be possible to distinguish SVT with aberrant conduction from VT (both will have wide-QRS). When in doubt, it is best to err on the side of treating such tachyarrhythmias as VT.

### Atrial Fibrillation (AF)

Next to premature beats this is perhaps the most common arrhythmia met within general practice. It is usually secondary to some organic heart disease such as rheumatic (especially mitral valve disease) or IHD, thyrotoxicosis, hypertension, and chronic corpulmonale. When the arrhythmia occurs in individuals less than 60 years of age without any known heart disease or other etiological factor, it is termed as idiopathic or lone atrial fibrillation. In AMI, it is usually encountered in patients with extensive anterior infarction, left ventricular failure, and right ventricular infarction. AF in such cases is generally transitory. It needs to be treated, if:
a. It is persistent or the paroxysms are very frequent
b. The paroxysm lasts for more than two hours, or
c. The ventricular rate is over 120/min

Atrial fibrillation can be intermittent or persistent. Both types are associated with a high risk of embolization and stroke. Other symptoms of AF are related to underlying heart disease, intensity of ventricular rate, and loss of atrial contraction with consequent decrease in stroke volume. Diagnosis is confirmed by ECG, which shows rapid asynchronous fibrillary waves with totally irregular ventricular response **(Fig. 1.9)**.

#### Treatment

There are ***four important aspects which should be considered in the management of AF:***
1. Control of ventricular rate
2. Prevention of recurrences
3. Prevention of thromboembolic episodes
4. Treatment of etiological factor

When AF with rapid ventricular rate complicates any chronic heart disease, it is usually associated with heart failure, and is best treated with digitalis. In acute situations such as AMI, rapid rate AF should be treated

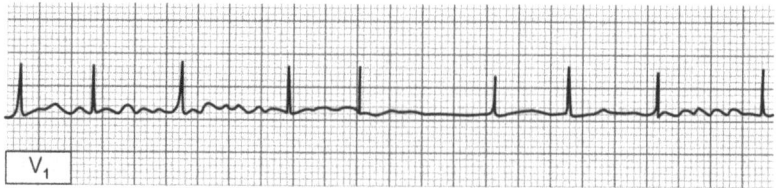

**Fig. 1.9:** Atrial fibrillation.

promptly since it may result in cardiac decompensation, hypotension, or increase in infarct size. **DC cardioversion** is the treatment of choice in such cases. In less urgent situations, **IV amiodarone** should be tried (IV digoxin if heart failure exists). Once sinus rhythm is restored, recurrences should be prevented with amiodarone.

Generally, only a short course of treatment (6-8 weeks) is required since the risk of recurrence of AF decreases rapidly with passage of time after infarction. Oral drugs such as digoxin, amiodarone, a beta-blocker, or CCBs usually suffice for long-term management of AF, the aim being to slow down the ventricular rate (between 60 and 80/min). Sometimes a combination of digitalis with beta-blocker or verapamil proves more effective in controlling ventricular rate than either drug alone. Class I drugs prescribed earlier for medium or long-term control of AF in patients with AMI are no longer used because of risk of pro-arrhythmias.

Prevention of thromboembolism
Atrial fibrillation, persistent or paroxysmal, carries a high risk of embolization. The risk is especially high in AF associated with mitral stenosis and a large left atrium. In nonvalvular AF, risk of stroke is increased in elderly people, in patients with diabetes, hypertension, CHD, and congestive heart failure, and in cases with past history of stroke/transient ischemic attack. In contrast, in younger patients (<60 years) with lone AF the risk of stroke is very low. All high risk cases of AF should receive lifelong prophylactic oral anticoagulation, if there is no contraindication. For stroke prevention, the aim should be to achieve an international normalization ratio (INR) of 2.0-3.0. When anticoagulation is not practical, some protection (albeit minimal) may be achieved with aspirin/clopidogrel therapy.

## *Atrial Flutter*

Though the etiopathogenesis of atrial flutter is similar to that of atrial fibrillation, it is a much less common arrhythmia. In fact in patients with AMI, it is the least common atrial arrhythmia. On bedside examination the main difference lies in the regularity of the pulse in atrial flutter in contrast to atrial fibrillation in which the rhythm is completely irregular. The atria beat at speeds around 250-350/min but the ventricular rate is usually between 75 and 150/min due to associated AV block of varying grade. ECG shows characteristic saw-tooth flutter waves (**Fig. 1.10**).

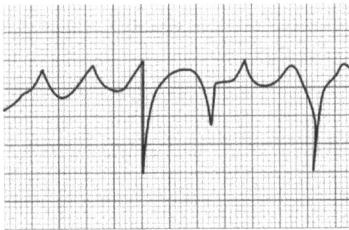

**Fig. 1.10:** Atrial flutter.

## Treatment

The treatment of atrial flutter is essentially similar to that of atrial fibrillation. However, atrial flutter is likely to prove more resistant to various pharmacological measures, and therefore, in acute cases, **cardioversion** may be considered at the very outset. In cases where immediate conversion of atrial flutter is not mandated by the clinical status of the patient, the ventricular rate should be slowed by a beta-blocker, CCB, or digitalis.

 ote

> The dosage of antiarrhythmic drugs in AF should be regulated by counting the heart rate at the apex, and not from the pulse.

## Ventricular Tachyarrhythmias

### Ventricular Premature Beats (VPBs)

These are characterized by wide QRS complexes that differ in morphology from normal sinus beats. A VPB is usually not preceded by a P-wave, and the ectopic beat is followed by a fully compensatory pause. VPB occurring after every second or thirds beat is termed as *bigeminy or trigeminy,* respectively. Depending upon the frequency of the ventricular ectopics/premature beats, the cardiac rate may be fast or normal. These are encountered in a variety of states such as infections, myocarditis or myocardial ischemia, and during hypoxia, anesthesia, or surgery. VPBs can also occur in anxiety states, and can be associated with a number of medications, **electrolyte** disturbances, and with excessive use of tobacco, alcohol, **and caffeine.** Occasionally no cause is obvious.

In AMI, VPBs **are encountered in at least three-quarters** of the **cases,** if properly **monitored. Ordinarily** of not much consequence, VPBs **have been considered** to presage VT or VF especially if—(1) fairly frequent, i.e., 5 or more/min, (2) occur in runs of two or more, (3) multifocal in origin or bigeminal, and (4) very premature, i.e., R-wave of the extra systole tends to fall on the T-wave of the preceding sinus beat. Such VPBs have been termed **"warning arrhythmias",** though more recent observations have thrown some doubt on their exact significance. It has been observed that such extrasystoles do not occur in about half of the patients who develop VF, while almost a similar number of patients who do develop VF do not have these so called "warning" extrasystoles.

### Treatment

The significance of VPBs depends upon the clinical setting. Asymptomatic and isolated VPBs in apparently healthy individuals do not usually carry any significance, regardless of their frequency or configuration. Longevity is not affected, nor any limitation of activity warranted. Exercise generally abolishes

VPBs in normal hearts. Any identifiable cause of ectopic beats should be removed.

Sometimes mild sedation or a beta-blocker may be required in patients conscious of irregular heart beat. Beta-blockers may be especially useful when VPBs occur in stressful situations, or are observed in cases with thyrotoxicosis or mitral valve prolapse.

In the presence of organic heart disease VPBs carry a higher risk of cardiovascular mortality/sudden death especially if their frequency increases during exercise. Any identifiable cause (vide supra) should be treated. Pharmacologic treatment is indicated only for symptomatic patients, and beta-blockers are the agents of choice. However, in acute medical or surgical setting (especially in cases of AMI), the drug of choice is lidocaine. If VPBs persist despite adequate doses of lidocaine, amiodarone should be tried. For long-term maintenance therapy, amiodarone is perhaps the safest. The need for prolonged antiarrhythmic therapy should be reviewed periodically.

Since the concept of warning arrhythmias is now suspect, ***prophylactic lidocaine therapy in AMI is not routinely recommended.***

## *Ventricular Tachycardia (VT)*

*Etiology*

It is a serious type of cardiac arrhythmia and is usually encountered in patients with structural heart disease, most commonly IHD with a background of MI. Other causes include cardiomyopathies, valvular heart disease, congenital heart disease, hypertension, metabolic disorders, and digitalis toxicity. Occasionally, no cause may be obvious.

*Clinical features*

Ventricular tachycardia is defined as ***three or more consecutive VPBs.*** It generally has an abrupt onset (often initiated **by** a VPB) with a rate of 120–250/min. The rhythm is usually regular but slight irregularity may exist **(Fig. 1.11)**. It may be **nonsustained** (when it lasts for <30 seconds) **or sustained.** The latter persists for >30 seconds, or requires earlier termination because of unstable condition of the patient. The symptoms depend upon the ventricular rate, the duration of tachycardia, and the presence and severity of underlying cardiac disease.

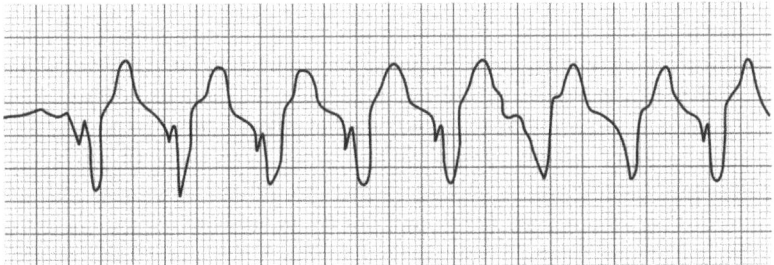

**Fig. 1.11:** Ventricular tachycardia.

Nonsustained VT is less often associated with organic heart disease and is generally asymptomatic. Some of these cases may, however, progress into sustained VT or even VF. Longer spells of VT are nearly always associated with organic heart disease, and can result in serious complications such as cardiac decompensation, severe angina, hemodynamic collapse, syncope, and terminal VF.

*Prognosis*

The prognosis of patients with VT depends upon the associated cardiac status. VT observed occasionally in patients without heart disease (e.g., during anesthesia, surgery) has a good prognosis with very low risk of sudden death. On the other hand, in patients with AMI, morbidity, and mortality is considerably enhanced even when VT is nonsustained.

*Diagnosis*

Ventricular tachycardia is diagnosed from an ECG recorded during the episode of tachycardia. It will show *wide-complex QRS tachycardia* at a rate >100 beats/min (**Fig. 1.10**). The morphology of QRS complexes may be uniform (**monomorphic**) or it may vary on a beat to beat basis, or over a series of successive beats (**polymorphic**). The latter is more likely to degenerate into VF. A special type of polymorphic VT with changing contour and amplitude of QRS complexes, and prolonged QT intervals (usually exceeding 0.50 seconds) is termed **torsade's de pointes**. On ECG it is characterized by successive runs of nonsustained VT in which peaks of QRS complexes appear first on one side and then on the other side of the baseline, imparting a typical twisting appearance. Such cases are invariably associated with recurrent syncope, and are at great risk of developing VF and sudden cardiac death.

*Treatment*

The management of VT varies according to whether it is sustained or non-sustained, is associated with underlying structural heart disease or not, and the nature of accompanying symptoms.

- ❖ **Nonsustained VT,** which is transitory, not associated with organic heart disease, and is asymptomatic, needs no special treatment. However, the predisposing factor should be identified and corrected rapidly to prevent a recurrence.
- ❖ **Sustained VT,** whether associated or not with cardiac disease, requires treatment. If the patient is ***hemodynamically stable, lidocaine or amiodarone*** may be used as primary therapy. If the arrhythmia does not quickly respond to pharmacological therapy, ***DC cardioversion*** should be considered. When a ***more rapid control of tachyarrhythmia*** is desired (as in patients with features of myocardial ischemia, hypotension, cardiac decompensation, or impairment of cerebral perfusion) the arrhythmia should be terminated at the earliest by ***synchronized cardioversion.*** Cardioversion should, however, be avoided if VT is digitalis induced. Such cases are best treated with IV phenytoin. After conversion of VT to

normal rhythm, IV maintenance infusion should be set up for 24–48 hours to prevent a recurrence (vide infra).

❖ **"Thumpversion"** (striking the patient's chest with a closed fist) can sometimes terminate VT, but carries the risk of provoking VF, if the chest stimulation occurs at the time of "vulnerable period".

*Prevention*

VT often recurs in patients with underlying heart disease, and therefore preventive measures are required in such cases. Commonly used drugs for this purpose include ***amiodarone and beta-blockers.*** The latter has the added advantage of reducing the risk of sudden death after MI.

In special circumstances patients of recurrent tachycardia will require implantable devices, which incorporate functions of pacing, cardioversion, and defibrillation.

*Other measures*

In all cases a thorough search should be made for ***acute reversible etiopathologic factors*** such as hypoxemia, hypokalemia, hypotension, heart failure, thyrotoxicosis, and drug toxicity (e.g., digoxin, amphetamines, phenothiazines, tricyclic antidepressants or alcohol). All patients with VT should receive mild sedation and oxygen therapy at fast rates. A close watch should be kept on blood pressure, and vasopressors used as required.

## *Ventricular Fibrillation*

Ventricular fibrillation is the most dangerous of all cardiac arrhythmias and is often a terminal event. It is characterized by extremely rapid uncoordinated and irregular fibrillary twitching movements of the ventricles which replace regular ventricular contractions **(Fig. 1.12)**. The cardiac output therefore falls to a naught, and the circulation of blood comes virtually to a standstill.

*Etiology*

The etiology of VF is similar to that of VT, and in fact, it may be preceded by spells of VT and/or ventricular ectopics. In patients with AMI, it is equally frequent in anterior and inferior wall infarctions, and may occur in three settings.

1. **Primary VF:** This is the usual type of VF encountered in cases of AMI. It occurs suddenly and unexpectedly, usually within 12 hours of onset of symptoms, and is not related to left ventricular failure.

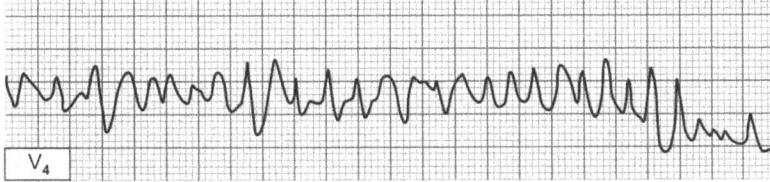

**Fig. 1.12:** Ventricular fibrillation.

2. ***Secondary VF:*** This occurs only in states of advanced left ventricular failure and cardiogenic shock complicating AMI.
3. ***Late VF:*** This may occur at any time between 1 and 6 weeks following AMI with anterior wall infarction, persistent sinus tachycardia, atrial flutter or atrial fibrillation in the early course, and intraventricular conduction defects are particularly at high risk of developing this type of VF.

*Treatment*

Primary VF is often very transitory and generally self limited. In high-risk cases, it may be prevented by prophylactic administration of lidocaine, amiodarone, or beta-blockers. The treatment of VF is **immediate non-synchronized electrical DC shock,** since the chances of restoration of proper cardiac rhythm decline rapidly with time. As a **first aid measure "thump version"** (one or two sharp heavy blow(s) in the middle of the chest over the sternum) should be tried, but if this fails, and in fact side by side, **CPR** should be started as described in the section on "Cardiac Arrest". Once sinus rhythm is restored, measures should be instituted to prevent a recurrence by IV lidocaine, amiodarone or procainamide. Metabolic acidosis quickly occurs following cardiovascular collapse, and should be corrected with 50 mL 7.5% sodium bicarbonate. Repeat doses should be given only according to plasma bicarbonate levels. The role of bicarbonate in such cases is, however, undergoing re-evaluation (*see* section on "Cardiac Arrest").

# BRADYARRHYTHMIAS

Bradyarrhythmia defines a cardiac rhythm with a rate less than 60 bpm. The defect in such cases may be in the SA node, AV node, or His bundle/Purkinje system.

## Sinus Bradycardia

This implies a heart rate slower than 60/min, with the rhythm still under control of SA node. It is usually due to increased vagal influence on the normal pacemaker, but can also result from organic disease of the SA node as in *"sick sinus syndrome"* (SSS). Slow heart rates are often seen in healthy young adults especially if they have an excellent physique, and also in patients suffering from hypothyroidism. Occasionally it is drug related (digitalis, verapamil, diltiazem, beta-blockers), or may be seen in the early stages of AMI (usually inferior or posterior).

In most of the cases, sinus bradycardia is asymptomatic. It becomes an emergency only when the heart rate drops to 40/min or less. Such cases may develop weakness, confusion, syncope, or even Stokes-Adams attack. Ectopic beats, both atrial and ventricular, are more likely to occur with slow sinus rates.

## Treatment

Any underlying factor, which is reversible should be identified and treated appropriately (e.g., related drugs, hypothyroidism). Severe bradycardia complicating AMI should be managed with *IV atropine. Pacing* may be required, if bradycardia persists and is symptomatic.

## Atrioventricular (AV) Block

This implies impaired conduction of the impulse from atria to ventricles. It may result from a variety of causes such as rheumatic, coronary, or congenital heart disease, calcific aortic stenosis, acute infections (rheumatic fever, diphtheria, etc.) and digitalis overdose. At times, the exact etiology is obscure.

AV **block can be of three types:** The *first degree AV block* is characterized by prolongation of conduction time (PR interval), but all atrial beats are conducted **(Fig. 1.13)**. The *second degree heart block* is of two types: *Mobitz type I* (Wenckebach type), and *Mobitz type II.* In the former **(Fig. 1.14)**, there is progressive increase in the conduction time until an impulse is not conducted.

Mobitz type II heart block denotes dropped beats occurring occasionally or at regular intervals, not preceded by progressive lengthening of conduction time **(Fig. 1.15)**. When two or more consecutive P-waves are blocked, it indicates advanced heart block.

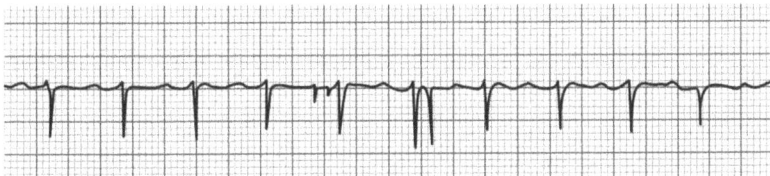

**Fig. 1.13:** AV-block.

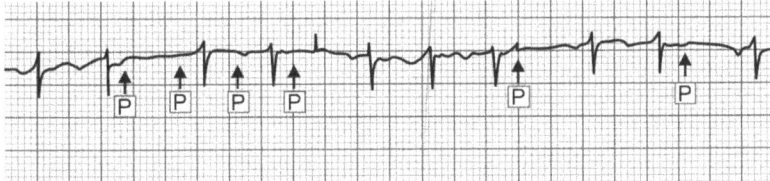

**Fig. 1.14:** Mobitz type I (2nd degree AV-block).

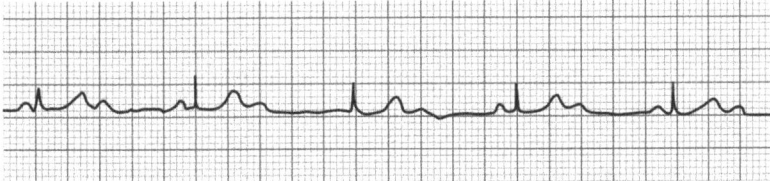

**Fig. 1.15:** Mobitz type II (2nd degree AV-block).

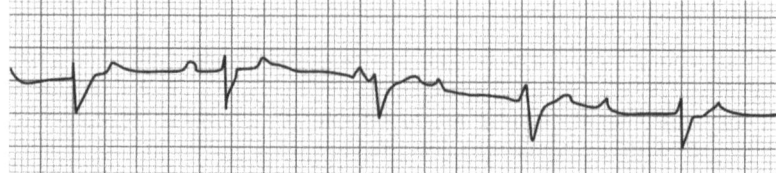

Fig. 1.16: Complete heart block.

The third-degree AV block (**Fig. 1.16**) is characterized by total blockade of the atrial pulses through the AV node/His bundle/Purkinje system (complete heart block). *Blocks that are proximal to bundle of His have normal QRS complexes, and heart rates of 40-60/min.* On the other hand, complete heart block of acute onset (as in AMI) has its origin, most commonly, *distal to bundle of HIS, and is slower in rate (usually <40/min) with abnormal wide QRS complexes.*

### Clinical Features

First degree, and type I second degree heart blocks are usually benign, and can occur in healthy individuals, especially well-trained athletes. In cases with AMI, such blocks occur more often in patients with inferior than anterior infarction, are usually transitory or intermittent, and rarely progress to complete heart block. Mobitz type II AV block is an uncommon type of block. When chronic and without any associated heart disease, it is usually asymptomatic. In AMI this type of heart block is almost always seen in anterior infarction, is invariably associated with wide QRS complexes, carries a bad prognosis, and often progresses (sometimes suddenly) to complete heart block.

Complete heart block may develop with either acute inferior or anterior MI (AV conduction system has a dual blood supply—from right coronary artery and left anterior descending artery). In the former setting (inferior MI), it often develops gradually, progressing stepwise from first degree and type I second degree block. In majority of such cases it is associated with QRS complexes of normal shape with a ventricular rate exceeding 40/min, and may be temporary. On the other hand, when complete heart block occurs in cases of anterior infarction, it often develops suddenly, usually within 12-24 hours after the onset of infarction. Occasionally, it may be preceded by *Mobitz* type II block. In such cases ventricular asystole may occur suddenly, and mortality is extremely high.

The *symptoms of advanced/complete heart block depend almost entirely on the ventricular rate.* Heart rates over 50 are generally well-tolerated. Slower rates (<45, especially <40/min) result in decreased cardiac output with consequent impairment of coronary and cerebral perfusion. The former may result in worsening of myocardial ischemia, hypotension, and ventricular arrhythmias. Cerebral features include light-headedness, giddiness, syncope, and seizures.

## Management

The gravity of heart block is related not only to its exact type but also to the rapidity with which it develops. It is usually the acute onset heart blocks (**as in AMI**) that present as medical emergencies. In such cases the prognosis also depends upon the extent and location of myocardial injury, the outcome being worse in patients of complete heart block associated with anterior MI because such cases usually have extensive myocardial damage.

- ❖ **Cardiac pacing:** In all cases of acutely developing complete heart block, whether associated with anterior or inferior MI, the only satisfactory treatment is cardiac pacing. The *pacing should be instituted on an emergency basis* when complete heart block is associated with (1) anterior MI and wide QRS complexes, (2) inferior MI and accompanying severe bradycardia (ventricular rate <45/min), and (iii) ventricular irritability or hypotension. A similar policy should be adopted in cases with advanced second degree AV block (vide supra). Pacing affords protection against sudden asystole and transient hypotension which may result in infarct propagation and ventricular arrhythmias. Pharmacological measures have little role to play except in a few cases of inferior MI in whom heart block in the very initial phases (within 6 hours after the onset of symptoms) may be due to excessive vagotonia, and may respond to atropine injections.
- ❖ **Drug therapy:** Notwithstanding the extreme usefulness of cardiac pacing in cases of advanced/complete AV blocks, it is not universally available or may take some time to be organized. In such circumstances **isoproterenol infusion** may be tried. This drug can be useful in all cases of complete heart block irrespective of the site of block. It increases cardiac rate, stroke volume and coronary blood flow, and causes peripheral vasodilatation (in contrast to norepinephrine which produces vasoconstriction). The drug is administered as IV infusion at a rate 2–16 µg/min starting with lower dose. If the block is at the level of AV node, atropine may also be useful.

Intravenous corticosteroids (hydrocortisone hemisuccinate) have little role, if any, in cases of complete heart block due to AMI.

## STOKES–ADAMS SYNDROME

### Etiology

Stokes-Adams syndrome is characterized by an abrupt but transitory loss of consciousness due to cerebral anoxia resulting from sudden decrease in cardiac output. The latter may be due to a marked decrease in ventricular rate, usually to 30/min or less (e.g., marked sinus bradycardia, sinus arrest or sinoatrial block, advanced or complete heart block), or serious ventricular rhythm disturbance (e.g., ventricular asystole, VT, or VF). The underlying disease in majority of cases is myocardial infarction, but SA attacks may also occur in cases of acute myocarditis, syphilitic cardio-aortic disease, and drug overdose.

## Clinical Features

In classical cases there is a history of attack(s) of sudden loss of consciousness, without any warning **("syncopal attacks")**. If standing, the patient falls down and may sustain injury. In attacks lasting more than 10 seconds there may be twitching followed by convulsions. If opportunity permits clinical examination during the attack, the patient will be found to be pale, limp, pulseless (or severely bradycardia), and virtually dead. However, his breathing continues and there is no cyanosis. The recovery usually occurs abruptly within a few seconds but if the arrhythmia persists for a minute or two, respiration may also cease, producing a picture of total cardiorespiratory arrest.

## Diagnosis

When the patient is seen in between Stokes-Adams attacks, the diagnosis will be based mostly on a characteristic history. Unlike epileptic fits, Stokes-Adams attacks are somewhat gradual in onset, very brief in duration, not preceded by an aura or cry, nor followed by any confusion, mental cloudiness, headache, or other postictal features. Cerebral ischemic attacks due to arteriosclerosis (transient ischemic attacks), on the other hand, are often recurrent, lasting usually for several hours, and are characterized by neurological deficits which are invariably identical in different attacks. A complete physical examination along with ECG and 24–48 hour Holter monitoring help in making a clinical diagnosis (*see* also section on "Syncope", Chapter 13).

## Management

### Treatment During the (Stokes–Adams) Attack

Treatment during the SA attack is on the same lines as for cardiac arrest. If a couple of blows on the middle of the chest fail to restore cardiac beat, external cardiac massage should be started at once. Meanwhile, an ECG should be obtained and drug therapy decided accordingly (see section on "Cardiac Arrest"). Most of the Stokes–Adams attacks are, however, so brief in duration that by the time the physician arrives at the site, the attack is already over and the patient has recovered consciousness. Treatment will then have to be planned to prevent recurrence of the attacks.

### Treatment in between the Attacks

Recurrent attacks of Stokes–Adams syndrome are most often due to acute onset cardiac disease (e.g., myocardial infarction), and are associated with advanced or complete heart block, transient asystole, VF, or marked brady-or-tachyarrhythmias. In most of such cases cardiac pacing is required urgently. However, in the interim period, isoproterenol infusion should be started (for

## Chapter 1: Cardiovascular Emergencies

details, see section on "Complete Heart Block"). Occasionally, symptomatic and advanced heart block may result from inappropriate use of calcium-channel blockers (verapamil and diltiazem), especially if used in combination with beta-blockers. Identification and removal of the cause coupled with supportive therapy usually suffice in such patients but (temporary) pacing may be required in some cases especially when **heart rate** is <40/min.

## ■ SUDDEN CARDIAC DEATH AND CARDIAC ARREST

### Definition

Sudden cardiac death (SCD) is defined as **natural death** usually from cardiac causes (in clinically stable patients) within 1 hour of the onset of acute symptoms, and heralded by abrupt loss of consciousness. Interventions in such cases may delay the biologic death but what is important is that the index event should have occurred as defined above. In *unwitnessed deaths this time-interval is extended to 24 hours after the victim was last seen to be alive and stable.* Sudden death can also be noncardiac in origin such as respiratory arrest (as in asphyxiation), trauma, or anaphylaxis but such events are distinct.

*Cardiac arrest* is a related term that refers to cessation of cardiac pump function, which may be reversible. Most often this follows VF, which itself is often due to some acute coronary episode, and may be preceded by VT.

### Etiology

Sudden cardiac death is most often due to acute myocardial infarction complicated by VF (often preceded by VT).

Less frequently SCD is associated with *left ventricular hypertrophy* (usually due to hypertension) which may as well, be accompanied by cardiac arrhythmias. Occasionally, sudden and unexpected stoppage of heart beat (SCD) may occur in complete heart block, severe low cardiac output states, cardiomyopathies, following anesthesia/surgical intervention, drug toxicity, certain diagnostic procedures (such as cardiac catheterization and angiography, endoscopic examinations, pericardial paracentesis), and electrocution, drowning, etc.

### Diagnosis

What matters in SCD and cardiac arrest is how quickly it is recognized since after about 3 minutes irreversible brain damage occurs as indicated by fixed dilated pupils. *Three most important features of cardiac arrest can be represented by acronym "APU".*
a. A: Apnea
b. P: Pulselessness (in big vessels such as carotid and femoral arteries)
c. U: Unconsciousness

Poor or absent respiratory efforts coupled with absent pulse are diagnostic of cardiac arrest. Respiratory jerks may persist for a minute or more after the onset of cardiac arrest. Pupils dilate and become unreactive to light after several minutes. Once cardiac arrest is suspected, treatment should be started immediately. Time must not be wasted on auscultation of heart, etc.

ote

Dilatation of pupils begins after cerebral blood flow stops for about 1 minute and becomes maximal in 2 minutes. However, pupillary and corneal reflexes may survive for as much as 10 minutes.

## Management

Management of SCD/cardiac arrest revolves around restoration of *effective* heart beat and respiration as early as possible (almost on war footing). The results greatly depend upon the awareness of the medical and paramedical personnel immediately near the patient, and their training in such a resuscitative procedure.

Since cardiac arrest and failure of respiration usually develop together, resuscitative efforts have to be directed to restore both circulation and respiration, and therefore, the **term CPR** is preferable to cardiac resuscitation. *Patients most likely to be successfully resuscitated by CPR include:*

❖ Hospitalized patients with acute ischemic heart disease and primary VF
❖ Cases with cardiac arrest in the absence of life-threatening comorbidities
❖ Cases with witnessed sudden arrest due to VF outside the hospital when electrical counter shock can be performed within approximately 7–8 minutes
❖ Patient with drug overdose, hypothermia, airway obstruction, or primary respiratory arrest.

**The sequence of resuscitation in CPR used to be ABC:** A (airway), B (breathing), C (circulation). However, American Heart Association in 2010 revised this sequence from **A-B-C to C-A-B,** thus changing the priority from "airway" and "breathing" to chest compressions (C) first, then airway (A) and breathing (B). This change has been based upon the fact that, (i) victims of cardiac arrest can go on for a minute or two (even longer) without taking a breath since they still have ample air in the lungs and blood, and chest compresses (cardiac massage) can keep blood flowing to the vital organs, (ii) rescuers are often worried about opening the airway and making an adequate mouth-to mouth seal which carries the risk of exposure to certain viral infections, and (iii) valuable time is likely to be lost in searching for a "barrier device" to avoid direct mouth-to-mouth contact. This change from A-B-C to C-A-B also makes it easier for untrained bystanders and medical personnel to begin CPR with chest compressions only. This advice applies to adults and children needing CPR, but not newborns and infants since majority of them collapse from breathing problems, and mouth-to-mouth breathing is essential for air to get into their system.

Even when fully trained personnel are available for CPR, the advice is to begin with 30 chest compressions in 18–20 seconds before checking the airway and giving rescue breaths.

ote

This "hands only CPR" was briefly mentioned in the last edition of this book (2009) after preliminary reports appeared in its favor. By now this _change in the priorities of "ABC of life support" is well established..

## Basic (Emergency) Measures

- ❖ **Initial Steps:**
  - Give a forceful thump on the lower part of the sternum with the inner side of the closed fist (Thumpversion). It may be repeated once or twice, if no response occurs. The aim is to convert VF to sinus rhythm, or to initiate electrical activity in an asystolic heart by mechanical stimulation. The maneuver should not take more than 1–2 seconds; if it is unsuccessful, one should immediately proceed to the next step.
  - If some help is available, elevate patient's legs by about 60 degrees and maintain this position for 20–30 seconds while the main rescuer goes ahead with chest compressions. This may increase the venous return to the heart by as much as 1,000 mL.
  - Extend the neck fully and tilt the head backward so that the tongue (which falls back in unconscious state) does not block the airway.
    These measures may be enough to restore cardiac activity but if not, then quickly go on to CPR as described below.
- ❖ **Cardiopulmonary Resuscitation Remember: C-A-B**
  **Compressions: Restore blood circulation external cardiac massage**
  - Put the patient on the back on a firm surface.
  - Kneel next to the person's neck and shoulder.
  - Place the heel of one hand (left hand in right handed subjects) parallel to, and over the lower half of sternum, and the heel of the other hand on the dorsum of the lower hand, interlocking the fingers **(Fig. 1.17)** to obtain a firm grasp between the two hands.
  - Use your upper body weight (not just your arms) as you push straight down (compress) the chest at least 5 cm. Push hard at a rate of about 100 compressions a minute, the movement taking place at the wrist joint—*"push hard and push fast"* **(Fig. 1.18)**.

*Effectiveness of cardiac massage* will be indicated by a palpable impulse over big vessels synchronous with each stroke over the sternum. Pressure should not be too hard nor applied over lower ribs or xiphisternum to avoid injury to ribs, lungs, liver, etc. External massage should not be interrupted for

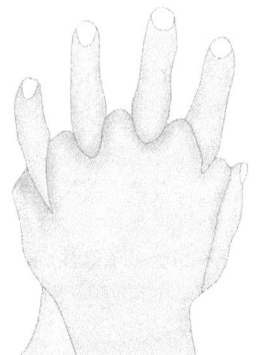

**Fig. 1.17:** Position of the hands—technique of interlocking the fingers.

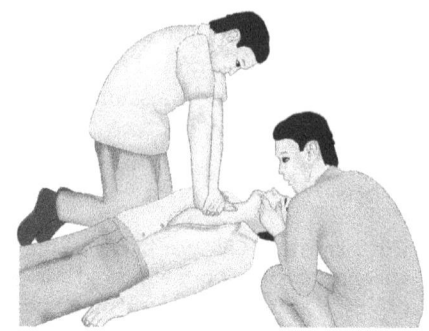

**Fig. 1.18:** Method of external cardiac massage by one rescuer and mouth-to-mouth ventilation by the other rescuer.

more than 5 seconds for any reason, and should be accompanied by artificial ventilation, as far as possible.

### Airway: Clear the Airway

- ❖ If the person performing CPR is well trained in the procedure, he should (after performing 30 chest compressions), open the victim's airway using the "head-tilt, chin-lift" maneuver (**Fig. 1.19**). This can be done by putting a small pillow or a rolled towel under the neck, and head tilted backwards. If another person is available he should position himself on one side of the patient, lift the neck with one hand and tilt the head backward with the other hand placed on the patient's forehead. Any denture or portion of food or any other material lying in the mouth should be quickly removed, and a clear airway ensured.
- ❖ The rescuer should check for normal breathing, taking no more than 5 or 10 seconds. If the person is not breathing normally, begin "mouth-mouth" breathing. If the person performing CPR is not well trained in this emergency procedure, he should skip mouth-to-mouth breathing and continue chest compression.

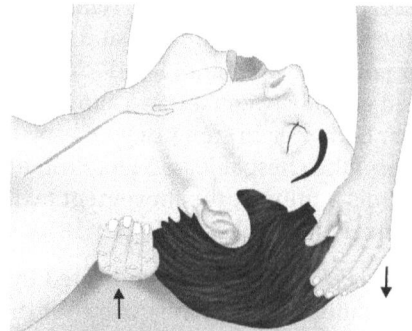

**Fig. 1.19:** Head- tilt neck-lift method of opening the airway.

## Breathing: Breathe for the Person

- With the airway open (using the head-tilt, chin-lift maneuver), the rescuer should pinch the nostrils shut, open his mouth wide and take a deep breath making a tight seal with his mouth around the patient's lips, either directly or through a gauze piece **(Fig. 1.20)**.
- He should then blow in as hard and as fast as possible delivering with each breath about 1,000 cc (double the average amount of air inhaled with each breath). After the first rescue breath (lasting 1 second) wait to see if the chest rises. If it does rise, give the second breath. These cycles should be repeated, 30 chest compressions followed by two rescue breaths constituting one cycle.
- Simultaneously with artificial ventilation another (trained) person should perform external cardiac massage. However, if there is only one rescuer he should combine the two procedures, interrupting cardiac massage every 10-15 seconds to ventilate the lungs two or three times. Three or four quick full breaths should be given initially without allowing full expiration. Later, artificial ventilation should be continued rhythmically at a steady rate of 12/minute.

The success or failure of emergency measures outlined above should be checked periodically by following signs—(1) return of pulsation in the femoral or carotid artery, (2) spontaneous respiratory efforts, and (3) palpable or recordable blood pressure.

*All this is possible only if a person properly trained in the art of CPR is available.*

ote

> Automated external defibrillators (AEDs) are currently available at prominent public places in many developed countries. When this facility is available, one shock should be administered, and CPR resumed—starting with chest compressions–for 2 minutes before administering a second shock.

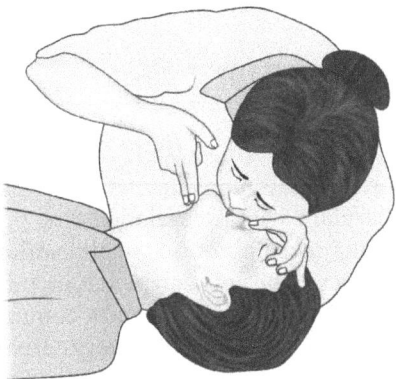

**Fig. 1.20:** Technique of mouth-to-mouth ventilation.

While this basic CPR is being continued, arrangement should simultaneously be made to transfer the patient to a facility with specialized intensive care for "advanced **life support**". This is not discussed here as it is beyond the scope of this text.

### Termination of Resuscitation

This is often a difficult decision and depends upon proper evaluation of cerebral and cardiopulmonary status as well as on any serious comorbidity. Fixed dilated pupils, deep unconsciousness, and absence of spontaneous respiration and cardiac activity after 15-30 minutes of adequate CPR usually indicate permanent cerebral damage and cardiac death. In such circumstances (and even earlier, if the patient has underlying critical disease) it may be appropriate for the doctor in-charge of the case to abandon further efforts at resuscitation.

### Prognosis

Despite several advances in recent years, outcome of patients experiencing sudden coronary death remains poor. A vast majority of cases of cardiac arrest occur outside the hospital setting and the death rate for such cases is at least 90%. Further, those who survive, over half have permanent brain damage.

### Factors Affecting Prognosis

- Chances of survival are poor in elderly, males and smokers.
- Associated comorbidities especially infection and renal failure have negative impact on patient's outcome.
- Prognosis is better if the first monitored rhythm of heart on ECG after cardiac arrest is VF/VT (because of effective defibrillation). For other rhythms chances of survival are very low.
- Patients with shorter duration of cardiac arrest (in VT/VT) have a better prognosis and chances of survival **than** those **with** a **longer duration** of arrest. Presence of these arrhythmias indicates that the arrest has begun **recently** as otherwise these, if untreated, would end up in asystole.

## ACUTE CARDIAC TAMPONADE

### Etiology

This is an uncommon medical emergency, which results from rapid collection of fluid in the pericardial cavity. Occasionally the process is slower, and a large amount of fluid may accumulate in the pericardial sac before features of cardiac tamponade appear. The fluid can be serous, purulent or hemorrhagic, and may be due to a variety of causes, the most common being tubercular, at any rate, in this part of the world. The circulatory embarrassment results from defective diastolic filling of the heart with corresponding drop in stroke output and blood pressure.

## Clinical Features

The onset may be acute (as in hemo-pericardium and purulent pericarditis) or gradual (e.g., tubercular effusion). In the former event, even small effusions of 200–250 mL may produce acute distension of the pericardium and interfere with flow of blood into the ventricles. On the other hand, with slowly developing effusions, large quantities (even over a liter) may accumulate without serious consequences, and then the patient may suddenly develop vascular collapse.

**Clinically** acute cardiac tamponade is suggested by a ***triad of signs comprising increasing venous pressure, falling arterial pressure, and a quiet heart.*** The patient is dyspneic, anxious, restless, appears pale, and has marked tachycardia. There is often evidence of ***paradoxical pulse,*** and BP is greatly reduced, pulse pressure being often 20 mm Hg or less. In severe cases shock may supervene.

When collection of fluid has been somewhat gradual, there may be additional evidence of systemic venous congestion indicated by engorged jugular veins, enlarged liver, and puffiness of face. In such cases examination of the heart will also reveal an increase in the area of cardiac dullness, and muffled heart sounds. The ECG is of further help and shows elevation of ST segment in all or any of the standard and/or precordial leads, without reciprocal depression or evolutionary changes in serial ECGs (as occurs in AMI). In chronic cases of pericardial effusion, T-waves may also be inverted in the standard leads. Echocardiography is diagnostic.

## Management

A rising venous pressure coupled with a falling arterial pressure (below 90 mm Hg) warrants immediate intervention.

### *Pericardiocentesis*

In patients with cardiac tamponade, draining even a small quantity of fluid can rapidly improve hemodynamics, and can thus be lifesaving.

The success of the procedure depends upon the size of the pericardial effusion, and the experience of the person performing the procedure. The availability of imaging methods such as echocardiography or ultrasonography to locate the effusion and guide needle insertion increases the success rate, and makes the procedure safe and reliable. The patient should be placed in recumbent position with the chest elevated by 30 degrees. Possible sites for needle insertion are shown in **Figure 1.21**.

Subxiphoid approach (2) is usually preferred. If the fluid withdrawn is bloody, it is essential to confirm the position of the needle to ensure that it has not penetrated the heart. A useful point to differentiate between intrapericardial blood and peripheral blood is that the former either does not clot or clots slowly because the whipping action of the heart tends to defibrinate it.

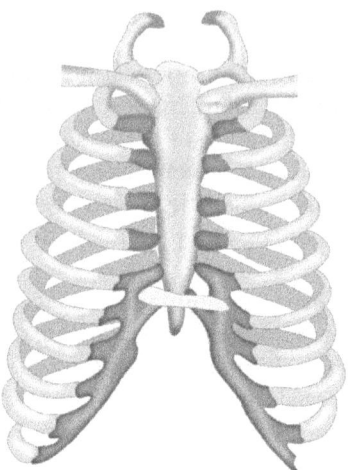

**Fig. 1.21:** Pericardiocentesis.

## Other Measures

In all cases of cardiac tamponade an attempt should be made to find out the cause of pericardial effusion, which should then be treated appropriately. When no cause is obvious and the effusion is serous (or even hemorrhagic), it should be presumed to be tubercular in origin (in this country, at any rate), and treated (accordingly).

# APPENDIX

| Table 1.13: Classification of blood pressure (for adults). | | |
|---|---|---|
| BP classification | SBP mm Hg | DBP mm Hg |
| Normal | <120 | <80 |
| Elevated | 120–139 | or 80–89 |
| Stage 1 Hypertension | 130–139 | or 90–99 |
| Stage 2 Hypertension | ≥140 | ≥90 |

As per recommendations of American Heart Association (2017).

| Table 1.14: Cardiovascular emergencies: Common drugs used in bolus form (in adults). | | |
|---|---|---|
| Drug | Supplied as | Dose (IV) |
| Adenosine | 3 mg/mL | 6 mg rapid IV; repeat 12 mg bolus after 2 min, if required |
| Amiodarone | 150 mg/3 mL | 150 mg over 1–2 min, followed by 0.5 mg/min for 18 hours |
| Atropine | 0.6 mg/mL | 0.6–1.2 mg; may be repeated every 5 min as required (for a total of 3 mg) |

*Contd...*

Contd...

| Drug | Supplied as | Dose (IV) |
|---|---|---|
| Calcium gluconate | 10% solution | 10 mL slow IV |
| Diltiazem | 5 mg/mL | 10–15 mg (0.15–0.25 mg/kg) over 2 min; repeat if required after 15 min |
| Epinephrine | 0.1 mg/mL | 0.5–1.0 mg every 5 min (diluted in 10 mL D5W) |
| Isoproterenol | 4 mg/2 mL | 100–200 mg IV push (diluted in 10 mL D5W) |
| Lidocaine | 2% solution | 1 mg/kg; can be repeated in half the dosage every 5–10 (20 mg/mL) min up to a maximum of 4 mg/kg |
| Metoprolol | 1 mg/mL | 2–3 mg slowly; may be repeated every 10 min up to 3 doses |
| Phenytoin | 100 mg/2 mL | 100–200 mg slow IV (not >50 mg/min); can be repeated after 10 min |
| Procainamide | 100 mg/mL | 1 mg/kg at a rate of 20 mg/min; not to exceed total dose of 1 g |
| Verapamil | 5 mg/2 mL | 5 mg slow IV; may be repeated once or twice every 5 min |

**Table 1.15:** Cardiovascular emergencies: Common drugs used in infusion form (in adults).

| Drug in infusion | Supplied as | For infusion, mix | Drug conc. | Dose |
|---|---|---|---|---|
| Amiodarone | 300 mg/2 mL | 300 mg in 250 mL D5W | 1–2 mg/mL | 5 mg/kg every 8 hours for 2–3 days along with oral therapy for prolonged use |
| Dopamine | 200 mg/5 mL | 200 mg in 250 mL D5W | 800 µg/mL | Small: 2–5 µg/kg/min<br>Moderate: 10–25 µg/kg/min<br>Large: >5 µg/kg/min |
| Dobutamine (Dobutrex) | 250 mg per vial | 250 mg in 250 mL D5W | 1 mg/mL | 2.5–5.0 µg/kg/min |
| Isoproterenol | 4 mg/2 mL | 4 mg in 500 mL D5W | 8 µg/mL | 2–16 µg/min |
| Lidocaine (20 mg/mL) | 2% solution | 1 g in 500 mL D5W | 2 mg/mL | 1–3 mg/min |
| Nitroglycerine | 50 mg per vial | 50 mg in 250 mL D5W | 200 µg/mL | Begin 10–20 µg/min, increase by 5 µg/min every 10 min till desired effect is reached |
| Noradrenaline | 2 mg/2 mL | 4 mg in 500 mL D5W | 8 mcg/mL | 8–32 µg/min |
| Procainamide | 100 mg/mL | 1 g in 500 mL D5W | 2 mg/mL | 1–4 mg/min |

# CHAPTER 2: Respiratory Emergencies

## LIFE-THREATENING HEMOPTYSIS

### Definition

Hemoptysis implies coughing up of blood from a focus in the respiratory passages below the vocal cords. Its intensity may vary from trivial, through mild, to *life-threatening*. The latter is defined by hemodynamic instability, abnormal gas exchange, or airway obstruction. The severity of hemoptysis (and therefore the prognosis) is related more to the *rate of bleeding* than the extent of pulmonary disease or the patient's age.

### Etiology

Hemoptysis can be associated with a large number of disease states **(Table 2.1)**. Rarely, hemoptysis is extremely severe and rapidly fatal within minutes, as with rupture of aortic aneurysm into the trachea or erosion of a large vessel in a lung cavity. In such instances the patient may die before medical aid can reach him.

### Pathophysiology

*The lungs have a dual blood supply* (pulmonary and bronchial circulation) and extensive anastomoses exist between the two. Pulmonary arteries arise from right ventricle, comprise a low-pressure circuit, and supply the lung parenchyma. The bronchial arteries arise from the aorta or intercostals arteries and carry blood under systemic pressure to the airways, the hila and visceral pleura. Life-threatening hemoptysis usually involves bleeding either from bronchial arteries or from pulmonary circulation exposed to high-

**Table 2.1:** Important causes of life-threatening hemoptysis.

| Hemoptysis | Causes |
|---|---|
| Infection | Tuberculosis, bronchiectasis, lung abscess, necrotizing pneumonia |
| Neoplasm | Bronchogenic carcinoma, metastatic carcinoma, mediastinal tumor, endobronchial polyp |
| Cardiovascular disease | • Mitral stenosis<br>• Pulmonary arteriovenous malformation |
| Miscellaneous | Swan–Ganz catheterization, exploratory needling |

pressure bronchial circulation through bronchopulmonary anastomoses. Such anastomoses are common in many chronic inflammatory states such as bronchiectasis. In some cases rupture of an ectatic pulmonary vessel (Rasmussen's aneurysm) is the cause of life-threatening hemoptysis (especially in tuberculosis).

## Diagnosis

Hemoptysis should first of all, be *differentiated from hematemesis and pseudohemoptysis*. The difficulty is likely to be encountered most in cases with severe hemoptysis where some of the coughed up blood is swallowed and later brought out as vomitus. In such a situation two points should be remembered: (1) hemoptysis is often preceded by cough whereas hematemesis is usually an abrupt phenomenon, and (2) in cases with hemoptysis, after the large bleed, patient usually continues to cough up small amount of blood mixed with sputum for a while unlike hematemesis, which occurs in well-defined episodes, each with a sharp beginning and a sharp ending.

Once it is confirmed that the blood brought out constitutes hemoptysis, a detailed relevant history and complete physical examination are mandatory to find out the cause of hemoptysis. *It is important to remember that hemoptysis is only a symptom and not a disease.*

A chest radiograph (**CXR**) is the basic investigation and may provide clues not only to the etiology of hemorrhage but possibly also about the site of bleeding within the lungs. However, CXR may be essentially normal in some cases of bronchiectasis, bronchial carcinoma or endobronchial polyp. **CT scan of the chest or an MRI** may be valuable in such cases. The gold standard in diagnosis of hemoptysis, however, is **bronchoscopy** which may not only reveal the site of bleeding but also establish etiopathologic **tissue diagnosis.** The timing of bronchoscopy is however, controversial. To obtain better results it should be performed as soon as hemoptysis has somewhat settled and the patient's condition is stable, preferably within 2–3 days of hospitalization.

## Management

All patients with life-threatening hemoptysis should be hospitalized. Cases with mild hemoptysis may be managed and observed at patient's home, if so desired. In such cases bleeding stops usually within 3-4 days. At any point of time, however, it may suddenly increase. **Hospitalization** becomes essential in such cases if: (1) hemoptysis continues for more than 72 hours, and (2) features of shock supervene or are impending.

A sudden large hemoptysis may occasionally be rapidly fatal, the patient dying before the doctor can reach him. The immediate cause of death in such circumstances is related, not to actual loss of blood, but to asphyxiation resulting from large amount of blood flooding the bronchial passages. More often, however, hemoptysis, even though large in volume, is not quite abrupt and allows time for management. The objectives of management are:

(1) prevention of airway obstruction, (2) support and maintenance of vital signs, and (3) control of bleeding.

- ❖ **Prevention of airway obstruction:** This is of paramount importance. When the area of lung disease is known, the patient should be put in lateral decubitus with the diseased side in dependent position so as to minimize the risk of aspiration into the uninvolved lung. If the doctor happens to be present at the time of actual massive bleeding, he should immediately put the patient in **semiprone position** on the edge of the bed and lower the head. This will facilitate the flow of blood out from the respiratory passages, and prevent asphyxiation. Such patients should ideally be admitted in intensive care units where constant monitoring is possible and facilities are available for suction and immediate endotracheal intubation if need arises.
- ❖ **Support of vital signs:** A good intravenous line should be established and IV fluids (crystalloids) started immediately. As soon as possible blood should be transfused to maintain the hematocrit >30, and supplemental oxygen started (arterial blood gases should be monitored in all cases of life-threatening hemoptysis and $PaO_2$ maintained above 55 mm Hg).
- ❖ **Cessation of bleeding:** Fortunately, in most of the cases of hemoptysis bleeding diminishes gradually over a period of 5-7 days and ceases spontaneously. Many drugs such as calcium gluconate, estrogens, clauden, vitamin K, etc. have been advocated to control bleeding, but their efficacy is doubtful. When bronchiectasis or pulmonary tuberculosis is considered as the cause of hemoptysis, appropriate broad-spectrum antibiotics or antitubercular treatment, respectively, should be instituted.

### *Other Measures*

While most patients of life-threatening hemoptysis can be managed conservatively, *emergency surgery* (lobectomy or pneumonectomy) may be warranted in cases who require multiple blood transfusions and in whom large hemoptysis continues for more than a week despite appropriate medical management.

A newer approach, in stable patients, is to localize the bleeding vessel(s) by bronchial arteriography and then *embolize the involved bronchial arteries*. This is possible only in specialized centers with experienced personnel. A major risk is embolic spinal cord injury.

### *Subsequent Measures*

After the immediate problems associated with hemoptysis are over, an attempt must be made to find out the cause of hemoptysis, and then treat it as best as possible. In majority of cases the cause is obvious from the clinical details of the patient coupled with CXR, CT scan and/or bronchoscopy. In a few cases, however, the etiology of hemoptysis may remain obscure even after comprehensive investigations. Such cases should be closely observed for the next few months and periodic CXR taken with a view to detect, at the earliest, any feature suggestive of neoplasm. However, majority of such cases, at any rate in India and other developing countries, will ultimately turn out to be suffering from pulmonary tuberculosis and hence, it may be desirable to put them on antitubercular treatment from the very beginning.

# FOREIGN BODY AIRWAY OBSTRUCTION

## Etiopathogenesis

Any foreign body in the mouth may slip back into the airway and produce obstruction. In children this could be a small toy or any other object held in the mouth. The most common object involved in all age groups, is **a fragment of food,** which may choke the victim while eating. The resultant obstruction may be partial or complete. In the latter situation the foreign body lodges in the throat like a cork in a bottle. The victim becomes severely asphyxiated, and may die or suffer permanent brain damage unless the obstruction is relieved **within 4 minutes.**

If the obstruction is partial, the situation may not be life threatening. However, serious complications may occur, if it is suddenly converted into a complete obstruction as may happen if forceful blows or taps are applied on the victim's back (a common house-hold procedure), which may drive the object deeper into the airway.

## Clinical Features

A victim choking on a foreign body may "try to swallow" or "cough it out" or "wash it down with water", but nothing may work. Often he is unable to speak, and may indicate that "I am choking" only by instinctively clutching his throat with his hand, or by nodding assertively when asked "are you choking"? There are *three signs which indicate complete obstruction of airway:* (i) inability to speak/breathe, (ii) pallor followed by increasing cyanosis, and (iii) loss of consciousness, and collapse. If the obstructing object is a fragment of food, the victim will be invariably found near an eating place.

## Management

Food choking may have been actually witnessed or may have to be inferred when, for no apparent reason, someone is found unconscious and not breathing near â **restaurant or eating place. In such a situation a diagnosis must be made at once and** resuscitation attempted immediately by **Heimlich maneuver** (HM).

### Principle of Heimlich Maneuver

This maneuver is based on the principle, that irrespective of the phase of respiration in which choking occurs, a considerable reservoir of air remains in the lungs (remainder of tidal volume and the expiratory reserve). When the diaphragm is raised with a sub-diaphragmatic thrust (employed in HM), this air is expelled with considerable force through the bronchi and trachea. It has been estimated that the volume of air expelled averages 0.94 L when the HM is applied during early expiratory phase and 0.35 L when performed at the end of forced expiratory phase. In either situation enough air pressure is generated to dislodge the obstructing object (whether associated with total or partial obstruction) and drive it out through the mouth.

The HM can be performed in several different ways depending upon the position of the victim. It can also be used by the victim to save himself.

*a. The victim is sitting or standing (Fig. 2.1)*

The rescuer should stand behind the victim, encircle his waist with his arms, placing the thumb side of the fist (made into a knob) against the victim's abdomen slightly above the naval but well below the tip of the xiphoid process (and not just a "bear hug"). With the other hand over it, he should press into patient's abdomen with a sharp inward and upward thrust. The obstructing object is usually thrown out of the mouth with force. If unsuccessful, the procedure should be repeated till free airway is established (up to 4–6 sub-diaphragmatic thrusts may be required).

*b. Victim is unconscious and lying on floor (Fig. 2.2)*

If the victim is lying face down on floor, the person should be rolled over on his back, face up. The rescuer should *kneel astride* the victim's hips (and not on one side), place the heel of one hand between the naval and xiphisternum put the other hand over it, and press into the abdomen toward the diaphragm with a quick upward thrust.

*c. The victim is alone and choking (self-save technique)*

The victim can perform the standard HM on himself by placing his hands in the same position as he would do if he were saving someone else. With the

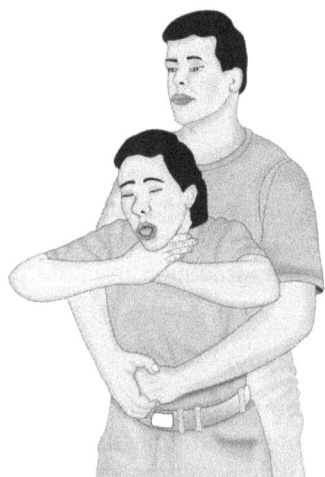

**Fig. 2.1:** Heimlich maneuver with the victim in standing position.

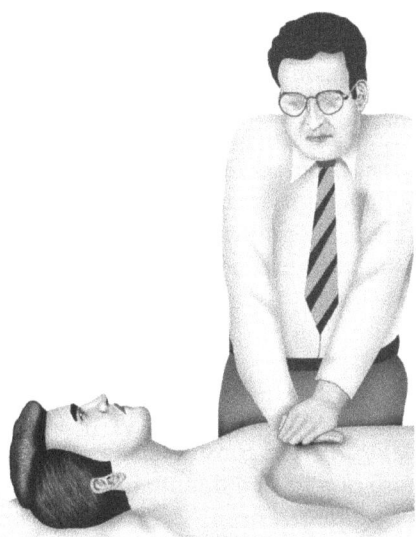

**Fig. 2.2:** Heimlich maneuver with the victim unconscious and lying on the floor.

knob of his fist directly against his own abdomen, he should use the other hand for inward-upward thrust. Alternatively, he can make use of a firm edge of a horizontal object (e.g., back of a chair or rounded corner of a table or sink) and press his abdomen against this edge with a quick forcible thrust. Several thrusts may be required to dislodge the foreign body and clear the airway.

### *Unsuccessful Attempts*

The procedure may be occasionally unsuccessful in dislodging the obstruction because of: (1) faulty technique; (2) when obstruction is tightly lodged in trachea or extends into bronchi; and (3) when foreign body has been aspirated into the lungs (for example, peanut).

### *Complications*

Surprisingly few complications have been reported when HM is properly applied. These are:
- Rib fracture
- Vomiting
- Abdominal soreness
- Gastric injury.

## ACUTE SEVERE BRONCHIAL ASTHMA

### Definition

Acute severe bronchial asthma or acute severe asthma (ASA) is defined as an exceptionally severe attack of bronchial asthma that does not respond to standard treatments of bronchodilators and corticosteroids. *It is a potentially fatal medical emergency, a feature not often recognized.* Since it is the intensity rather than the duration of the acute episode (of bronchial asthma), which is more critical in such cases, the term "ASA" is preferred over "Status Asthmaticus". However, the latter term *"Status Asthmaticus"* is useful to describe cases of *prolonged* severe attack of bronchial asthma continuing for more than 24 hours that are difficult to treat/therapy-resistant. Unusually severe form of acute asthma is the *"sudden asphyxia asthma"* in which the patient may even die due to respiratory arrest within 1 or 2 hours of what appears to be an ordinary attack of asthma.

## Pathogenesis

Bronchial asthma is generally caused by a combination of *genetic and environmental factors:* Earlier considered a purely allergic disorder it is now thought to be more of a reversible inflammatory condition of the airways associated with *heightened bronchial reactivity of both large and small airways to multiple stimuli.* Physiologically, acute asthma has two components —an acute early bronchospastic component and a later inflammatory response.

- ❖ **Early bronchospastic response:** Immediately upon exposure to allergens, mast cell degranulation occurs along with release of inflammatory mediators such as histamine, leukotrienes, bradykinin, and cytokines. These products cause airway smooth muscle contraction, increase capillary permeability (microvascular leakage) and mucus secretion, and activate neuronal reflexes. This early asthmatic response is characterized by bronchoconstriction that is generally responsive to conventional bronchodilators (beta-2 agonists).
- ❖ **Later inflammatory response:** The inflammatory mediators activate inflammatory cells in the airways such as mast cells, eosinophils, basophils, and neutrophils. These cells attach to the epithelium and endothelium, and subsequently migrate into the tissues of the airway. Desquamation of the airway epithelium occurs, and nerve endings are exposed. This inflammatory interaction further promotes airway hyper-responsiveness, which may persist long after the triggering event is over and acute phase subsides. This inflammatory component may occur in individuals with even mild asthmatic exacerbation resulting in prolonged spells of irritating cough (mostly dry), often resistant to antibiotics and various cough syrups.

The bronchospasm along with mucus plugging and edema in the peripheral airways together result in airway occlusions which lead to development of extensive alveolar areas in which ventilation (V) is severely reduced but perfusion (Q) is maintained (areas with very low V/Q ratios). And this forms the basis of gas exchange abnormalities observed in acute severe asthma.

## Precipitating Factors

Bronchial asthma has a strong genetic predisposition, and is often an expression of the atopic state which comprises a family history of asthma, hay fever, or dermatitis. *In sensitive patients,* an acute attack of bronchial asthma can be triggered by a number of allergens, which increase airway inflammation and bronchial responsiveness. These can be:

- **Inhaled allergens** such as seasonal pollens, domestic mites (often found in mattresses, pillows, stuffed furniture and pet dog/cat), environmental pollutants (ozone, nitrogen oxide, sulfur dioxide, etc.), tobacco smoke (active or passive), and chemical irritants in the work place.
- **Respiratory infections** including viral infections of the upper respiratory tract, chronic sinusitis often with postnasal drippings. Not infrequently intermittent or persistent wheezing and cough (presumably because of sensory nerve irritation) persist long after the triggering event is over. The dry cough is often a troublesome symptom *(cough-variant asthma),* and may last for days and weeks, sometimes resulting even in syncope *(cough syncope).*
- **Pharmacological agents:** Important drugs include aspirin, beta-adrenergic blockers, and nonsteroidal anti-inflammatory drugs (NSAIDs).
- **Exercise-induced:** In certain individuals, especially children, exercise may induce bronchial constriction and precipitate an attack of asthma. *Typically, the attacks do not occur during exercise but follow it* within a few minutes, peak at about 10–15 minutes, and subside by 60 minutes after the exercise. The attacks are severer with higher ventilatory effort (e.g. more likely with running than with walking), and in dry and cold environment (than in hot and humid air). Bronchial constriction is the result of airways' attempt to warm and humidify an increased volume of inspired air during exercise, and is associated with temperature related hyperemia and capillary leakage in the airway wall. The long-term prognosis is guarded, and many patients develop recurrent episodes of airway obstruction independent of exercise.
- **Contributory factors:** Many factors can precipitate a severe attack of bronchial asthma such as acute emotional stress, food additives, cold temperature, gastroesophageal reflux disease and sudden discontinuation of medicines.

## Clinical Features

Asthmatic exacerbations may be acute or subacute and are characterized by episodes of breathlessness, cough, wheezing, chest tightness, or any combination thereof. The time course of such exacerbations may vary greatly. On one extreme are patients in whom airway obstruction measured by PEF (peak expiratory flow) worsens over several days before the appearance of severe symptoms. Such cases are so-called *"slow-onset **asthma exacerbation**",* and are chiefly due to faults in **management such as inadequate treatment, inappropriate** use of **hand-held inhalers,** and psychosocial stress factors. On the other extreme are patients with *"sudden onset asthma exacerbation"* in whom lung functions deteriorate rapidly and severely in a matter of hours. The triggering factor(s) in these instances are massive exposure to common allergens, sensitivity to NSAIDs or food allergens. Without prompt and appropriate treatment these cases invariably progress to ventilatory failure and death.

## Physical Examination

A patient with ASA is often found to be agitated, and even confused or drowsy. He is unable to recline, has marked tachycardia (heart rate over 120/min), and noisy respiration with wheezing in both phases of respiration. If the attack is severe or prolonged, accessory respiratory muscles become active, and paradoxical breathing (retractions of intercostal and sub-costal muscles) can be observed. At this stage pulsus paradoxus (significant reduction of arterial systolic pressure in inspiration) may also develop. A variation greater than 12 mm Hg in systolic blood pressure between inspiration and expiration represents asthmatic crisis. In advanced stages, when ventilatory muscle fatigue sets in, pulsus paradoxus may decrease or disappear. An important feature to remember is that *as the severity of attack increases and respiratory fatigue develops, the air entry decreases progressively, the chest becomes more and more silent, and wheezing sounds may decrease giving a false impression about the gravity of the attack.*

## Differential Diagnosis

Bronchial asthma can be easily diagnosed, but the adage *"all that wheezes may not be asthma"* should not be forgotten. The greatest difficulty is likely to be encountered when acute dyspnea occurs in a middle-aged or elderly person in whom acute left heart failure (LHF) is a genuine possibility. A past history of bronchial asthma is helpful, but not infrequently it may appear for the first time in a middle-aged subject. On the other hand, myocardial infarction with LHF may occur in a known asthmatic patient. It is worth emphasizing that diffuse rhonchi, the hallmark of bronchial asthma, are not uncommon in acute LHF. However, mistakes can be avoided by careful attention to details of history, a thorough **cardiovascular** checkup including ECG, and when possible, an echocardiogram.

Bronchial narrowing and wheezing with consequent respiratory difficulty can also result from *partial bronchial obstruction* due to a foreign body or tumor, or from external pressure on the bronchus. Wheezing, in such cases is unilateral and often localized over the site of the obstructed bronchus. Another possible source of confusion arises when sudden and persistent dyspnea develops in a case of COPD, either because of superadded acute chest infection or pneumothorax. A CXR and other laboratory investigations,

## Chapter 2: Respiratory Emergencies

should decide the issue. Such cases often present as acute respiratory failure (ARF) (see section on "Acute Respiratory Failure").

### Assessment of Severity of Acute Asthmatic Attack

An attack of bronchial asthma seldom causes much anxiety, at any rate not in the mind of the physician, because of the availability of highly effective drugs.

However, *deaths are known to occur during acute attack of asthma* and may be due to: (i) inadequate perception of severity of attack by the patient and thus delay in seeking treatment, and (ii) failure on the part of the attending physician to properly assess the severity of disease and treat the patient aggressively. It is therefore, always desirable to **grade the severity of acute exacerbation (Table 2.2)** of the attack **at the very start of therapy** and also periodically thereafter, not only to serve as a guide to intensity of treatment required but also to evaluate its efficacy.

### Diagnostic Evaluation

**Exacerbations** in asthmatic patients are best assessed by *peak expiratory flow (PEF)* determined by simple hand-held devices. These become more meaningful when expressed as percentage of normal, or of the patient's best obtainable value during remission and while on optimal treatment. During an acute attack of asthma PEF is usually between 20% and 30% of the predicted value. Following treatment symptoms generally resolve when PEF reaches about 50% of normal, and wheezing subsides at a PEF about 60% and 70% of normal.

Another investigation of great value is **pulse oximetry,** since it provides a continuous evaluation of oxygen saturation which is vitally important because the primary cause of death in status asthmaticus is hypoxia. Pulse oximetry is

| \multicolumn{2}{l}{**Table 2.2:** Grading of severity of acute asthma.} | |
|---|---|
| Grades | Severity |
| **Grade I** (Mild attack) | Normal pulse rate or minimal tachycardia (<100/min), but no evidence of respiratory distress or cyanosis; diffuse wheezing; peak expiratory flow 50–80% predicted |
| **Grade II** (Moderate attack) | Moderate tachycardia (100–120/min), visibly active accessory respiratory muscles, diffuse loud wheezes, mild cyanosis, $PaCO_2$ less than 42 mm Hg (because of alveolar hyperventilation), $PaO_2$ >60 mm Hg |
| **Grade III** (Severe attack) | Marked sinus tachycardia (over 120/min), pulsus paradoxus, respiratory rate >30/min, markedly increased activity of accessory respiratory muscles, loud expiratory (and later also inspiratory) wheeze, normal or elevated $PaCO_2$ with $PaO_2$ <60 (at room air) |
| **Grade IV** (Very severe attack) | Patient exhausted, dehydrated, little air movement, absent or minimal wheeze, altered sensorium, $PaCO_2$ elevated (due to alveolar hypoventilation), terminal peripheral circulatory failure |

preferable over arterial blood gas (ABG) study as it is readily available and is non-invasive. ABG study may not always be available and serial estimations are cumbersome. It is usually utilized to assess hypercapnia during the patient's initial assessment. Oxygen saturation is then monitored via pulse oximetry throughout the treatment.

At least one CXR should be obtained in all patients with ASA. Hyperinflation is generally observed, but additional findings may be revealed such as pneumonia, atelectatic patches (due to mucus plugging) and pneumothorax. Other useful investigations include a complete blood count, blood sugar analysis, an ECG, and renal function tests especially in elderly patients.

## Management

The secret of successful treatment of ASA seems to lie in instituting intensive and full medication at the earliest opportunity. Acute severe asthma is one emergency in which over-treatment is seldom harmful, but under-treatment can be hazardous. With increasing duration of severe bronchial spasm, inspissated and tenacious plugs of mucus form which block the terminal bronchi with consequent focal atelectasis. The resulting hypoxia increases pulmonary vascular resistance and aggravates bronchial spasm thus creating a vicious circle.

After confirming the diagnosis and assessing the severity of ASA, the treatment should be directed toward controlling both bronchoconstriction and inflammation. The mainstays of treatment are beta-agonists, corticosteroids, and theophylline.

### Specific Measures

- ❖ **Beta-2 agonists:** It is to be noted that airway smooth muscle has only beta-2 adrenergic receptors, and therefore these drugs (salbutamol/albuterol) constitute the first line of therapy in ASA being both selective and specific. Beta-2 agonists act by relaxing smooth muscle of all the airways, from trachea down to terminal bronchioles through stimulation of cyclic adenosine monophosphate (AMP)-mediated bronchodilation **(Fig. 2.3)**. One ampoule of salbutamol *(Salsol)* containing 2.5 mg of the drug should be nebulized every 3–4 hours or even more frequently. Once some relief is observed, the frequency of nebulization should be decreased

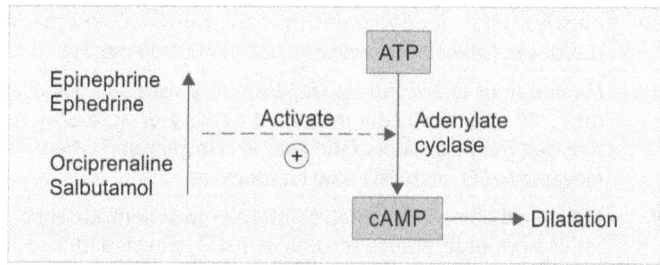

**Fig. 2.3:** Mechanism of action of adrenergic stimulants.

to every 4-6 hours. However, some patients with severe, refractory status asthmaticus may benefit from the addition of these drugs parenterally (salbutamol IV in a bolus dose of 500 mg over 3 minutes followed by a continuous infusion at a rate of 8-10 ng/minute for 24-48 hours).

❖ **Glucocorticoids:** Steroids are the most important treatment of ASA as these counter both inflammatory cell recruitment and the release of inflammatory mediators into the airways. These drugs also prevent late phase reaction and subsequent bronchial hyper-responsiveness. *In ASA, corticosteroids are lifesaving although their effect may not be evident for 4-6 hours.* These should therefore, be given early and in high doses. Hydrocortisone hemisuccinate is used initially in a loading dose of 3-4 mg/kg followed by 100 mg every 6-8 hourly. After 24-48 hours, patient should be switched over to oral prednisolone starting with 40-60 mg daily. *Nebulized corticosteroids have little role, if any, in the treatment of status asthmaticus.*

❖ **Bronchodilators ipratropium bromide** (anticholinergic) has a weak bronchodilator effect but may be particularly useful when bronchospasm is induced by beta-blockers, in patients with COPD, or when acute asthma is exceptionally severe. It is best nebulized along with beta-2 agonists, and the two drugs when combined may produce better results in such cases.

❖ **Antibiotics:** Despite the fact that many cases of ASA are triggered by viral infections, broad spectrum antibiotics are routinely given to such cases as superadded infections are not uncommon. When the infection is overwhelming or the results of bacteriological studies (of sputum) disclose Gram negative infection, a third generation cephalosporin should be used either alone or in combination or with an aminoglycoside or newer quinolones.

❖ **Other measures:** Oxygen therapy is essential in all cases of ASA since hypoxia is the leading cause of death in such cases. Oxygen therapy can be delivered via a nasal cannula or naso-oral mask. The aim should be to keep the patient's oxygen saturation above 92% (above 95% in patients with associated cardiac disease). When respiratory failure is threatened tracheal intubation and mechanical ventilation are indicated.

**Magnesium sulfate** infusion has also been recommended since magnesium can relax smooth muscle and therefore may cause bronchodilation. Usually 1-2 g may be considered during initiation of therapy.

## *Discharge from Hospital*

To avoid risk of early relapse, patients admitted to the hospital with ASA, especially those who required some type of mechanical ventilation, should be discharged only when: (1) able to walk comfortably, (2) there is no waking during night, (3) clinical examination of the chest is normal or near normal, (4) short acting inhaled beta-2 agonist is required no more frequently than every 4 hours, and (5) PEF (after inhaling short acting beta-2 agonist) is more

than 70% of the predicted or personal best effort. *Discharge medications should be carefully planned keeping in view the following guidelines:*
- Prednisolone tablets 30–40 mg daily should be given for 1–3 weeks with very gradual tapering
- Inhaled steroids are often required at a higher dosage than before admission
- Inhaled short acting beta-2 agonists should be used 3 or 4 times a day or as often "as necessary"
- Patient should be explained the *difference between preventive and symptomatic treatment of asthma*. A peak expiratory flow meter should be prescribed, its proper usage explained, and the patient advised how to recognize exacerbations early (and institute prompt treatment).
- **Leukotriene modifiers** *(singular, montair)* are useful for long-term control of asthma, and may be considered as alternative/additive to low dose inhaled corticosteroids in patients with persistent asthma.
- Appropriate use of hand-held multi-dose inhalers must be explained to the patient.

### General Measures

Bronchial irritants of all types (such as smoke, dust, drought, etc.) should be avoided. Patients in acute severe asthma may lose as much as 2 L of fluid through hypercapnia and perspiration. Adequate fluid intake should be ensured in such cases to prevent inspissation of tracheobronchial secretions. Expectorants are of no proven value.

### Prognosis

In general, unless a complicating illness such as heart failure or chronic obstructive airway disease is present, ASA has a good prognosis. Of course, appropriate therapy consonant with the severity of the disease, must be administered immediately upon hospitalization. A delay in initiating treatment, especially in using corticosteroids, is probably the worst prognostic factor. All the three essential drugs (beta-2 agonists, corticosteroids, and bronchodilators) should be used in full dosage from the very start, and not increased in a step-wise manner.

Fatalities in ASA, though quite uncommon are not unknown. Death from asthma can be sudden and unexpected *(sudden asphyxic asthma)*. Affected individuals rapidly develop severe hypercapnic respiratory failure with acidosis, and succumb to asphyxia. Early and intensive medical treatment combined with expert mechanical ventilation may be able to salvage such patients.

### Caution

- Never use morphine or its derivatives, barbiturates, and even antihistamines to allay anxiety, as all such drugs depress respiratory center and may lead to respiratory arrest.

- Do not use epinephrine, if there is the least possibility of the case being one of LHF.
- The initial intensive treatment should not be reduced abruptly.

## Summary

- Acute bronchial asthma has two components—an acute bronchospastic component and a later inflammatory component. The latter promotes further airway hyper-responsiveness in asthma.
- Acute attacks are triggered by stimuli (such as exposure to an allergen) that produce bronchoconstriction, and then are perpetuated in the setting of chronic airway inflammation.
- Management of acute asthma revolves around reducing bronchial constriction with beta-2 agonists and bronchodilators, and controlling inflammation with rapidly acting corticosteroids and a short course of antibiotics.

# SPONTANEOUS PNEUMOTHORAX

## Etiology

Pneumothorax (PTX) implies leakage of air from the lungs into the pleural cavity with associated collapse of the lung. When it occurs without any preceding trauma, it is defined as **"spontaneous"** and may be primary or secondary. *Primary spontaneous PTX occurs without any apparent cause and in the absence of any significant lung disease, whereas secondary type is associated with some underlying pulmonary disease.*

**Primary (spontaneous) pneumothorax:** The cause of primary spontaneous PTX is unknown but is very likely due to rupture into the pleural cavity of one or more thin subpleural blebs or bullae (dilated peripheral air sacs) usually located in the apical portion of the lung. Less commonly, primary PTX is encountered in inhalational drug abusers (cocaine, marijuana), during pregnancy, in weight lifters and in individuals exposed to sudden changes in atmospheric pressures such as pilots and scuba divers.

**Secondary (spontaneous) pneumothorax** occurs in association with a large number of lung diseases **(Box 2.1)**, most common being chronic obstructive pulmonary disease (COPD) which accounts for about two-thirds of the cases.

## Pathophysiology

The parietal and visceral pleurae are normally separated by a potential intrapleural space with a negative pressure between (-) 10 to (-) 12 mm Hg during inspiration, and (-) 2 to (-) 4 mm Hg during expiration. Negative pressures as high as (-) 80 to (-) 100 mm Hg may be generated during coughing, sneezing or straining. Any break in the alveolar/pleural barrier allows air to escape into pleural space. Consequently, the normally negative intrapleural

> **Box 2.1: Conditions associated with secondary spontaneous pneumothorax.**
> 
> - **Airway disease:** Chronic obstructive pulmonary disease (chronic bronchitis, emphysema, asthma), cystic fibrosis.
> - **Infections:** Pulmonary tuberculosis, bacterial (lung abscess, especially thin walled) staphylococcal abscesses (pneumatocele), fungal and parasitic pneumonia; acquired immune deficiency syndrome (AIDS) often associated with *Pneumocystis carini* pneumonia.
> - **Interstitial lung disease:** Pneumoconiosis, sarcoidosis, idiopathic pulmonary fibrosis.
> - **Connective tissue diseases:** Rheumatoid arthritis, ankylosing spondylitis, polymyositis and dermatomyositis.
> - **Cancer:** Lung carcinoma, sarcomas involving the lung.

pressure (which keeps the lungs expanded) increases (becoming less negative/or even positive) allowing the pulmonary elastic recoil pressure to collapse the lung. The result is an **impairment of ventilation** with decrease in total lung capacity and vital capacity. Along with these ventilatory changes, blood is shunted through the unventilated portions of the lung resulting in **hypoxemia**.

## Clinical Features

*Primary spontaneous PTX* occurs usually in young subjects (20-40 years), more often in males, and without underlying lung problems. Symptoms are usually limited, and onset may be marked only by some chest pain and/or mild breathlessness. Tension pneumothorax seldom occurs in such cases.

In *secondary spontaneous pneumothorax* (which by definition, occurs in patients with significant underlying disease) symptoms tend to be more severe and depend upon (a) the *amount of air in the pleural cavity,* (b) the *speed with which it collects, and* (c) *the state of the collapsed as well as the* uninvolved lung. The loss of function in the affected lung(s) results in hypoxemia and may be observed as cyanosis. In more severe cases hypercapnia may be encountered with consequent altered sensorium.

**Tension pneumothorax:** In such cases the air in the pleural cavity continues to increase, so that ultimately it develops a pressure much greater than that of the atmosphere. This is because the tear in the lung is of the ball-valve type which permits the air to enter the pleural space during inspiration, and especially during bouts of coughing and straining, but does not allow the air to escape from the pleural cavity into the tracheobronchial tree during expiration **(Figs. 2.4A and B)**. As a result thereof, the mediastinum is shifted to the opposite side, the lung underneath is completely collapsed with significant impairment of respiration and/or blood circulation. Unless quickly relieved, acute respiratory distress develops rapidly as revealed by intense breathlessness, cyanosis, perspiration, hypotension, and terminal shock.

The physical signs depend upon the type of PTX. When the amount of air in the pleural cavity is minimal (occupying 1/3 or less of the hemithorax),

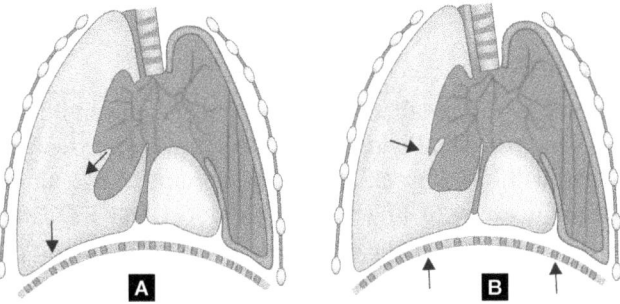

**Figs. 2.4A and B:** (A) Inspiration; (B) Expiration.

there may be hardly any physical sign. In most of such cases the tear in the pleura seals off soon after some air leaks into and distends the pleural cavity (closed PTX). When the tear is bigger and there is a larger amount of air in the pleural cavity, the pleural air communicates freely with the tracheobronchial tree and is thus at atmospheric pressure (open PTX). On the affected side the chest moves less, vocal fremitus and vocal resonance are decreased and percussion note is hyperresonant. The breath sounds are diminished in intensity, and occasionally, distant bronchial breathing is heard, which may be of the amphoric type.

Physical examination in patients with tension pneumothorax reveals classical signs. On the affected side the hemithorax appears full and moves very little, if at all. Resonance of the lung is markedly increased, vocal fremitus and vocal resonance are diminished and the breath sounds are totally absent though occasionally distant bronchial or amphoric breathing may be heard. There are usually no adventitious sounds. In some cases pneumomediastinum and subcutaneous emphysema may also occur.

## Diagnosis

Open and tension PTX can be easily diagnosed from the typical clinical features described above, the most important being diminished air entry coupled with increased lung resonance. However, a small (closed) PTX may remain undetected, especially if its onset is not associated with chest pain or if there is preexisting chest pathology such as emphysema. In the latter situation PTX should be suspected whenever there is a sudden increase in dyspnea. A CXR (in upright position) is of great help not only to confirm the diagnosis of PTX but also to know its extent, the degree of pulmonary collapse, and any associated lung disease. PTX with a partial or completely collapsed lung and shift of the mediastinum suggests tension PTX.

## Caution

The patient should never be sent to radiology department, if there is even the least suspicion of tension PTX; only portable CXR should be arranged.

## Management

### Specific Measures

Small spontaneous pneumothorax is generally a benign condition and usually requires only *monitoring*. Invariably it resolves without treatment and the air is absorbed within 1-2 weeks. When the volume of free air in the pleura (and therefore the extent of lung collapse) is more (large PTX), the treatment comprises tube drainage. Tube drainage becomes mandatory when there is a fistulous communication between the bronchial tree and pleura *(open pneumothorax)*. If tube drainage is unsuccessful, surgical intervention may be required.

**Tension pneumothorax** is a medical emergency and requires prompt treatment. As an emergency measure a sterile large bore needle (16-18 gauge) should be inserted plunged into the PTX cavity through second or third intercostal space in the midclavicular line with the patient in sitting position. This first-aid measure can be lifesaving. The needle should be properly strapped and fixed to the chest wall.

As soon as possible an intrapleural catheter should be inserted and connected to water seal drainage. Further treatment should be planned in accordance with the underlying pathology.

**Recurrent pneumothorax:** About a quarter of all cases of primary spontaneous PTX will experience a recurrence, often on the same side, and usually within the first two years. After the first recurrence, subsequent episodes are more frequent. Recurrent pneumothorax should also be treated as described above but this should be supplemented with attempt to produce pleurodesis by intrapleural instillation of some sclerosing agent.

### General Measures

All cases of spontaneous PTX should be kept under medical supervision, and their physical activities restricted until the air is absorbed and the lung fully re-expanded as observed on serial CXR. Oxygen therapy will be required to relieve hypoxemia in tension PTX and in patients with secondary PTX. Inhaling a high oxygen mixture probably results in faster absorption of air.

## ACUTE SEVERE PNEUMONIA

Pneumonia implies infection (with inflammation) of the pulmonary parenchyma, and can occur due to a variety of organisms, and in two different settings.
1. In the community at large *(community-acquired pneumonia)* from normal social contact.
2. In hospitalized or nursing home patients *(hospital-acquired infection)*.

## A. Community-acquired Pneumonia (CAP)

As the name suggests this is a type of pneumonia that is acquired infectiously from normal social contact (in the community at large). CAP is a common illness and can affect people of all ages. Most of such cases (>95%) are ambulatory, have low mortality, and can be treated as outpatients. Severe infections occasionally occur due either to high virulence of the infecting agent or poor host defense. Independent risk factors for CAP include alcoholism, bronchial asthma, and immunosuppression.

### Etiology

Pathogens frequently encountered in cases of CAP are listed at **Table 2.3**. The *most frequent pathogen in adults is Streptococcus pneumoniae* followed by *K. influenzae,* and respiratory viruses. In infants and children below 5 years, the most common pathogens are *Chlamydia trachomatis*, respiratory syncytial virus, and *H. influenzae.* In elderly people and/or those with coexisting illness, besides *S. pneumoniae,* infection with more virulent pathogens or polymicrobial infections *(such as S. aureus, M. catarrhalis,* and aerobic gram-negative bacilli) are more common.

### Clinical Features

Community-acquired pneumonia is a common illness, its clinical picture varying according to age of the patient, virulence of infecting organisms and host resistance. The severity of pneumonia has been variously defined, but the most *useful clinical signs of severe CAP are a respiratory rate >30/min, followed by confusion and hypotension.* CAP has been classified as "typical" or "atypical". However, the distinction between the two types is medically insufficient.

**Table 2.3:** Commonly encountered pathogens in patients with CAP.

| Mild and moderately ill patients (Outpatient treatment) | Severely ill patients (Requiring hospitalization) |
|---|---|
| **Major pathogens** | **Major pathogens** |
| • S. pneumoniae<br>• M. pneumoniae<br>• H. influenzae<br>  Respiratory viruses<br>• C. pneumoniae<br>• Aerobic Gram-neg bacilli<br>  (except P. aeruginosa) | • S. pneumoniae<br>• H. influenzae<br>• Polymicrobial (including anaerobic bacteria)<br>• Aerobic Gram-neg bacilli<br>  (including P. aeruginosa)<br>• S. aureus<br>• Legionella spp |
| **Miscellaneous pathogens** | **Miscellaneous pathogens** |
| • M. catarrhalis<br>• Legionella spp<br>• S. aureus<br>• M. tuberculosis<br>• Endemic fungi | • M. pneumoniae<br>• H. influenzae<br>• M. catarrhalis<br>• M. tuberculosis<br>• Endemic fungi |

For the treatment of pneumonia, it is more important to know the causative organism though it is difficult (if not impossible) on the basis of all the clinical, radiological, and laboratory data.

**Atypical pneumonia** is also known as *"walking pneumonia".* When it develops independently from another disease it is called *"primary atypical pneumonia".* Atypical pneumonia is caused by atypical organisms (other than *Streptococcus pneumoniae, H. influenzae, and Moraxella catarrhalis*). These atypical organisms include special bacteria, viruses, fungi, and protozoa, most common being *Mycoplasma pneumoniae, Chlamydia pneumoniae, and Legionella pneumoniae.*

In addition, this form of CAP is atypical in presentation with only moderate amounts of sputum, no consolidation, only small increase in white cell count, and no alveolar exudate. Atypical cases of CAP have a varying combination of certain common symptoms such as moderate to high fever, headache, cough with purulent sputum sometimes with hemoptysis, pleuritic chest pain, arthralgia, and myalgia, and rapid shallow breathing. It is to be remembered that the clinical presentation of CAP is often more subtle in elderly patients who may not always exhibit classic symptoms. They may instead experience predominantly new or worsening mental confusion, hypothermia and falls.

### Diagnosis

The aim is twofold: (1) to establish the diagnosis, and (2) to identify causative pathogenic organism(s).

*Diagnosis of pneumonia*

Physical examination of the chest may reveal crackles on auscultation, impaired percussion, and bronchial breathing. Such classic findings suggestive of consolidation are seen more often in patients with typical rather than atypical CAP in whom chest findings are likely to be rather non-specific.

**Radiography:** Chest skiagram is a critical component in diagnosing pneumonia. It will help to establish the diagnosis and also identify complications. The extent of radiographic findings will define the severity of illness, and can be a useful in choosing between domiciliary and inpatient treatment. Serial chest radiography will help in studying the progression of CAP

Chest skiagram may reveal a lobar consolidation, which is common in typical pneumonia; or it could show **bilateral,** more diffuse **infiltrates** often seen in atypical pneumonias. Rapid cavitation is not a typical feature of CAP (except in community acquired, methicillin-resistant *S. aureus*). Occasionally chest radiography performed early in the course of the disease could be negative in CAP but a repeat X-ray after 24 hours will always reveal the diagnosis. Chest radiographic findings can worsen rapidly, and require a significant period to improve. Clinical resolution **occurs long before radiologic resolution.**

Repeat chest skiagram should be done after 48–72 hours and will show improvement, if treatment is appropriate. Very frequent chest X-rays are unnecessary since complete resolution may take 3-4 weeks.

A CT scan of the chest should not be done routinely in cases of CAP. It is suggested when an underlying **bronchogenic carcinoma** is **suspected or** if any **abnormalities are observed not consistent with the diagnosis of pneumonia only.**

*Identification of causative pathogens*

- **Sputum** should be **examined** by Gram stain and (in selected cases) by culture. Collection of proper/adequate sputum specimen may not be possible in cases with atypical CAP, in the elderly, or when patient's sensorium is altered. Bronchoscopy and bronchoalveolar lavage may be considered in such cases especially if the patient is very sick, **unusual organism** is **suspected,** or the results of initial therapy are not satisfactory. It is a paradox that in clinical practice Gram stain which can be useful in initiating antimicrobial therapy is seldom used while sputum culture is often done even though its sensitivity and specificity are poor. In fact *routine sputum cultures are not recommended except in complicated cases of CAP.*
- **Blood cultures** are also not very useful except perhaps in very serious cases of CAP. In such cases two blood culture samples should be taken (one from each arm) before starting antibiotic therapy. Serologic tests are not helpful in the initial evaluation.
- A comprehensive evaluation of the patient also requires complete blood counts and estimation of blood sugar, electrolytes, and hepatic and renal functions. Additionally, patients requiring hospitalization will need ABG studies, and if elderly, an electrocardiogram, and in selected cases also an echocardiogram.

## *Management*

There is no optimal therapy for CAP. Initial treatment should be based on findings of physical examination, laboratory results, and outpatient characteristics (age, comorbidities, history of smoking, etc.). An important decision is to choose between outpatient and inpatient treatment. Factors that increase the need for hospitalization include:

- **Clinical parameters:** (a) Age greater than 65 years, (b) underlying chronic illness, (c) respiratory rate >30/min, (d) temperature less than 35°C or greater than 400°C, (e) heart rate >130 beats/min, (f) systolic blood pressure less than 90 mm Hg, and (g) altered sensorium.
- **Laboratory parameters:** (a) Severe anemia (hematocrit <30%), (b) white cell count <4,000 or >30,000/mm$^3$, (c) absolute neutrophil count <1,000/mm$^3$, and (d) creatinine greater than 1.4 mg%.
- **Radiologic findings:** Involvement of more than one lobe of the lung or bilateral disease; (b) presence of a cavity; and (c) presence of pleural effusion.

### Antibiotic Therapy

Since exact causative organism is not identified (or identification is delayed), treatment is usually empiric. This approach is also justified by repeated observations that in patients with CAP the symptoms, physical findings, and laboratory test results have a poor correlation with specific etiology.

- ❖ **Domiciliary treatment:** Most of the patients of CAP qualifying for outpatient treatment will be young, free from significant comorbidity, with stable cardiorespiratory functions, normal vital signs and mental status, and a temperature between 360°C and 400°C. The most common organism in such cases is *Streptococcus pneumoniae followed by Haemophilus influenzae, especially in elderly people.* Oral monotherapy for CAP is no longer preferred. The recommended empiric agents are amoxicillin and a macrolide or doxycycline. This is the most cost-effective way to optimally treat CAP. Empiric monotherapy with a macrolide (azithromycin, clarithromycin) is ineffective due to high macrolide resistance rates among *Strep. pneumoniae* strains. For outpatients with comorbidities, extended release amoxicillin-clavulanate plus a macrolide (or doxycycline) should be used.
- ❖ **Hospitalized patients:** Cases requiring hospitalization often have multiple risk factors **(Box 2.2)** but should still be treated empirically for *S. pneumoniae,* unless they have risk factors for *S. aureus* or *Pseudomonas pneumonia,* which include recent hospitalization or use of IV antibiotics in the last 90 days, mechanical ventilation, septic shock.

Adequate therapeutic response, both clinical and radiological, should be obvious within 3–5 days (blood counts returning toward normal, afebrile phase on two consecutive days, improvement in breathlessness). Antibiotic therapy should then be switched over from intravenous to such oral agents that are readily absorbed from the gut **(Table 2.4)**.

---

**Box 2.2: Factors adversely affecting the course of CAP.**

- ❑ **Historical:**
    - ➢ Age >60 years
    - ➢ Comorbid diseases, e.g., diabetes, congestive heart failure, chronic liver, kidney, and pulmonary diseases
    - ➢ Suspicion of aspiration
    - ➢ Chronic alcoholism
- ❑ **Physical examination:**
    - ➢ Altered mental status
    - ➢ Respiration rate >30
    - ➢ Temperature >40°C or <35°C
    - ➢ Systolic blood pressure <90 mm Hg
    - ➢ Evidence of sepsis or coexisting disease(s) stated above
- ❑ **Laboratory findings:**
    - ➢ White cell count >20,000 or <4000, Hemoglobin <9 g% or hematocrit <30, serum creatinine >1.5 mg%, $O_2$ saturation <90%, or $PaCO_2$ >50 on room air
    - ➢ *CXR:* Involvement of multiple lobes, and presence of cavitation/pleural effusion

**Table 2.4:** Antibacterial spectrum of commonly used drugs in CAP.

| Antibiotic | S. pneumoniae | H. influenzae | Gram(-) aerobes | Atypical pathogens | Anaerobes |
|---|---|---|---|---|---|
| Amino-penicillins | + | + | + | – | – |
| Macrolides | + | – | – | + | – |
| Cefuroxime | + | + | + | – | – |
| Quinolones | + | + | + | + | + |
| Ceftriaxone/ Ceftazidime | + | + | + | + | – |

❖ **Duration of therapy:** Traditionally patients with CAP are treated for 5-7 days. In hospitalized patients intensive antibiotic therapy should be given until the patient shows signs of clinical improvement and stability, at which time, regimen can be switched to oral antibiotics and should be administered for a total of 7 days.

### Prevention

Pneumococcal vaccination is recommended for all persons older than 65 years, and before age 65 years in chronic smokers, and in adults with comorbidities. Additionally, influenza vaccines should be given yearly to all individuals who receive vaccination against *S. pneumoniae.*

## B. Hospital-acquired Pneumonia

Hospital-acquired pneumonia (HAP) or nosocomial pneumonia (NP) is a common infection in critically ill hospitalized patients. The term "HAP" refers to any pneumonia developing in a hospitalized patient 48-72 hours after being admitted. It is thus a distinctly different from "community-acquired pneumonia".

### Etiology

Hospital-acquired pneumonia is more often caused by bacterial (80-90%) than viral infections (10-20%).

**Bacterial pneumonia:** The most important pathogens are *Pseudomonas aeruginosa* and *S. aureus*, both methicillin-sensitive and methicillin-resistant *S. aureus* (MRSA). Other important pathogens include enteric gram-negative bacteria (mainly *Klebsiella pneumoniae, Escherichia coli, Serratia marcescens, Proteus* sp, *and Acinetobacter* spp).

Methicillin-sensitive *S. aureus, Streptococcus pneumoniae, and H. influenza* are the most commonly implicated pathogens when pneumonia develops within 4-7 days of hospitalization, whereas *P. aeruginosa*, MRSA, and enteric gram-negative organisms become more common with increasing duration of hospitalization/intubation.

Another adverse factor is prior antibiotic factor (within the previous 90 days) as it increases the likelihood of polymicrobial infection and antibiotic-resistant organisms (particularly MRSA and *Pseudomonas* infection).

**Viral pneumonia:** These include influenza and respiratory syncytial virus and, in the immunocompromised host, cytomegalovirus

### Pathogenesis

Microaspiration of bacteria that colonize the oropharynx and upper airways in seriously ill patients plays the most important role in pathogenesis of HAP. On the other hand seeding of the lung due to bacteremia or inhalation of contaminated aerosols is of lesser pathogenetic significance.

*Endotracheal intubation* (with or without mechanical ventilation) is the single most important risk factor in HAP. The risk is especially high in the first 10 days of intubation. The detrimental effects of endotracheal intubation arise from several factors: (a) normal airway defenses are bypassed; (b) cough and mucociliary clearance is impaired; (c) aspiration of bacteria-laden secretions that pool above the inflated endotracheal tube is facilitated.

Other risk factors which have relatively greater significance in non-intubated patients include previous antibiotic therapy reduced gastric acidity (high gastric pH) by various drugs to prevent stress ulcers, age >70 years, and some coexisting cardiac, pulmonary, renal, or hepatic illness.

### Clinical Features

In non-intubated patients signs and symptoms of HAP are generally the same as those for CAP, and include fever often with chills, cough, dyspnea, and chest pain. All such symptoms are more intense in mechanically ventilated patients who may also have tachycardia disproportionate to pyrexia, purulent secretions, and worsening hypoxemia.

### Diagnosis

It is often difficult to make a diagnosis of HAP with certainty since the symptoms and signs are nonspecific. However, one or more of clinical findings ordinarily associated with pneumonia (such as fever, cough, purulent sputum, and leukocytosis) are often present. The problem is confounded by **the fact** that such features may be due to pre-existing pulmonary disease or other comorbidities. Suspicion of HAP may be raised by new onset of chest pain, a pleural friction rub, a sudden unexpected deterioration in clinical status, or appearance of new or progressive infiltrates on CXR. Differential diagnosis in such patients will include atelectasis, pre-existing lung disease, severe congestive heart failure, pulmonary thromboembolism, and acute respiratory distress syndrome (ARDS).

**Laboratory work up,** other than radiological studies, is generally not rewarding. Sputum examination has the same limitations as in CAR blood cultures are positive in only a minority of cases but are more specific. Positive culture(s) are associated with a more severe illness.

Gram stain and culture of endotracheal aspirates are of uncertain benefit because of frequent contamination with bacteria that may be colonizers as well as pathogens, and a positive culture may or may not indicate infection. Bronchoscopic sampling of lower airway secretions is more reliable since it can differentiate colonization from infection, and can thus be helpful in choice of antibiotic(s).

Blood oxygenation saturation by pulse oximetry should be regularly monitored, and may be supplemented periodically by arterial blood gas (ABG) analysis. Additionally, all cases of HAP should have routine laboratory testing as described in the section on CAP.

### Treatment

As in patients of CAP, treatment is with antibiotics that are chosen empirically, keeping in view local sensitivity factors and time of onset of pneumonia. Early-onset pneumonia occurs within the first 4 days of hospitalization, whereas late-onset pneumonia usually occurs 5 or more days after hospitalization. An early and adequate empiric treatment is a major determinate of favorable outcome. As a general rule, treatment must begin with two or more broad-spectrum drugs which are then changed to narrowest regimen possible based on clinical response and results of culture and sensitivity tests.

- **Early-onset HAP:** Any one of the following antibiotics may be used: Ceftriaxone/cipro or levofloxacillin/ampicillin-sulbactam.
- **Late-onset HAP:**
  - An antipseudomonal cephalosporin *(cefepime or ceftazidime)* OR an antipseudomonal carbapenem *(imipenem, meropenem)* OR A beta-lactamase inhibitor *(piperacillin, tazobactam)*
  - An antipseudomonal fluoroquinolones *(cipro or levofloxacin)*
  - Linezolid or vancomycin.

### Prognosis

**HAP** carries a high mortality (25–50%) despite the availability of effective antibiotics. However, much of this mortality may not be attributable to pneumonia itself, but may be related to patient's comorbid conditions. Infection with antibiotic resistant bacteria worsens prognosis. The outlook is relatively better if the initial antibiotic therapy is successful.

### Prevention

- One of the simplest and most effective preventive measures for HAP is proper positioning of the patients who are on mechanical ventilation. All such patients should be nursed as far as possible, in semi-upright position (unless contraindicated), to reduce the risk of aspiration.
- Limit use of endotracheal and nasogastric tubes. Whenever possible non-invasive ventilation using bi-level positive airway pressure (BiPAP)

or continuous positive airway pressure (CPAP) should be used since it prevents the breach in airway defense that occurs with endotracheal intubation.
- ❖ Rotate antibiotic administration according to culture reports.
- ❖ Maintain gastric acidity.

## Summary

- ❖ Hospital-acquired pneumonia includes *ventilation-acquired pneumonia, postoperative pneumonia and pneumonia that develops in unventilated patients who have been hospitalized for at least 72 hours.*
- ❖ Predictors of severe illness include advanced age, coexisting pulmonary and other morbidities, immunocompromized state, tachypnea (>30/min), multilobar involvement, altered mental status, impending shock, associated sepsis, and altered blood gases ($O_2$ saturation <90% or $PaCO_2$ >50 mm Hg).
- ❖ Precise bacteriologic diagnosis is difficult; culture of potential pathogen from blood (or pleural effusion) is the most specific finding.
- ❖ Initial empiric therapy must be quick, adequate, and comprise two or three broad-spectrum drugs in different pharmacological groups. Depending upon clinical response and repeat culture results, the antibacterial cover should be changed to narrowest regimen.

## ■ PNEUMONIA IN IMMUNOCOMPROMISED PATIENTS

### Etiology

Pneumonia in "immunocompromised patients" (ICP) is often caused by unusual pathogens but may also be due to those accounting for CAP and HAP. Likely pathogens depend to a large extent on the type of defect in the immune system defenses **(Table 2.5)**.

**Table 2.5:** Types of defect in immune system defenses.

| Human immune system defect | Clinical disorder/therapy associated with defect | Likely pathogens |
|---|---|---|
| Neutropenia | Acute leukemia, aplastic anemia, cancer chemotherapy | Gram-negative bacteria, S. aureus, Candida, Aspergillosis spp. |
| Defective Chemotaxis | Diabetes mellitus | S. aureus, gram-negative aerobes |
| Defective intracellular killing | Chronic granulomatous disease | S. aureus |
| Defective cell-mediated immunity (T-cell deficiency) | Hodgkin's lymphoma, cancer chemotherapy, corticosteroid therapy | Mycobacteria, viruses (e.g., herpes simplex virus, cytomegalovirus), Aspergillosis and other fungi |

## Clinical Features

Most of the symptoms and signs apparently resemble those seen in CAP or HAP in immunocompetent patients, and may include fever with or without chills, cough, dyspnea, and chest pain. However, pneumonia in ICP is less likely to have purulent sputum or significant signs, if they are neutropenic. In some patients, the only sign is fever.

## Diagnosis

Pneumonia should be suspected in ICP on the basis of suggestive symptoms (vide supra) and confirmed by chest skiagram coupled with assessment of oxygenation (usually by pulse oximetry), (induced) sputum cultures and/or bronchoscopic secretions), and blood cultures.

## Treatment

The nature of immune system defect and risk factors for specific pathogens determine the precise antibacterial therapy. Generally, broad-spectrum antibiotics effective against gram-negative bacilli *S. aureus,* and anaerobes are required (as in HAP). If the clinical picture does not improve within 5 days of antibiotic therapy (in patients with conditions other than HIV infection), addition of antifungal therapy should be considered.

An important constituent of treatment of pneumonia in ICP is to adopt measures to *enhance immune system function.* Examples will include administration of granulocyte-colony stimulating factor (G-CSF) in patients with chemotherapy-induced neutropenia, and IV gamma globulin in patients with hypogammaglobulinemia (e.g., in leukemia, multiple myeloma). *Vaccination* against *Pneumococcus* and *H. influenzae* should also be considered in all ICP patients at risk of developing pneumonia.

# RESPIRATORY FAILURE

## Definition

Respiratory failure is a medical emergency in which the respiratory system fails in one or both of its gas-exchange functions, namely oxygenation and carbon dioxide elimination.

Biochemically it is recognized by lowered arterial oxygen ($PaO_2$ <50 mm Hg) with or without raised carbon dioxide ($PaCO_2$ >60 mm Hg). **The fundamental disturbance is hypoxemia.** When inadequacy of gas exchange mechanism is evident only during activities of daily life, the condition is labeled as **respiratory insufficiency.**

## Pathophysiology

In accordance with the definition, respiratory failure can be classified as *hypoxemia or hypercapnia.*

- ❖ **Hypoxemic or Type 1 respiratory failure** is defined as a state with low level of oxygen in the blood ($PaO_2$ <60 mm Hg) with a normal or low arterial carbon dioxide tension ($PaCO_2$ <50 mm Hg). It results primarily from inadequate gas exchange. *Hypoxemia is the primary abnormality* while $PaCO_2$ remains normal or may even be decreased (due to hyperventilation in response to hypoxemia). The condition can develop with or without lung disease. This is the most common type of respiratory failure and can be associated with virtually all acute diseases of the lungs. Various conditions that affect oxygenation are:
    - Ventilation-perfusion mismatch (parts of the lung receive oxygen but not enough blood to absorb it, e.g., pulmonary embolism).
    - Diffusion problem (oxygen cannot enter the capillaries due to parenchymal disease, e.g., pneumonia, pulmonary edema).
    - Low ambient oxygen (e.g., at high altitude).
    - Alveolar hypoventilation (due to reduced respiratory muscle activity, e.g., in acute neuromuscular disease); this can also cause type 2 respiratory failure, if severe.
    - Shunt (oxygenated blood mixes with nonoxygenated blood (e.g., right-left shunt).
- ❖ **Hypercapnia or type 2 respiratory failure** results from inadequate alveolar ventilation and is characterized by *hypoxemia* ($PaO_2$ <60 mm Hg) with hypercapnia ($PaCO_2$ >50 mm Hg). In simple form it can be defined as the build up of carbon dioxide ($PaCO_2$) that has been generated by the body but cannot be eliminated. A large number of conditions can result in this type of respiratory failure **(Box 2.3)**, the most common being severe airway disorder, e.g., asthma and COPD.

---

**Box 2.3: Causes of hypercapnic respiratory failure.**

- ❑ **Alveolar hypoventilation**
    - ➢ *Respiratory drive abnormality*
        - ♦ Overdose of sedatives, narcotics, tranquilizers, anesthetics
        - ♦ Head injury, brain tumor, and vascular accidents
        - ♦ Excess oxygen administration in patients of COPD
        - ♦ Obesity-hypoventilation (Pickwickian) syndrome
        - ♦ Severe myxedema
        - ♦ Severe alkalosis
    - ➢ *Neuromuscular disorders*
        - ♦ Infections: Poliomyelitis, tetanus
        - ♦ Neurologic diseases: Amyotrophic lateral sclerosis, myasthenia gravis, multiple sclerosis, Guillain-Barre syndrome
        - ♦ Muscular dystrophies
        - ♦ Phrenic nerve injury
        - ♦ Drug-induced neuromuscular paresis: Curare and congener, and anticholinesterase inhibitors
- ❑ **Ventilation-perfusion abnormalities**
    - ➢ Chronic obstructive pulmonary disease (COPD)
    - ➢ Severe thoracic deformity

## Clinical Picture

Manifestations of respiratory failure may appear in an acute or chronic form. In the acute type clinical features are dominated by life-threatening derangement in blood gases and acid-base status, while in chronic respiratory failure, the manifestations are less dramatic and may not be as readily apparent.

Basically the symptoms and signs are those of the underlying disease coupled with those of hypoxemia or hypercapnia. The *cardinal features of hypoxemia* include disorientation, restlessness, tachycardia, tachypnea, arrhythmias, and (in later stages) cyanosis. Pulmonary vasoconstriction occurs resulting in pulmonary hypertension, which may finally lead to right ventricular failure (**chronic corpulmonale**).

*Hypercapniac respiratory failure presents* with somnolence, headache, and dyspnea with varying degrees of tachycardia, tachypnea, impaired sensorium, confusion, and asterixis. These features are due to the potent vasodilator effect of carbon dioxide both peripherally and centrally. Peripheral vasodilatation accounts for full and bounding pulse and warm skin, while in the central nervous system such vasodilatation results in increased intracranial pressure and *cerebral edema* which account for neurological features such as headache, impaired memory, flapping tremors, irritability, confusion, and agitation.

It must, however, be remembered that the symptoms and signs of ARF are both insensitive and nonspecific, and therefore the physician must maintain a high index of suspicion, and order arterial blood gas analysis whenever respiratory failure is suspected.

ote

Central cyanosis is a common feature in cases of ARF. However, its absence does not exclude ARF since cyanosis may become obvious only when respiratory failure becomes grave and $PaO_2$ drops dangerously below 40 mm.

## Precipitating Factors

In cases of COPD, ARF is usually precipitated by superimposed chest infection which is often subtle. *Sedatives, and narcotics,* inadvertently prescribed to control confusion, agitation, and insomnia in patients with hypercapnia, can impair ventilatory drive. Even antiallergics should be avoided. In patients with chronic pulmonary disease(s), ARF may also be precipitated by massive exposure to air pollution or allergens, and non-compliance with medication (e.g., bronchodilators in asthmatics).

## Diagnosis

Whenever a patient with respiratory failure is encountered, *three factors should be clearly defined for a rational therapeutic approach:*
- Basic etiology of respiratory failure
- Precipitating factor(s), and

❖ Severity of respiratory failure.

Attention to clinical details coupled with chest radiography and ECG will usually reveal the first two factors. The intensity of respiratory failure is best assessed by ABG studies.

## Management

Besides specific therapy directed toward the underlying disease (not discussed here), management of ARF primarily comprises: (1) respiratory care to maintain adequate gas exchange; and (2) general supportive care.

1. **Respiratory support:** This comprises both non-ventilatory and ventilatory measures.

    a. *Non-ventilatory aspects* oxygen therapy, since hypoxemia constitutes the principal threat to life in cases of ARF, oxygen therapy is the cornerstone of management. The aim should be to reverse hypoxemia and stabilize the patient with **$PaO_2$ >60** mm Hg (oxygen saturation >90%). Higher arterial oxygen tensions are of no proven benefit. Continuous oxygen therapy should be given at low flow rates by nasal cannula (1-3 L/min) or Venturi mask (24-40%). Higher concentrations of oxygen are necessary to **correct hypoxemia** in patients with **acute respiratory distress syndrome (ARDS), pneumonia and other parenchymal lung diseases.**

    Throughout oxygen therapy, and especially during the first 24 hours, a close watch should be kept on the patient's clinical status and on blood gases. This is because due to prolonged hypercapnia and (compensatory) bicarbonate retention in ARF, the normally powerful stimuli to ventilation ($CO_2$ and acidosis) are lost, and hypoxemia becomes the dominant source of respiratory drive. By relieving hypoxemia, oxygen therapy may weaken this ventilatory stimulus, further depressing respiration and worsening hypercapnia. Some increase in $PaCO_2$ can be expected but should not be a cause of alarm provided the patient remains alert. If the rise in $PaCO_2$ is excessive (>10 mm Hg), oxygen delivery should be reduced, titrating oxygen saturation to 5-10% below the previous level. *However, oxygen therapy should not be withheld because of such fears.* Inadequate reversals of hypoxia or continuing increase in $PaCO_2$ are indications for instituting mechanical ventilation.

    b. *Ventilatory aspects:* Ventilatory support aims at maintaining patency of the airway and ensuring adequate alveolar ventilation. This can be provided by noninvasive ventilatory assistance **(NIVA)** or through tracheal intubation and **mechanical ventilation.** The former (NIVA) provides continuous positive airway pressure (CPAP) or variable positive airway pressure (VPAP) through an occlusive nasal or face mask. NIVA is generally used for short-term ventilatory support in patients with hypercapnic ventilatory failure not responding to pharmacological intervention, but not considered to be in need of immediate intubation.

It has the following advantages: (1) no need for anesthesia, sedation and paralysis, (2) reduced incidence of nosocomial infections, (3) improved patient comfort, and (4) safety from complications associated with intubation.

**Indications for tracheal intubation and mechanical ventilation:**
1. Persistent hypoxemia despite supplemental oxygen
2. Impaired airway protection
3. Inability to clear secretions
4. Respiratory acidosis, and
5. Progressive general fatigue or mental status deterioration.

Several modes of positive-pressure ventilation are available including: (1) Controlled mechanical Ventilation (CMV), (2) Synchronized intermittent mandatory ventilation (SIMV), and (3) positive end-expiratory ventilation (PEEP). Their discussion is beyond the scope of this text.

The aim should be to restore $PaO_2$, $PaCO_2$ and pH to safe (not normal) limits (i.e., $PaO_2$ between 55 and 60 mm Hg, $PaCO_2$ between 60 and 65 mm Hg, and pH above 7.2). Attempt should never be made to suddenly reverse $PaCO_2$ to normal levels. It is to be realized that patients of ARF with $CO_2$ narcosis have enormous bicarbonate retention brought about by renal compensation to chronic hypercapnia. Any attempt to suddenly reverse this hypercapnia will invariably result in acute alkalosis which may precipitate hypokalemia, seizure, and cardiac arrhythmias.

2. **General supportive care:**
   a. Adequate nutrition should be provided preferably through conventional oral feeding.
   b. Proper hydration must be ensured to avoid inspissations of bronchial secretions and maintain optimal urine output.
   c. Sedatives, hypnotics, and opioid analgesics frequently employed during mechanical ventilation should be used carefully to avoid over-sedation, leading to prolongation of intubation.
   d. Meticulous care should be taken to avoid nosocomial infection, and complications associated with central venous lines, and indwelling catheters.
   e. Attention must also be paid to prevent complications associated with serious illness, e.g., stress ulcers, deep venous thrombosis (DVT), and pulmonary embolism (PE). Since $H_2$-receptor antagonists and proton pump inhibitors (which raise gastric pH) increase risk of nosocomial pneumonia, sucralfate may be preferred. The risk of DVT and PE may be reduced by subcutaneous administration of low molecular weight heparin.

## Summary

Acute respiratory failure may develop in three different situations: (1) ventilation-perfusion abnormalities accompanied by excessive breathing workload due to underlying pulmonary disease (most commonly COPD), (2) ineffective muscular contraction, and (3) deficient central drive. Defining the particular mechanism in a given case is essential for proper management.

Many patients with COPD have underlying heart disease. Atrial arrhythmias are also frequent in such cases. All patients with COPD and ARF warrant admission in ICU and majority will require ventilatory support. The essential steps in management are:
1. Adopt specific therapy to treat underlying disease.
2. Control bronchospasm as quickly and effectively as possible.
3. Ensure patency of airways and oxygen therapy.
4. Institute "controlled" continuous oxygen therapy at low flow rates.
5. Ensure adequate nutrition and hydration especially in patients on mechanical ventilation.
6. Consider NIVA in the early stages of management.

## ACUTE RESPIRATORY DISTRESS SYNDROME

### Definition

**Acute respiratory distress syndrome (ARDS) is a type of acute lung injury characterized by diffuse damage to alveolo-capillary membrane, in the absence of any pre-existing lung disease. An international consensus conference has suggested that the original term "acute" rather than "adult" respiratory distress** syndrome should be used, since ARDS is not limited to adults.

### Etiology

**Acute respiratory distress syndrome** can result from a number of diverse conditions that cause acute lung injury either by inhalation/aspiration **(bronchial side),** or hematogenous route **(blood side) (Box 2.4).** Some of the more frequent causes of the syndrome, in decreasing order of frequency, are aspiration of gastric contents, disseminated intravascular coagulation, pneumonia (in ICU), fractures, sepsis, burns and cardiopulmonary bypass. The risk of ARDS increases sharply when multiple risk factors operate as in patients with burns or fractures.

### Pathogenesis

As already stated, ARDS is not a disease by itself but a serious disorder, which may develop in a variety of acute medical/surgical conditions. Increased membrane permeability resulting from diffuse lung damage allows seepage of protein-rich fluid into the interstitial and alveolar spaces. Such fluids inhibit surfactant (which prevents collapse in normal lungs), resulting in widespread atelectasis. This *functional surfactant deficiency* is a key factor in the pathogenesis of the syndrome.

> Box 2.4: Conditions which may be associated with ARDS.

- **Direct lung injury (through bronchial side)**
  - Liquid aspiration (e.g., gastric contents, near drowning).
  - Pulmonary infections (usually diffuse pneumonia).
  - Inhalation of smoke and noxious fumes (e.g., chlorine, nitrous oxide, ammonia, phosgene, high concentration of oxygen).
  - Pulmonary contusion.
- **Indirect lung injury (through blood side)**
  - Severe or prolonged shock due to any cause
  - Gram-negative septicemia
  - Severe pancreatitis, multiple fractures, burns
  - Massive blood transfusion
  - Immunologically mediated conditions (e.g., Goodpasture's syndrome, systemic lupus erythematosus)
  - Fat embolism, amniotic fluid embolism
  - Cardiopulmonary bypass (pump lung)

Once the destructive sequence of ARDS begins, it is likely to be self perpetuating. Hyaline membranes form in respiratory passages, and finally interstitial fibrosis supervenes. Those who survive the acute phase gradually **recover pulmonary functions** from second week onward (from lysis of interstitial fibrosis by alveolar microphages.

## Clinical Features

Signs and symptoms of ARDS develop acutely usually within 12–72 hours of the triggering event. Clinically, the course of ARDS progresses through four stages.

**Stage I:** Earliest clinical features comprise severe respiratory distress and variable tachycardia. Examination of the lungs is usually non-contributory at this stage, and CXR is normal. Because of some interstitial edema at this stage ventilation-perfusion abnormalities may be present with decrease in $PaO_2$ (and normal or low $PaCO_2$).

**Stage II:** The changes observed in stage I worsen, rales are widely heard, and symbolize presence of fluid in pulmonary alveoli. Diffusion abnormalities occur, hypoxemia increases, and cyanosis appears. These two stages may progress over 2–7 days.

**Stage III:** As the condition worsens profound hypoxemia supervenes, rales may be heard all over the lungs, and areas of tubular breathing may be present. Radiologically, alveolar collapse is a prominent feature and results in right to left shunt, so that conventional oxygen therapy is not of much use at this stage.

**Stage IV:** Finally, respiratory failure sets, which may be nonresponsive to conventional oxygen therapy, terminally, acidosis develops and death occurs due to cardiorespiratory arrest.

It may be added that patient may present in any of these stages and progression may or may not occur depending upon the nature and severity of acute lung injury, treatment provided, and the host response.

## Diagnosis

There is no single diagnostic test or marker of ARDS. It should be suspected whenever any catastrophic event is followed, after a delay of a few days, by rapid onset and progression of respiratory failure. Clinically, there will be evidence of respiratory distress with dyspnea, tachypnea, and hypoxemia that is relatively refractory to administration of oxygen. Radiological appearance of diffuse pulmonary infiltrates (predominantly in the dependent areas of the lungs) is highly suggestive, but these may be absent in the early stages of the disease. The best investigation under the circumstances is study of blood gases, which will invariably reveal $PaO_2$ less than 55 mm Hg. Other physiological abnormalities seen in these cases include reduced respiratory compliance, increased shunt fraction and increased dead space ventilation.

## Management

Acute respiratory distress syndrome should be constantly kept in mind whenever dealing with any of the clinical disorders listed at **Box 2.4**, since delay in diagnosis may mean all the **difference** between life and death. **Once the complication is suspected** the patient should be **referred,** at the earliest, to a hospital with an intensive respiratory care unit, as the management is highly skilled and needs great expertise.

**Unfortunately,** increased understanding of the pathogenesis of ARDS has not yielded desired therapeutic benefits. The disease still carries a mortality of 50–60% or even more depending upon the intensity of the disease and efficacy of management. No specific pharmacological intervention has yet been **known** to significantly alter the outcome of ARDS.

### *Specific Measures*

A detailed discussion of all the measures employed for management of ARDS is beyond the scope of this book. It should be adequate for this text to enumerate the principles of management. These are as follows:

- ❖ **Reversal of hypoxemia:** This invariably requires mechanical ventilation which is the basic life-saving therapeutic modality in such cases. The aim should be to maintain $PaO_2$ between 55 and 60 mm Hg. *A low tidal volume (6 mL/kg body weight) ventilation compared to conventional tidal volume (11 mL/kg body weight) ventilation is recommended. Most cases will require positive end-expiratory pressure (PEEP)* to minimize alveolar collapse.
- ❖ **Control of infection:** While routine prophylactic administration of antibiotics is controversial, an empirical antibiotic therapy should be

started early especially if sepsis is suspected. In the later phases of ARDS, when evidence of infection may be clearer, appropriate culture, and sensitivity tests should guide the antibiotic therapy.
- ❖ **Treatment of precipitating cause(s),** most frequent being infection.
- ❖ **Appropriate management of fluid and electrolyte balance** coupled with judicious use of diuretics is essential. Both hypovolemia and fluid overload are to be avoided by *central hemodynamic monitoring.*

The most important of all these measures is reversal of hypoxemia. In the earliest stage administration of 100% oxygen may be adequate. However, as the condition advances, *some form of mechanical ventilation* is required. Its indications are: (a) respiratory rate >35/min, (b) vital capacity <15 mL/kg, (c) $PaO_2$ <55 mm Hg (with patient breathing 100% oxygen); and (d) pH <7.25.

Several forms of mechanical ventilation are available; however in patients with ARDS **PEEP** ventilation is most appropriate. PEEP improves oxygenation by increasing the volume and diameter of the terminal air passages, and by preventing the collapse of small airways and alveoli. A lower opening pressure is thus required during the following inspiratory phase. Correspondingly, the lung compliance increases, cost of breathing is decreased, ventilation perfusion improves and right-to-left intrapulmonary shunt decreases. Additionally, PEEP often results in shift of the edema fluid from air passage and alveoli to interstitial tissue of the lung.

### Other/Newer Measures

Corticosteroids have been tried extensively but have not been found to generally benefit patients with ARDS, either in the early or the **late phase of the disease.** *Exogenous surfactant therapy* has been studied as an exciting therapeutic modality but the results have been disappointing. Likewise, the beneficial role of ketoconazole (which inhibits the biosynthesis of leukotrienes), nitric oxide (a selective pulmonary vasodilator), nonsteroidal anti-inflammatory drugs (inhibitors of prostaglandin pathways), pentoxyphyllin (a phosphodieterase inhibitor), and antiendotoxin therapy is yet to be established.

### General Measures

Throughout the course of the disease, which may stretch over 4–8 weeks certain general measures should be instituted to help recovery. For this purpose, a five point protocol has been outlined:
1. **Exercise**—respiratory and whole body
2. **Nutrition**—attain anabolism by adequate caloric intake
3. **Fluid administration**—maintain optimally dry state
4. **Emotional support**
5. **Good sleep.**

Their discussion is beyond the scope of this book.

## Complications

A number of complications may occur during the course of the disease. These are likely to be overlooked on account of variety of symptoms and signs already existing and related to several events occurring simultaneously. Various complications can be:

- ❖ Bacterial infection
- ❖ Pulmonary thromboembolism
- ❖ Left ventricular failure
- ❖ Disseminated intravascular coagulation
- ❖ Bronchial obstruction
- ❖ Pneumothorax.

# 3 CHAPTER

# Gastrointestinal Emergencies

## ACUTE VOMITING

### Etiology

Causes of vomiting are variable, ranging from primary gastrointestinal (GI) etiologies to an associated symptom of neurologic, rheumatologic, oncologic, endocrine, or renal pathologies. Occasionally, vomiting may have a psychogenic basis as in bulimia or cyclic vomiting syndrome.

Acute vomiting may also be a predominant symptom of gastric outlet or upper gut obstruction. Occasionally, vomiting is iatrogenic, mostly medication related.

### Management

#### General Considerations

Though aspiration pneumonia and hematemesis *(Mallory-Weiss syndrome)* occasionally complicate acute vomiting, it is the fluid and electrolyte disturbances, which usually call for an urgent treatment. Besides dehydration, prolonged severe vomiting may produce starvation, weight loss, marked loss of potassium, and chloride (hypochloremic alkalosis), and even ketosis, which may by itself perpetuate vomiting.

#### Specific Measures

- ❖ Cause of vomiting should be determined by detailed history coupled with relevant investigations, and treated appropriately.
- ❖ In mild cases, oral feeds should be continued but restricted to light drinks, such as plain water, lemonade, diluted fruit juice, and weak tea.
- ❖ When vomiting is severe, intravenous fluids (D5W/Normal saline) may be required. Oral rehydration solutions should be substituted when oral intake becomes possible.
- ❖ In cases with severe and prolonged vomiting, serum electrolytes should be estimated, and any significant disturbance treated accordingly (*see* Chapter 5).
- ❖ Antiemetics, such as prochlorperazine *(Stemetil)* 12.5 mg and/or ondansetron *(Emeset)* 4 mg IM can be of help.

- Vomiting resulting from motion sickness is best controlled by antihistamines, dimenhydrinate *(Dramamine),* and promethazine *(Avomine),* which block stimuli from vestibular apparatus to the vomiting center. One to two tablets of any of these drugs should be prescribed 30–60 minutes prior to journey. Therapy given after vomiting has begun is generally ineffective.
- **Antiemetics:** Vomiting may be troublesome in some cases of severe acute GE. Intravenous fluid therapy generally helps to reduce emesis in such cases. In patients with uncontrollable, protracted vomiting, antiemetics may be considered, such as prochlorperazine *(Stemetil)* or ondansetron *(Emeset).*

## ACUTE DIARRHEAL DISEASES

### Definition

Passage of at least three watery or loose stools lasting more than 24 hours (but of less than 2 weeks duration) is termed as *acute diarrhea.* Accompaniments may include vomiting, gripping pain in abdomen, and blood and/or mucus in the stool. In the former setting, the condition is termed as *acute gastroenteritis (GE),* and in the latter, *dysentery.*

### Etiology

A large number of conditions can produce the syndrome of acute diarrhea. Although a majority of cases are infectious in nature and usually self-limiting, the differential diagnosis is broad **(Box 3.1)**. It is important to differentiate between bloody and non-bloody diarrhea, as that may help discern, which bacteria or virus is the cause of the patient's illness. Certain pathogens require antimicrobial treatment, while others are self-limited and some may even get worse, if treated with antibiotics.

### Clinical Features

*Bacterial agents* may produce either inflammatory or secretory diarrhea. The latter is caused by preformed toxins and therefore has a rapid onset, as with *Staphylococcus aureus* **food poisoning,** or *when toxins are formed after bacterial colonization,* as with *Vibrio cholera.* In contrast inflammatory diarrhea results from direct bacterial invasion of the intestinal mucosa, most notably by *Salmonella, Shigella,* and *E. histolytica* (acute amebiasis).

The area of the intestines predominantly affected in the two types of diarrhea varies. The secretory type affects the upper small bowel, and therefore, generally produces *watery diarrhea.* On the other hand, direct bacterial invasion usually affects the distal small bowel and colon, which results in release of water, electrolytes, blood, protein, and mucus into the intestinal lumen. The clinical presentation is dysentery and may include abdominal

**Chapter 3:** Gastrointestinal Emergencies 125

> **Box 3.1: Etiological agents for acute infective diarrhea.**
>
> - **Bacterial:**
>   - V. cholerae
>   - Salmonella*
>   - **E. coli:**
>     - Enterotoxigenic Escherichia coli (ETEC)
>     - Enteropathogenic Escherichia coli (EPEC)
>     - Enteroinvasive Escherichia coli (EIEC)
>   - Shigella*
>   - Campylobacter jejuni*
>   - Yersinia enterocolitica*
>   - C. difficile
> - **Parasites:**
>   - E. histolytica
>   - Giardia lamblia
>   - Ascaris lumbricoides
> - **Viruses:**
>   - Rotavirus
>   - Norwalk and Norwalk-like agents
>   - Adenovirus
>   - Enterovirus

*Denotes organisms which are known to cause bloody diarrhea.

pain, bloody diarrhea, and myalgias. Severe cases may result in bacteremia, sepsis, and death.

**Viral agents** and their cytotoxins lead to an increased cellular permeability leading to secretion of water and electrolytes into the intestinal lumen *(secretory diarrhea)*. Viral gastroenteritis (unlike invasive dysentery) is generally not associated with fever, abdominal pain, or other systemic symptoms. Viral acute diarrhea is usually due to *rotavirus infection* in children and *Norwalk virus* in adults. The former affects mainly infants and young children, has a subacute onset, and is often accompanied or even preceded by vomiting. In adults, acute diarrhea due to *Norwalk virus,* related agents, and adenoviruses usually occurs in small epidemics in localized communities or institutions. Some cases of *"travellers' diarrhea"* also belongs to this group.

In majority of cases of acute GE, irrespective of the etiology, the illness is mild to moderate in severity, short-lived, and usually self-limited. However, sometimes profuse diarrhea and vomiting occur with explosive suddenness rapidly leading to dehydration, *hypovolemia, metabolic acidosis, and oliguria with circulatory collapse. In fact, volume depletion is the key factor* to be looked into in such cases. In moderately severe cases of dehydration, the patient becomes irritable, eyes appear sunken, the nose is pinched, and the tongue and the inner side of the cheeks appear dry. As volume depletion and electrolyte losses worsen, abdomen may become distended (due to *hypokalemia),* breathing becomes deep and rapid (due to *acidosis),* pulse appears to be weak and thready, blood pressure falls, and *oliguria* develops.

## Diagnosis

In every case of acute diarrhea, it is useful to try to determine, if it is due to small or large bowel involvement **(Table 3.1)**. Some pathogens like *Salmonella* and *Yersinia* can involve both small and large gut. A good clinical history coupled with naked eye and microscopic examination of the stool is all that is required in most of the cases. *Proctoscopy* may be done in doubtful cases and will reveal ulcerated, hemorrhagic and friable mucosa when acute diarrhea is due to colonic pathology. Stool culture and other special tests to identify specific pathogens are seldom required or practical in general practice.

## Management

This is common to all cases of acute GE, and should be especially directed to patient's *hydration status*. For many patients, this may be the only treatment necessary. Oral rehydration with liberal use of standard oral rehydration solutions (ORS) should be sufficient for cases with mild to moderate dehydration. Patients with severe acute GE may lose most of the 8-10 L of GI fluids normally secreted daily, and therefore, intravenous fluid resuscitation should be started. There is no simple method to determine the amount of fluid loss. A rough estimate of volume depletion however, can be made on the basis of 0.25-0.5 L of fluid loss per loose stool or vomit + the amount of urine passed + 1 L for insensible loss (this may increase considerably in hot summer weather especially if patient is febrile).

The *rate of fluid administration* is important. One-third of the total calculated fluid (or about 2 L in adults) should be rushed in the first 2-3 hours. This should result in clinical improvement judged by parameters, such as blood pressure, skin turgor, and urine output. The remaining amount of fluid should thereafter be infused slowly, during the next 12-24 hours. In majority of cases, it should be possible by then to discontinue IV fluids. Thereafter, oral replacement therapy (ORT) **should be instituted and continued for another 1 or 2 days till the** patient is able to resume a more or less normal diet.

**Table 3.1:** Diagnosis of acute diarrhea.

| Site of involvement | Pathogens | Stool volume | Cellular exudate* | Location of pain | Proctoscopy |
|---|---|---|---|---|---|
| Small bowel | V. cholerae, E. coli†, Norwalk, rotavirus, giardia | Large | Rare | No pain or peri-umbilical | Normal |
| Large bowel | Shigella, E. coli†, Campylobacter, E. histolytica | Small | Common | Lower abdomen/rectal pain | Abnormal |

*Cellular exudate comprises pus cells, red blood cells and macrophages.
†Different strains of *E. coli* can involve both small and large bowel.

## Chapter 3: Gastrointestinal Emergencies

**In children,** the rate of fluid administration should be 30 mL/kg during the first 1 hour and 20 mL/kg for the next 2 hours. If the child does not pass urine within 3 hours of such IV hydration, acute renal failure should be suspected. This is, however, rare. Most of the children will begin to pass urine within 2 hours, and in them IV fluids should be continued for another 2-3 hours. ORT should be started simultaneously. Finally, as the condition improves and the child starts taking ORS. IV fluids can be discontinued. In fact, it should be possible to remove IV line in almost all cases within 6 hours as rehydration will be completed by then. Thereafter, ORT should suffice for maintenance as well as for any continuing fluid loss.

The *type of fluid* to be administered also merits consideration. Since GI fluids contain sodium, potassium, and hydrogen ions or bicarbonate in large amounts, acute GE is usually associated with significant Na⁺ and K⁺ depletion, and acidosis or alkalosis. Many types of fluids have been recommended for IV infusion in such cases. These are, however, not always available. A simple regimen is to administer $D_5W$ and isotonic saline (which are universally available) in a ratio of 2:1. Alternatively, Ringer's lactate may be used.

### *Specific Measures*

- ❖ **Chemotherapy:** Most of the acute diarrheal illnesses are self-limited, and therefore, antibiotic therapy is not indicated as a routine. However, antibiotics should be administered in cases of suspected acute invasive bacterial process and severe diarrhea, systemic symptoms, fever, or abdominal pain. Majority of cases, especially young, healthy adults, can be treated as outpatients provided they are able to tolerate oral intake.
  Since precise bacteriological diagnosis is usually unavailable in acute setting, antibiotic treatment must be empiric. Currently, quinolones (in one form or the other) are the treatment of choice (e.g., ciprofloxacin 500 mg orally twice daily for 3-5 days). If there is any concern for Shiga toxin-producing *E. coli*, antibiotics should be avoided as they could precipitate the onset of hemolytic uremic syndrome. In most settings, a rapid PCR is available to aide in differentiating the types of diarrhea. If oral medication is not possible, ciprofloxacin may be given intravenously. Azithromycin is an option in children and pregnant women. If *C. difficile* infection is suspected, stool should be tested for *C. difficile* toxin and treatment initiated with metronidazole. If amebic dysentery is of concern, a combination of metronidazole and ciprofloxacin will provide best results as bacterial infection is often coexistent.
- ❖ **Antidiarrheal agents:** Antimotility and antisecretory agents, such as *loperamide (Imodium)* or diphenoxylate with atropine *(Lomotil)* should be avoided in children and in febrile parents with dysentery because of risk of constipation and bloating (and even toxic megacolon in patients with inflammatory bowel disease). They may be used carefully in afebrile patients who have non-bloody diarrhea. Antidiarrheal agents should only be initiated after *C. difficile* has been excluded. If used in *C. difficile*, they

may cause an acute bowel obstruction or toxic megacolon. Even pectin-kaolin suspension containing codeine should be avoided.

### General Measures

Hospitalization is seldom required in cases of acute GE but may be considered in patients with extreme of ages, severe toxemia, massive diarrhea or extreme dehydration, and severe vomiting preventing oral replenishment.

Abdominal cramps, if troublesome, may be relieved by use of anticholinergic drugs, such as propantheline bromide *(probanthine)* or injection *pentazocine*. Routine use of antispasmodics is not recommended because of risk of inducing intestinal paresis and masking fluid loss by trapping fluid and electrolytes in the intestinal lumen.

### Complications

- ❖ Peripheral circulatory failure
- ❖ Acute tubular necrosis

## GASTROINTESTINAL PERFORATION

Though acute perforation can occur in any part of the GI tract, the most common sites are duodenum and small intestines where a peptic ulcer or a typhoid ulcer, respectively, may perforate. The latter is covered in Chapter 8.

### Perforation of Peptic Ulcer

#### Clinical Features

In peptic ulcer disease, perforation usually complicates a **chronic ulcer** which may be gastric, **duodenal** or stomal, the most common being duodenal. A past history of ulcer pain or indigestion is usually available. It is an acute emergency characterized by sudden excruciating and constant pain initially localized to the epigastrium (may radiate to either shoulder) but later becomes diffuse, as *generalized peritonitis* sets in. Sometimes, *the pain is milder or may even be absent,* if the perforation: (1) is very small and is immediately sealed off, (2) occurs in the lesser sac, or (3) is complicated by gastro-duodenal hemorrhage.

**Physical examination** usually reveals signs of *generalized peritonitis* often with a varying degree of shock. The abdomen shows board like rigidity and is extremely tender. The diagnosis is confirmed clinically by finding partial *obliteration of hepatic dullness,* and radiologically by the presence of *free air under the diaphragm* in a plain X-ray of the abdomen taken in the sitting or standing position.

### Management

**The following principles should be observed:**
- ❖ The patient should be hospitalized immediately.

- Injection morphine/pethidine/pentazocine should be given in adequate doses to relieve pain.
- **Shock,** if present, should be treated appropriately.
- **Gastric contents** should be aspirated every half hour and all oral feeding suspended during acute stage.
- **Antibiotics** infection of the peritoneum invariably occurs in such cases and is generally polymicrobial including both aerobic and anaerobic organisms. Aggressive parenteral antibiotic therapy should be administered for first few days including metronidazole (to cover anaerobic organisms), newer generation cephalosporins and ciprofloxacin. Aminoglycosides may also be used.
- **Surgical measures** like suturing of the perforation, peritoneal lavage, vagotomy and antrectomy, or vagotomy and pyloroplasty should be considered. The final decision should be left to the surgeon who should be involved in management from the very start.

# ACUTE GASTROINTESTINAL BLEEDING

## Etiology

Causes of acute GI bleeding can be broadly divided into upper and lower GI bleed (**Box 3.2**) depending upon whether the site of bleeding is proximal or distal to ligament of Teitz. Such cases can usually be diagnosed by upper or lower GI endoscopy. *GI bleed is defined as obscure when both upper and lower endoscopic results are negative.*

## Clinical Features

The mode of presentation depends upon the *amount and rapidity of blood loss.* Gradual blood loss may result only in progressive anemia. Acute bleeding manifests either as hematemesis or melena. With *significant acute bleeding* (loss of about 0.5–1 L or more of blood) volume depletion occurs, which may impair vital organ perfusion, and cause tachypnea, tachycardia, and blurred

---

**Box 3.2: Causes of significant gastrointestinal bleeding.**

- **Upper GI bleed:**
  - Erosive gastritis—esophagitis, esophageal varices, Peptic ulcer disease Mallory—Weiss tear
  - Rare causes including vascular malformation
- **Lower GI bleed:**
  - Angiomas
  - Polyps/carcinoma
  - Diverticular disease
  - Upper GI source
  - Ischemic/inflammatory colitis
  - Other causes (including bleeding hemorrhoids)

vision. More severe GI hemorrhage, approaching 40% of blood volume, is often associated with pallor, cold extremities, and hypotension. Shock may supervene, if the blood loss is brisk.

Alterations in sensorium, or onset of confusion/semi-stupor early in the course of upper GI bleeding should suggest **hepatic encephalopathy.** In such cases, other features of portal hypertension/hepatic cirrhosis should be looked for, such as jaundice, palmer erythema, gynecomastia, and ascites.

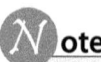ote

- Patient may occasionally have massive GI bleeding without any external appearance of blood for some time.
- A single black stool (melena) signifies loss of at least 100 mL of blood.

### General Management

- **Hospitalization:** Ideally, every patient with acute GI bleeding should be hospitalized because of unpredictability regarding the course of events (the situation is almost similar to acute coronary pain). However, the patient may be treated at home, if he is comparatively young, has only melena, and is hemodynamically stable. Urgent hospitalization should be advised, if variceal bleeding is suspected since such cases are at risk of developing hepatic encephalopathy.
- **Fluid replenishment:** Regardless of the site or source of bleeding, immediate aim of treatment in cases with significant blood loss should be volume replenishment by isotonic crystalloids. *Colloid solutions offer no special advantage and are expensive.* Blood transfusions should be given as required maintaining hemoglobin near 10.0 gm% and hematocrit between 30 and 35%. A satisfactory hemodynamic state is suggested by blood pressure reaching low normal level and a urine output of about 50 mL/hour. Associated thrombocytopenia and coagulopathy, if detected (often in patients with liver failure), should be corrected appropriately.
- **Intubation:** If continual upper GI bleeding is suspected, a nasogastric tube should be gently passed and gastric lavage done to empty the stomach of all blood. Repeated lavage should be done with small aliquots of tap water (150 mL in adults and 5 mL/kg in children) at room temperature, and the fluid removed after 3–5 minutes. A pink or red effluent persisting after 3–4 lavages suggests continuing bleeding. The value of gastric lavage with iced saline or the usefulness of adding norepinephrine is not proven.

ote

Hematocrit determined immediately after massive bleeding may not accurately reflect the amount of blood loss, since equilibration with extravascular fluid (and hemodilution) require several hours.

## Upper Gastrointestinal Bleeding

*Etiology*

Important causes of upper GI bleeding are listed at **Box 3.2**. The source of bleeding is commonly in the esophagus, stomach, or duodenum. An examination of vomitus (for bright red blood) or gastric aspirate (for "coffee-ground" material), and a look at the stool for melena (black, tarry, and often foul-smelling) will confirm bleeding from upper GI tract. The presence of melena indicates that blood has been present in the GI tract for >12 hours. *Hematochesia* (passage of bright red or maroon blood per rectum) from an upper source usually indicates severe hemorrhage.

*Initial Assessment (TRIAGE)*

A preliminary assessment of the severity of bleeding should be made from factors already described. *Hematemesis, usually, implies greater blood loss (usually >1 L) than melena alone and the mortality with former is about twice that of the latter.* The risk of rebleeding and mortality are also higher in patients with comorbid conditions, and in the elderly. Risk stratification is, usually, based on the following criteria:

- ❖ **Very low risk:** These cases have no evidence of hematemesis or melena within past 12–24 hours, are free from any comorbid condition especially liver disease, have a normal nasogastric aspirate, and normal hemodynamics and laboratory tests. Such cases can be managed at home, but endoscopy should be performed, preferably within 24 hours.
- ❖ **Moderate risk:** Such patients have active bleeding (manifested by hematemesis or bright red blood on nasogastrip aspirate) and moderate tachycardia (heart rate >100/min). However, systolic pressure is reasonably maintained (>100 mmHg). They are also free from any serious co-morbid illness. Such patients require hospitalization and a semi-urgent endoscopy.
- ❖ **High risk:** This sub-group comprises patients with severe active GI bleed with *hemodynamic alterations,* such as low-systolic pressure (<90 mm Hg), and oliguria. Such patients are usually elderly (age over 65 years), and often have serious coexisting medical illness or evidence of advanced hepatic disease. These cases need *emergent endoscopy.*

*Diagnosis*

A precise etiological diagnosis is difficult on clinical grounds but may be suspected by a history of non-steroidal anti-inflammatory agents (NSAID) ingestion, peptic ulcer disease, chronic alcoholism, and when hematemesis follows severe retching.

All patients with upper GI bleeding, except very low risk cases, should have routine blood chemistry (including renal and hepatic profile), hematocrit, coagulation studies, and blood typing. Additionally, CXR and ECG should be obtained as baseline parameters. The most specific diagnostic tool is esophageal-gastric-duodenal endoscopy, which is helpful in both diagnosis and management of the pathology.

## Erosive Gastritis—Esophagitis

Upper GI bleeding due to acute gastroesophageal erosions is generally due to use of **NSAIDs,** aspirin being the most ulcerogenic. The risk of bleeding is generally dose related but erosions are known to occur with aspirin in doses as low as 75 mg/day. The risk is especially high in *chronic alcoholics,* in elderly patients, and with *concomitant administration of corticosteroids, SSRIs, and COX-2 inhibitors.*

### Clinical Features

Erosive gastritis is usually asymptomatic or associated with only dyspeptic symptoms. The most striking symptom is upper GI bleeding, which may present as *hematemesis* containing "red colored material", or as *coffee-brown aspirate* (in intubated patients), or as *melena*. Fortunately, the bleeding is hemodynamically insignificant, and usually self-limited.

### Diagnosis

Even though bleeding from gastric erosions is small, it may be difficult to distinguish it from more serious pathologies, such as esophageal varices and peptic ulcer. **Endoscopy** should, therefore, be performed in all cases, as early as possible. The (endoscopic) findings include erosions, petechiae, and subepithelial hemorrhages. These are generally superficial, and vary in size and number. Associated inflammation is either minimal or absent.

### Treatment

Once bleeding occurs, all incriminating drugs should be discontinued. Patients should receive *sucralfate suspension* (1 g orally every 4–6 hours) and *proton-pump inhibitors* (PPI). Since bleeding from gastric mucosa is generally diffuse, endoscopic hemostatic techniques are not helpful.

## Bleeding Peptic Ulcer

### Diagnosis

Upper GI endoscopy (UGIE) is the best procedure for the diagnosis and assessment of a bleeding peptic ulcer. Certain endoscopic findings also help in predicting the outcome of GI bleed in such cases. The *risk of re-bleeding* is higher in cases with large ulcers (ulcer size >2 cm), and those with high gastric ulcers, or posterior duodenal ulcers. About half the cases with peptic ulcers have an *H. pylori* infection.

### Management

The principal aim should be to arrest active bleeding and prevent re-bleeding. Fortunately, in majority of patients bleeding stops **spontaneously with**

**supportive** care and reduction in gastric acidity. *Therapeutic intervention* may be required in patients with *active* ongoing bleeding.

*Specific measures*

The most important aspect of management is to stabilize a hemodynamically fragile patient. Two large bore IVs should be placed and fluid resuscitation started immediately. Laboratories should be drawn to check liver function, CBC, coagulation factors, and blood type/cross match.

Since low pH gastric juice can impair platelet function and decrease hemostasis, PPIs are given routinely. PPIs reduce mortality in those with severe disease, and also decrease risk of re-bleeding. Endoscopic therapy with epinephrine injection or application of endoscopic clips is generally not favored. More recently *octreotide* (a synthetic analogue of somatostatin) has been used and may reduce continual bleeding from actively bleeding peptic ulcer (though it is more effective in controlling variceal bleeding).

The patient should be evaluated immediately for the need for endoscopy to diagnose and treat the blood loss.

In hemodynamically stable patients without evidence of active large volume blood loss, the peptic ulcer may be managed in the outpatient setting. A combination of PPIs and sucralfate can assist with managing symptoms and repairing the lining of the GI tract. Regardless, plans should be made for endoscopy.

Patients with a bleeding ulcer should be evaluated for causes of the ulcer so as to prevent recurrence. This will include a thorough evaluation of medications, alcohol and tobacco use, stress, and also testing for *H. pylori*. Please note, the *H. pylori* testing is less sensitive when the patient has active GI blood loss and when the patient has taken PPIs.

Emergency surgery is seldom required in peptic ulcer bleeding. Nevertheless, an **urgent surgical intervention** may have to be considered in following situations:
- Acute blood loss sufficient to reduce hemoglobin to <8 g and hematocrit to <24
- Recurrent bleeding (after endoscopic procedure) requiring more than 1 L of blood daily for 2 or 3 consecutive days
- An episode of massive hemorrhage, which may require more than 10 units of blood transfusion to combat shock
- Non-availability of adequate amounts of blood
- Age above 50 years.

## Mallory–Weiss Syndrome

This is characterized by non-penetrating mucosal lacerations at the gastroesophageal junction, which usually arise from events that suddenly increase transabdominal pressure (such as forceful retching and/or vomiting, coughing, and heavy weight lifting). Less common causes include pregnancy and upper GI endoscopy. Alcohol abuse is a significant risk factor.

Mallory-Weiss tears are much more common in men than in women, and result in *hematemesis* with or without melena. The bleeding may vary in extent from mild to massive, but almost always stops spontaneously. The diagnosis is confirmed by UGIE which reveals tears in the lower esophageal mucosa and submucosa.

### Treatment

The *bleeding is usually self-limited* but occasionally fluid resuscitation and blood transfusion may be required. Supportive treatment includes antiemetics, and use of sucralfate and PPIs to reduce acid that may impair healing of the mucosal tear. In the rare situation, when bleeding does not subside spontaneously, endoscopic epinephrine injection or thermo-coagulation may be required. Prognosis is good and most patients stop bleeding spontaneously with healing of the mucosal tear in 48-72 hours.

## Bleeding Esophageal Varices

Varices are fragile, dilated, bulbous, submucosal venous channels that develop in patients with portal hypertension. Though both esophageal and gastric varices may be found, bleeding usually occurs in the distal 5 cm of the esophagus. Approximately 40% of patients with varices will experience bleeding with mortality rates of 30-50%. The risk of bleeding is extremely high in alcoholic cirrhotics who continue to drink.

It is to be noted that signs and symptoms alone are not sufficient to diagnose varices as the cause of upper GI bleeding since in nearly half the cases with known varices bleeding is from a source other than the varices.

### Specific Measures

After initial management and stabilization of hemodynamics (usually within 6-12 hours), endoscopy should be performed to confirm esophageal varices as the cause of bleeding. In many cases, bleeding will stop spontaneously. However, endoscopic variceal treatment must be done in all cases, since over half of these patients will re-bleed within 1 week. Any *associated coagulopathy* due to underlying liver disease must also be taken note of in the overall management of such cases.

- **Pharmacologic agents:** *Somatostatin* is the first-line drug in patients with variceal hemorrhage but has been largely replaced by *octreotide* (a synthetic analogue of somatostatin). It decreases splanchnic and hepatic blood flow as well as transhepatic and variceal pressure. Because of a very short half-life, it is typically given as bolus of 50-100 mg followed by an infusion of 25-50 mcg/hour and continued for 4-5 days. The immediate use of octreotide has proven effective in controlling bleeding in majority of cases. *Terlipressin* appears to be more effective than octreotide, but may not be easily available. It is the only medication that has been shown to reduce mortality in acute variceal bleeding.

*Non-selective beta-blocking agents* decrease splanchnic blood flow and are therefore useful in prevention of re-bleeding but have no role in the management of active variceal bleeding. *Propranolol* should be started, unless contraindicated, in a low dose **(10–20 mg twice** daily) and **then increased stepwise, with a close watch on heart rate and blood pressure. The aim should be to reduce the heart** rate by 25% of the basal value (but not less than 55/minute).

- **Endoscopic therapy:** Endoscopic sclerotherapy (EST) involves the injection of various sclerosing agents to promote thrombus formation. Another procedure is endoscopic *band ligation* by placing rubber bands which block blood flow and promote thrombus formation. Both therapies achieve control of bleeding in about 90% of patients, but band ligation is associated with fewer complications. When combined with octreotide, endoscopic procedures are more effective in controlling acute bleeding, early re-bleeding, and in improving survival.
- **Balloon tamponade:** With the availability of pharmacological and endoscopic measures to control variceal bleeding, balloon tamponade (by *Sengstaken-Blakemore or other similar tubes)* is rarely used, and usually reserved for patients in whom octreotide therapy fails to control active bleeding, or as an emergency procedure till endoscopic intervention becomes available. Balloon tamponade is often associated with life-threatening complications. It should, therefore, be used only by an experienced team and for a period not exceeding 24 hours.
- **Other measures:** Antibiotics are prescribed empirically to cirrhotic patients with bleeding varices as they are at great risk of developing *hepatic encephalopathy* and severe infections. Some degree of *coagulopathy* is not uncommon in cirrhotic patients, and may be a contributory factor in GI bleeding. This can be assessed by prothrombin index (INR >1.5) and platelet counts. Appropriate therapy with vitamin K, fresh frozen plasma, and platelet concentrates often helps to mitigate bleeding in such cases.

Some patients, who have recurrent bleeding and/or continue to bleed despite pharmacologic and endoscopic measures, may require emergency portal decompression by *transjugular intrahepatic portosystemic shunt (TIPS)*. This is best considered in patients with reasonably good hepatic functions.

## LOWER GASTROINTESTINAL BLEEDING

Lower GI bleeding is much less common than bleeding from upper GI tract, often involves a much larger anatomic area of the gut, and can be due to diverse pathologies **(Box 3.2)**. The severity of bleeding can vary from mild anorectal ooze to severe hematochezia, but is generally less profuse, and often intermittent compared to upper GI hemorrhage. It subsides spontaneously in majority of cases, blood transfusions are seldom required, and hospital mortality is very low.

## Etiology

The cause of lower GI bleed depends to a large extent on the patient's age. In younger patients Meckel's diverticulum, inflammatory bowel disease, infectious colitis, and polyps are the most likely causes. In adults up to 60 years, diverticulosis, inflammatory bowel disease, and neoplasms are the more common cause. In the elderly patients, angiodysplasia, diverticula, and neoplasms predominate. It may be added that in this country diverticulosis is much less common than in Western countries, probably because of difference in dietetic habits.

## Diagnosis

The appearance and color of the stool is of great help in locating the site of lower GI bleeding, especially when observed by the physician. Diarrheic stool containing blood (especially when associated with gripping pain or tenesmus) is characteristic of inflammatory bowel disease and infections. Streaking of stool with blood or bleeding per rectum in the form of drops/small jet is highly suggestive of anorectal bleeding especially hemorrhoids. Large volumes of bright red blood suggest left colonic or rectal neoplasm. On the other hand, maroon-colored stool suggest a lesion in right colon or small intestine. Clots in the stool indicate a lower GI source while melena is always indicative of upper GI bleed.

The investigation of choice is *colonoscopy* performed after thorough bowel preparation. In the hands of the experienced endoscopist, it can reveal the site of bleeding in of all cases. When results are not conclusive and the bleeding continues or recurs, *angiography and technetium-labeled red blood cell scans* may be considered. Barium enema is no longer used as a diagnostic study in lower GI bleeding; rather it interferes with endoscopic visualization.

## Summary

- ❖ GI bleeding can arise from upper or lower gut depending upon whether the pathology is located above or below the ligament of Teitz, respectively.
- ❖ Vomiting of blood (hematemesis) is seen only in upper GI bleeding whereas hematochesia generally (but not always) indicates lower GI bleeding. Black stool (melena) is characteristic of upper GI hemorrhage.
- ❖ Initial treatment in massive GI hemorrhage should focus on volume replacement by crystalloid solutions until blood transfusions are arranged.
- ❖ Esophago-gastroduodenal endoscopy is essential for precisely defining the cause of upper GI bleeding. It also provides various therapeutic options for control of bleeding in such cases.
- ❖ NSAIDs, corticosteroids, COX-2 inhibitors, and alcohol are important risk factors for upper GI bleeding, especially in elderly and hypoxic patients.

❖ Significant lower GI bleeding is less common than bleeding from a source in upper GI tract. Colonoscopy is the investigation of choice. However, a precise etiological diagnosis is more difficult in such cases because of the large area involved, and also because bleeding is often self-limited.

# ACUTE HEPATIC FAILURE

## Definition

Acute liver failure (ALF) is a condition characterized by rapid development of hepatocellular dysfunction, marked specifically by coagulopathy **and alteration in mental status** *(encephalopathy)* **in** *patients who do not have pre-existing liver disease.*

## Etiology

A large number of conditions can result in ALF **(Table 3.2)**, most common being acute viral hepatitis, especially hepatitis B virus, which accounts for almost half of all cases. Most of these patients are young adults. Hepatitis A and C virus infection seldom lead to fulminant hepatic failure. *Drug-induced liver injury* is the second major cause of ALF, which occurs most often in individuals older than 40 years of age. This can be of two types: predictable and idiosyncratic. The former occurs in a dose-dependent fashion, while idiosyncratic liver injury is unrelated to the administered dose. The classical example of predictable acute liver injury is paracetamol (acetaminophen) overdose, seen more often in Western countries where vaccination and improved sanitation have reduced the incidence of viral infection. Excessive alcohol consumption (severe alcoholic hepatitis) also accounts for a significant number of cases of ALF.

## Clinical Features

Acute liver failure is a broad term that encompasses both "fulminant" and "sub-fulminant" (or late-onset) hepatic failure. Hepatic failure is usually defined as *fulminant* when encephalopathy sets in within 6-8 weeks of first hepatic symptoms, and as *subfulminant* when encephalopathy develops after

| Table 3.2: Causes of acute hepatic failure. | |
|---|---|
| **Viruses:** Hepatitis A, B and E, Varicella-Zoster, Cytomegalovirus, and Epstein-Barr | **Chemical agents:** Ethanol, carbon tetrachloride, benzene phosphorus, and ethylene glycol |
| **Drugs:** Acetaminophen, halogen, anesthetics, isoniazid, rifampicin, methyldopa, phenytoin, anabolic steroids, and sulfonamides | **Miscellaneous:** Autoimmune hepatitis, Reye's syndrome, fatty liver of pregnancy, Wilson's disease, toxic mushrooms, Budd-chiari syndrome, and multiorgan failure |

8 weeks but before 26 weeks. The interval (between the onset of symptoms and the development of encephalopathy) provides clues to the likely cause of the disease and the prognosis with medical care alone. In *hyperacute* cases, this interval is a week or less, and the cause is usually viral hepatitis or acetaminophen toxicity. More slowly evolving or subacute cases may represent exacerbations in chronic liver diseases, or result from idiosyncratic drug-induced liver injury. It is to be noted that patients with subacute causes, despite having less coagulopathy and encephalopathy, have a consistently worse prognosis with medical care alone than those in whom the illness has a more rapid onset.

Clinical manifestations of ALF can affect many organs and systems resulting in a varying degree and combination of *encephalopathy, coagulopathy, renal failure, and infection/sepsis*. These are described later in this section. The most striking feature, of course, is encephalopathy with different grades of impairment of consciousness **(Table 3.3)**. Jaundice is invariably present but may be minimal. When ALF supervenes in patients with chronic liver disease, often there are also other signs of underlying hepatic disease, such as splenomegaly, ascites, prominent collaterals, palmer erythema, etc.

## Diagnosis

In all patients suspected of moderate to severe acute hepatitis, prothrombin time should be measured, and mental status carefully evaluated. A prolonged prothrombin time (INR >1.5) and/or any evidence of altered sensorium should immediately suggest a diagnosis of ALF prompting urgent hospitalization. Thorough laboratory investigations should then be carried out in order to evaluate both the etiology and severity of ALF.

### Laboratory Diagnosis

These should include:
- Complete blood count
- Prothrombin time (INR)
- **Chemistries:** Liver function tests (including transaminases, alkaline phosphatase, albumin, and total bilirubin)
- Renal function tests (creatinine, urea, electrolytes)
- Blood glucose level (which may be dangerously low), and lactate (often elevated)
- Arterial blood gas (may reveal hypoxemia)
- Serum ammonia level (arterial, if possible)
- **Viral hepatitis serologies:** Anti-HAV IgM, $HB_sAg$, anti-HBc IgM, anti-HCV
- Other tests, such as (suspected) drug toxicity levels (e.g., acetaminophen), ceruloplasmin level, HIV status, autoimmune markers (for diagnosis of autoimmune hepatitis), immunoglobulin levels, and (in women) pregnancy test.

## Management

**Management of** ALF **should comprise:** (1) **Supportive care,** (2) **Specific therapy of dominant presenting feature(s), and** (3) **If possible treatment of cause of liver failure.**

### Supportive Measures

Life-threatening complications are common in ALF, and therefore, all such patients should be managed in an intensive care unit to watch for unpredictable development of multiorgan failure. Proper oxygenation should be ensured and suitable measures taken to assess and stabilize all vital functions. These should include *management of fluids, metabolic alterations, cardiovascular abnormalities, and infections.* Adequate nutrition should also be ensured both by oral and intravenous routes, taking care to restrict protein intake in patients with features of hepatic encephalopathy.

- **Fluid therapy:** Fluid therapy should be rationalized by continuous recording of intravascular volume by pulmonary capillary wedge pressure (PCWP) or if that is not possible, by central venous pressure (CVP). As far as possible, normovolemia should be maintained. Fluid overload will increase portal pressure and may precipitate or worsen cerebral edema. On the other hand, hypovolemia with consequent hypotension will adversely affect hepatic, renal, and other vital organ functions.
- **Metabolic derangements:** Hypoglycemia is a common complication of ALF. Hence, blood glucose levels should be monitored every 4 hours throughout the course of illness. Simultaneously, a continuous IV infusion of 10% dextrose should be started, with a reasonable goal of maintaining blood glucose levels between 80 and 160 mg/dL. Significant alterations are common in *both sodium and potassium* levels. Marked *hypokalemia* develops often in the early stage of the disease and may be accompanied by metabolic alkalosis, both of which can worsen mental status. In later stages, however, metabolic acidosis may supervene due to accumulation of lactic acid and other metabolites resulting from severe anoxemia. *Hyponatremia* is an almost universal finding due to water retention and a shift in intracellular sodium transport.
- **Cardiovascular abnormalities:** Complex circulatory derangements can occur in ALF. These include a *low systemic vascular resistance* and a compensatory increase in cardiac output (a hemodynamic profile similar to that seen in septic shock). *Arterial hypotension* occurs in the later stages of ALF, and may be contributed by hemorrhage and *sepsis*. Norepinephrine infusion may be required, if fluid restoration fails to maintain blood pressure.
- **Infections:** Bacteremia is a common problem especially when patients are comatose and have numerous indwelling catheters. Additionally, phagocytosis is impaired and complement production is decreased. However, fever and leukocytosis may be minimal or even absent. Both Gram positive and Gram negative infections can occur, and so also fungal

infections. Other recognizable infections in such cases include subacute bacterial peritonitis and aspiration pneumonia.

## Hepatic Encephalopathy

Encephalopathy has a central place in the clinical picture of ALF, has a key prognostic importance, and constitutes a life threatening, but potentially reversible, medical emergency. Essentially, it implies inability of the liver to remove toxic substances which accumulate in the blood stream and result in loss of functions/impairment of consciousness in varying degree.

### Etiology

Broadly speaking hepatic encephalopathy (HE) may occur in three types of cases:
1. Patients with acute severe liver disease as in ALF. This accounts for a small number of cases of HE.
2. In patients with chronic liver disease (e.g., cirrhosis) where HE is caused or aggravated by an additional cause. This is the most common cause of encephalopathy.
3. Patients who have portal-systemic shunting (in portal hypertension) often without any active liver disease—an unusual but obvious cause of HE.

### Pathogenesis

There is no single or uniformly accepted mechanism as to how liver dysfunction or portosystemic shunting might lead to encephalopathy. Central to the pathogenesis of HE is the role of nitrogen-containing compounds from the intestine, generated by gut bacteria from food, and transported by the portal vein to the liver where most of it is metabolized (through the urea cycle), and excreted immediately. Irrespective of the etiology, this process is grossly impaired in all cases of HE either because hepatocytes are incapable of metabolizing the waste products or because portal venous blood bypasses the liver through collateral circulation or a medically created shunt. Nitrogenous waste products thus accumulate in the systemic circulation (hence the old terminology *"portosystemic encephalopathy"*).

The most important of such waste products is **ammonia ($NH_3$)**. This small molecule crosses the blood-brain barrier and is absorbed and metabolized by neuronal cell astrocytes (which constitute about 30% of the cerebral cortex). Astrocytes use ammonia when synthesizing glutamine from glutamate. Excessive production of ammonia* results in **increased levels of glutamine** that leads to increase in osmotic pressure in the astrocytes which become swollen *(cytotoxic brain edema)* resulting in increased intracranial pressure. Unfortunately, signs of elevated intracranial pressure, such as papilledema and loss of pupillary reflexes are not reliable and occur late in the disease. CT imaging of the brain is also unhelpful in detecting early cerebral edema.

Some other toxic products implicated in the **pathogenesis** of HE **include:** (1) Increased activity of the **(inhibitory) gamma-aminobutyric acid** *(GABA),* **which** inhibits neurotransmission, (2) *Mercaptans* (metabolites of methionine), (3) *Short-chain fatty acids,* and (4) Increase in *false neurotransmitters* (such as octopamine and histamine), which interfere with normal neurotransmitters (dopamine, serotonin, and norepinephrine).

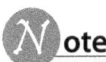ote

It is a common observation that ammonia levels don't always correlate with the severity of encephalopathy. In such cases, it is suspected that more ammonia has already been absorbed into the brain in cases with severe symptoms (and thus relatively low serum levels).

## Clinical Features

The hallmark of ALF is a change in mental status, which may vary from altered behavior and sleep rhythm to impairment of consciousness in varying degree **(Table 3.3)**.

As already stated, encephalopathy can develop in two types of cases: (1) Subjects with initially normal or apparently normal liver *("primary group"),* and (2) Patients with chronic liver disease, usually cirrhosis *("secondary group").* Patients in the former group usually develop encephalopathy abruptly, often without any apparent cause. In the "secondary group" however, several factors may precipitate encephalopathy. These include:

- Gastrointestinal bleeding which provides a protein-rich meal
- Infections
- Alcohol ingestion
- Dehydration and electrolyte abnormalities especially hypokalemia which may result from excessive vomiting, paracentesis, or use of diuretics
- Surgical intervention
- Medicines that suppress central nervous system, such as barbiturates or benzodiazepines.

**Signs and symptoms** of HE may begin slowly, and worsen gradually, or begin suddenly and be severe from the start. **Early symptoms** are difficult to detect but may be observed if looked into carefully in susceptible patients. Such symptoms can be forgetfulness, mild confusion, and irritability. With advancing degree of encephalopathy these worsen in proportion to the degree of hepatic disease **(Table 3.3)**. Basically, the **first stage of encephalopathy** is characterized by inverted sleep pattern (sleeping by day and awake at night), **second stage** by lethargy and personality changes, **third stage** by worsened confusion, and the **fourth stage** by progression to coma.

A *"liver flap"* (asterixis) is often demonstrable in the early stages of coma, and is ascribed to impaired inflow of joint and posture information to the reticular system in the brain stem resulting in lapses in posture. Flapping

**Table 3.3:** Clinical grading of hepatic encephalopathy.

| Grades | Symptoms |
|---|---|
| Grade I | Trivial lack of awareness, euphoria or anxiety, episodic drowsiness, disturbed sleep rhythm, liver flap |
| Grade II | Increased drowsiness, disorientation for time and place, lethargy or apathy, liver flap |
| Grade III | Somnolence to semistupor but responsive to verbal stimuli, aggressive, gross disorientation, incoherent speech |
| Grade IV | Coma, unresponsive to verbal or painful stimuli. |

tremor is, however, not specific to hepatic failure and can also be observed in patients with severe cardiac, respiratory and renal failure.

Other signs and symptoms of chronic liver disease are often present and include a variable degree of icterus, peripheral edema, ascites, and gynecomastia. In severe encephalopathy, the tendon reflexes may be exaggerated and plantar reflex extensor (Babinski's sign). A particular smell *(fetor hepaticus)* may be detected in urine and breath due to the presence of mercaptans.

### *Diagnosis*

The diagnosis of HE is largely a clinical one based on the development of confusion, altered sensorium, and coma in a patient with confirmed liver disease. Many disorders can manifest in a manner similar to HE. These include: (1) Cerebral hemorrhage, (2) Subdural hematoma, (3) Meningitis, (4) Sedative overdose, and (5) Alcohol intoxication or alcohol withdrawal. Most of these conditions can be suspected on clinical grounds and excluded by laboratory investigations, such as complete blood count, liver function tests, prothrombin time, **serum ammonia** level, **serum** electrolytes, **and** kidney **function** tests. A CT scan of the brain may be required to exclude neurological disorders.

### *Management*

A high level of suspicion should be maintained whenever hepatic encephalopathy is a possibility. With early diagnosis and proper management, it may be possible to save two out of every three cases in the "precoma" stage compared to over 90% mortality when deep coma supervenes. The prognosis is intimately related to the severity of liver damage.

Patients with more than minimal encephalopathy should be managed in ICU since intubation of the airway is often necessary to prevent life-threatening complications, such as aspiration, or respiratory failure. Appropriate steps should be taken to help with breathing and blood circulation if patient is in coma.

The first step in management is to **identify and treat any factor(s) that may have caused hepatic encephalopathy.** Given the *frequency of infection* *as the underlying cause,* antibiotics are often administered empirically both to suppress intestinal flora as well as to control possible bacterial infections (clinical or subclinical, **and usually gram negative**). *Appropriate antibiotics effective against both gram-positive and gram-negative bacteria should be given intravenously.* To suppress **generation** of **ammonia and** other **waste** products by **intestinal flora, neomycin, and** metronidazole are often prescribed but neomycin and other aminoglycoside antibiotics carry risk of renal failure, and metronidazole could cause peripheral neuropathy. A safer and probably more effective antibiotic is the newly introduced drug *rifaximin,* a non-absorbable antibiotic but without the complications attached to neomycin and metronidazole. However, the drug is expensive.

- **Diet:** In the past, protein consumption was restricted (often completely) for risk of worsening encephalopathy. This has been shown to be rather harmful especially since many patients with chronic liver disease are malnourished. Currently, a diet with moderate protein content (30-40 g) is recommended initially, which may be gradually increased as recovery sets in. Dietary supplementation with branched-chain amino acids and probiotics has also been recommended but results are not proven.

- **Lactulose:** This is a non-absorbable synthetic disaccharide which reaches the lower git unchanged (there is no enzyme "lactulase" in man). In the colon lactulose is hydrolyzed by bacteria into lactic and acetic acids, which promote bowel transit, reduce pH of the stool, and decrease ammonia levels. About 10-30 mL may be given thrice a day, the dose being adjusted so as to result in 2-3 loose motions a day. Overzealous treatment may result in considerable fluid loss through osmotic diarrhea. Treatment with lactulose is beneficial in encephalopathy associated with chronic hepatic failure; its role in encephalopathy of fulminant hepatic failure is not established.

- **Miscellaneous measures:** Colonic bacterial activity should be decreased by bowel wash once or twice a day unless the patient already has lactulose-induced diarrhea. Blood losses, if any, or associated *severe anemia* (hemoglobin <8 g%) should be corrected by blood transfusion, and fresh frozen plasma, if there is overt bleeding. Platelet transfusions are indicated when platelet count falls below 50,000/mm$^3$. Various vitamins, especially vitamin K, should be administered daily. The risk of gastric erosions is increased in patients with AHF (as in any critically ill patient). Corticosteroids are contraindicated in all types of AHF, especially since they increase the risk of gastric erosions. Such gastric erosions are more likely to result in upper GI bleeding in these cases because of associated coagulopathy. Intragastric pH should, therefore, be reduced by adequate doses of PPIs given intravenously.

- **Treatment of cerebral edema** (an important cause of altered mental status) is rather unsatisfactory, and patients of AHF respond poorly to treatment that is effective in other forms of cerebral edema. A rapid IV infusion of 100 mL of 20% mannitol may be tried, and repeated after 6-8 hours if neurological improvement is observed. Mannitol therapy is contraindicated in the presence of renal failure since fluid overload may worsen cerebral edema. Corticosteroids, surgical decompression, or hyperventilation seem to be of little benefit.

### General Measures

Patients should be nursed with the head of the bed elevated to about 20-30 degrees to decrease the risk of both aspiration and cerebral edema. Extreme flexion, extension, or rotation of the head must be avoided, since these positions reduce venous return from the head and may worsen cerebral edema. Delirium and restlessness should, as far as possible, be controlled by physical measures. However, if the patient is violently restless, oxazepam *(Serepex)* may be given orally in a small dose (10-15 mg). Benzodiazepines, phenobarbitone, and even antihistamines are to be avoided.

### Coagulopathy

Since liver plays a central role in the synthesis of almost all coagulation factors, *Coagulopathy* is another cardinal feature of ALF. Plasma concentration of fibrinogen and prothrombin are especially impaired in ALF, and platelet count may also be decreased, usually related to DIC. In fact, because factors V and VII have a rapid turnover, *serial estimation of prothrombin time is the best measure to periodically assess hepatic function.* Treatment comprises administration of fresh frozen plasma, and platelet transfusions (if platelet count falls below 50,000/mm$^3$)

## Renal Failure

Renal failure can develop in approximately half of the patients with ALF and worsens the prognosis. The renal failure is oliguric and typically functional (altered hemodynamics) but acute tubular necrosis may also occur (e.g., paracetamol overdose). Intra-renal vascular resistance is increased (with consequent decrease in GFR) due to activation of sympathetic and renin-angiotensin system aimed at restoring arterial pressure. This is in contrast to systemic circulation where vascular resistance is decreased and cardiac output increases.

The renal vasoconstriction is initially counterbalanced by intra-renal hyper-production of vasodilators, such as prostaglandins. When this balance is lost, for whatever reasons, renal vascular resistances dramatically increase and renal failure develops **(hepatorenal syndrome).** This is diagnosed by: (1) Very low urinary sodium values (<10 mEq/L) due to avid sodium retention, and (2) Increase in serum creatinine level above 1.5 mg/dL. Once developed, hepatorenal syndrome responds very poorly to treatment (including volume replacement), and has a high mortality.

## Prognosis

There has been some improvement in the prognosis of ALF over the years due no doubt to awareness and better management of **life-threatening complications.**

However, the disease **still carries an unacceptably high mortality. Prognosis is better in younger patients between 10 and 40 years of age. Markers of unfavorable prognosis include:**
- Type B hepatitis
- Development of coma Grade III or more
- Laboratory data showing bilirubin level >15 mg/dL, arterial pH <7.30, and prothrombin INR >3.5
- Associated pregnancy, especially in third trimester
- Rapid shrinkage of liver as documented by imaging
- Sepsis and other associated organ failure, such as acute renal failure or acute respiratory distress syndrome.

*When a patient has Grade IV encephalopathy and is dependent on mechanical ventilation, it is usually too late.*

## Summary

Acute liver failure, especially the fulminant type, is associated with severe impairment of multiple liver functions especially detoxifying, hemostatic, and phagocytic properties. Hemodynamic and renal status is also precarious in such patients. Detection of patients of ALF in the precoma stage coupled with immediate hospitalization and skilled management in ICU offer a fair chance of recovery. In all cases of hepatic failure presenting with impaired mental status, causes of coma other than encephalopathy must be excluded (e.g., hypoglycemia, sepsis, intracranial pathology, drug intoxication).

There is no specific treatment for ALF, and appropriate supportive therapy forms the basis of management in such cases:
- Hospitalize the patient at the earliest and ensure proper oxygenation
- Restrict daily protein intake to 30–40 g
- Monitor PCWP/CVP and maintain proper fluid balance with 10% dextrose and normal saline infusions; acid-base and electrolyte balance should be maintained as best as possible
- Suppress intestinal bacteria with neomycin and metronidazole; rifaximin is preferable. Intravenous broad-spectrum antibiotics should be used empirically since ALF is invariably associated with infections.
- Lactulose therapy is beneficial only when hepatic encephalopathy complicates patients with chronic liver disease
- Efforts should be made to maintain adequate circulating volume, and preserve all vital functions including adequate urine output
- All vitamin supplements should be provided; anemia (hemoglobin <10g%) and coagulopathy should be managed appropriately

❖ Antihistamines, tranquilizers, sedatives, and narcotics in any form must be avoided. Corticosteroids also serve no useful purpose, and may be actually harmful.

*Special Measures*

A new drug—IV *acetylcysteine* has been found to be beneficial in both acetaminophen toxicity and non-acetaminophen-related liver failure, especially the latter.

*Liver transplantation* is the definitive treatment in liver failure. In selected patients for whom no allograft is immediately available, one should consider support with bioartificial liver. This is a short-term measure that only leads to survival, if the liver spontaneously recovers or is replaced. Nonbiologic extracorporeal liver support systems, such as hemodialysis, hemofiltration, charcoal hemoperfusion, plasmapheresis, and exchange transfusions permit temporary liver support until a suitable donor liver is found. However, long-term benefit has not been confirmed.

# ACUTE PANCREATITIS

Acute pancreatitis (AP) implies sudden inflammation of the pancreas characterized by abdominal pain and distension (ileus), nausea and vomiting, and associated elevation of pancreatic enzymes. Most of the cases (~ 85-90%) recover fully with conservative measures. The remaining 10-15%, however, have a severe form of the disease, which carries high morbidity and mortality. The course of AP is in fact always uncertain, and many patients who start with mild disease may end up in severe pancreatitis.

## Etiopathogenesis

Various causes of AP are listed in **Table 3.4**. The two most important causes are **gallstones and alcohol.** Other causes of AP are much less common. The apparently *idiopathic acute pancreatitis is often due to occult biliary microlithiasis.*

| Table 3.4: Causes of acute pancreatitis. ||
|---|---|
| **Common causes** | **Rare causes** |
| • Gallstones<br>• Ethanol | Infections: Mumps, hepatitis B, coxsackie virus, ascaris penetrating duodenal ulcer hypercalcemia |
| **Uncommon causes** ||
| Drug-induced*<br>Abdominal trauma<br>Idiopathic | Hypertriglyceridemia, end-stage renal failure, carcinoma of the head of pancreas, ampullary stenosis, pregnancy |

*Various medicines incriminated in the causation of AP include: corticosteroids, HIV drugs (didanosine and pentamidine), diuretics, valproic acid, azathioprine, and atypical antipsychotics, such as clozapine, risperidone, and olanzapine.

Two types of pancreatitis are recognized—mild and severe (acinar), depending upon whether their predominant response to cell injury is inflammation or necrosis, respectively. Eighty percent of patients with AP have the milder form, and these patients recover without any sequel. On the other hand, severe pancreatitis is characterized by organ failure (hypoxemia, hypovolemia, hypotension, and kidney failure) or complications, such as necrosis, vessel damage (hemorrhage) or fluid collection. Due to the pancreas lacking a capsule, the inflammation and necrosis can extend to include facial layers in the immediate vicinity of the pancreas.

Gallstone-induced pancreatitis is probably related to gallstone obstruction within the main pancreatic duct or reflux of bile into the pancreatic duct owing to impaction of the stone at the ampulla. The pathophysiology of alcoholic pancreatitis is unknown but is likely related to direct toxic injury of alcohol to pancreatic acinar cells.

## Clinical Features

The chief symptom of AP is acute, severe upper abdominal or left upper quadrant pain often radiating to the back, and associated with nausea and vomiting. Fever and/or mild icterus may be present and occasionally, pleural effusions may occur as a result of capillary leak syndrome. The clinical picture in patients with severe AP is more complex as the pancreatic pathology may evolve over 2-4 weeks beginning with acute interstitial pancreatitis and followed by necrosis, infection, and finally pancreatic abscess formation. Patients recovering from acute stage may later develop chronic pancreatitis, which can lead to diabetes or pancreatic cancer. Some cases may also experience unexplained weight loss due to lack of pancreatic enzymes hindering digestion.

**Physical examination** often reveals upper abdominal tenderness (mostly epigastric) with or without local guarding. Abdomen may be distended and bowel sounds reduced from reflex bowel paralysis. A mild icterus is not uncommon. Bluish discoloration can sometimes be noticed in the periumbilical region *(Cullen sign)* or in the flanks *(Grey-Turner sign)*, indicative of retroperitoneal hemorrhage. These are however, uncommon signs. In severe cases, *tachycardia* often develops and even features of *shock* may supervene. The latter is due to hypovolemia (resulting from exudation of plasma protein into the retroperitoneal space), increased vascular permeability (due to increased formation and release of various kinins), and sepsis **(Box 3.3)**.

## Diagnosis

Acute pancreatitis is diagnosed by the presence of at least three of the following: (1) Typical clinical symptoms, (2) Elevated serum amylase and/or lipase levels greater than three times the upper limit of normal, (3) Typical findings on radio-imaging. However, the degree of rise in amylase/lipase does not help in assessing the severity of the disease. Amylase level increases within 6-24 hours

> **Box 3.3: Complications of acute pancreatitis.**
>
> ❑ **Local (Abdominal)**
>   ➢ Pancreatic necrosis, pseudocyst and abscess obstructive jaundice
>   ➢ Involvement of adjoining organs (e.g., bowel infarction, GI bleed, portal-splenic vein thrombosis)
> ❑ **Systemic**
>   ➢ *Metabolic*: Hypocalcemia, hyperglycemia, hypertriglyceridemia, acidosis
>   ➢ *Cardiac*: Pericardial effusion, arrhythmias, shock
>   ➢ *Pulmonary*: Atelectasis, pneumonia, pleural effusion, adult respiratory distress syndrome
>   ➢ *Renal*: Azotemia, oliguria
>   ➢ *Miscellaneous*: Encephalopathy, fat necrosis, disseminated intravascular
>   ➢ Coagulation

of onset, remains high for only a short period, and then returns to normal in 2-7 days. It is to be remembered that false positive elevated serum amylase can occur in a number of conditions including salivary gland disease, bowel obstruction, cholecystitis, and a perforated ulcer. Serum lipase estimation is more sensitive and specific than serum amylase in the diagnosis of AP. Its level rises within 4-8 hours after the onset of symptoms and remains elevated longer than amylase (up to 7-14 days).

**Imaging and radiological studies** are extremely valuable. Abdominal ultrasound is generally performed first as it is simple and non-expensive. It may show an inflamed pancreas but its main utility is for the diagnosis of gallstones, and alcoholic fatty liver (combined with a history of alcohol consumption). A chest skiagram *(CXR)* is also desirable and may show elevated diaphragm, linear focal atelectasis in the lower zones, or pleural effusion. Diffuse infiltrates provide a warning of acute respiratory distress syndrome.

*CT scan* of the abdomen is an important investigation for assessment of pancreatitis. It is especially useful when the diagnosis of pancreatitis is uncertain or there is abdominal distension. However, CT abdomen may be normal or show only equivocal findings, if performed within the first 12 hours of the onset of symptoms. CT scan will also reveal the true extent and nature of pathology (pancreatic edema or necrosis, or peri-pancreatic fluid collections). Subsequent scans allow a **more rational follow up of** the case and may detect complications, such as abscess **and pseudocyst. *Magnetic resonance imaging* (MRI) may be considered for the visualization of pancreas, particularly of pancreatic fluid collections, and necrotized** debris. However, CT scan is considered the gold standard in diagnostic imaging for acute pancreatitis.

### *Other Investigations*

Complete assessment requires several **laboratory investigations.** These include white cell count, hematocrit, estimation of blood glucose, blood urea nitrogen (BUN), serum glutamic oxalacetic transferase (SGOT), lactic dehydrogenase (LDH), calcium, and when possible arterial oxygen and base deficit. Based on the results of these investigations, criteria have been defined for *predicting the severity of acute pancreatitis* (vide infra).

## Prognostic Indices

**Clinical prediction:** Many scoring indices have been used to assess the prognosis and survival rates in acute pancreatitis. One of the commonly used parameter is Ranson score for predicting the severity of acute pancreatitis **(Box 3.4)**.

The criterion for point assignment is that a certain break-point be met at any time during that 48 hour period, so that in some situations, it can be calculated shortly after admission.

> *Interpretation*
> - **Score <3:** Severe pancreatitis unlikely; >3: severe pancreatitis likely
> - **Score 0–2:** 2% mortality; score 3–4: 15% mortality; score 5–6: 40% mortality; score 7–8:100% mortality
> - Prognostic scoring based on CT abdomen results have also been defined **(Table 3.5)**. Using this score, prognosis is good with scores of 0–3 (mortality <5%), but becomes progressively worse with increasing score (mortality: 5–20% with scores of 7–10).

The CT criteria score has a maximum of 10 points, and is the sum of degree of pancreatitis and pancreatic necrosis grade points.

## Management

Acute pancreatitis is potentially a multiorgan disease with a variable and unpredictable course. While a great majority of the cases have a simple benign course and a self-limited disease, about 10–15% patients develop severe AP, which may be associated with necrosis, infected necrosis, abscess formation, and pseudocyst. The difficulty lies in identifying this subset of patients especially since many cases with an initial mild onset may suddenly and unexpectedly turn into severe disease. It is, therefore, wise to treat every patient with AP as if the disease is likely to develop into severe AP. Within 72 hours patients with acute severe pancreatitis can usually be identified through appearance of features of an organ failure. Periodic assessment of severity of the disease based on criteria mentioned above **(Box 3.4 and Table 3.5)** help in this process.

Since, there is no specific etiology, the treatment of AP is largely symptomatic and supportive. Even in the severe form of the disease no medical treatment/intervention has been conclusively shown to be beneficial. The main principle of treatment is to put the gland at rest thereby allowing it time to heal while maintaining vital functions as near normal as possible.

> **Box 3.4: Ranson's criteria for assessing severity of acute pancreatitis.**
> 
> ☐ **On admission**
>   ➢ Age >55 years
>   ➢ White cell count >16,000/cu.mm, Blood glucose >200 mg/dL, SGOT >250 IU, LDH >350 IU
> ☐ **During subsequent 48 hours**
>   ➢ Fall in hematocrit by more than 10%
>   ➢ Increase in BUN >5 mg/dL after IV fluid hydration
>   ➢ Serum calcium below 8 mg/dl
>   ➢ $PaO_2$ <60%
>   ➢ Base deficit >4 mEq/L
>   ➢ Estimated fluid sequestration >6 L.

**Table 3.5:** Grading of severity of acute pancreatitis—CT scan criteria.

| Degree of pancreatitis | Grade points |
|---|---|
| Normal pancreas | 0 |
| Enlarged pancreas | 1 |
| Inflamed pancreas | 2 |
| Single fluid collection/phlegmon | 3 |
| Multiple fluid collections | 4 |
| *Extent of pancreatic necrosis* | |
| No necrosis | 0 |
| Necrosis of one-third pancreas | 2 |
| Necrosis of one-half pancreas | 4 |
| Necrosis of >one-half pancreas | 6 |

### *Specific Measures*

- **Relief of pain:** Pain should be controlled with pethidine or pentazocine, and vomiting with promethazine *(Phenergan)* or ordansetron *(Emeset)*. Morphine should be avoided as it may induce ampullary spasm.
- **Nasogastric intubation:** In all cases of AP oral feeding should be stopped initially for 2-4 days and nasogastric suction done frequently. The latter reduces acid stimulus to the duodenum, and thereby inhibits pancreatic secretion. Nasogastric intubation also reduces abdominal distension in the early stages of the disease and helps in identifying any gastrointestinal bleed. In majority of cases abdominal distension subsides in 2-3 days when the tube should be removed and oral feeding resumed in a graduated manner. Longer periods of intubation may be required in patients with severe AP.
- **Intravenous fluids:** Fluid requirement is greatly increased in severe AP since these patients lose a lot of high protein exudates into the peritoneal cavity as well as retroperitoneal space. This leads to hypovolemia (increase

in hematocrit) with consequent decrease in pancreatic blood supply, which in turn, promotes pancreatic necrosis.

Aggressive hydration should, therefore, be provided at a rate of 5-10 mL/kg/h of normal saline or lactated Ringer's solution, unless cardiovascular, renal or related comorbid factors preclude aggressive fluid replacement. Fluid requirement should be reassessed and adjusted at frequent intervals during 24-48 hours after admission based on clinical parameters, hematocrit, and blood urea nitrogen (BUN). Central venous pressure (CVP) monitoring should help fluid administration.

- **Antibiotics:** Prophylactic use of antibiotics is controversial. Antibiotics do not affect initial febrile reaction which is due to non-bacterial pancreatic inflammation. However, in cases of severe AP associated with pancreatic necrosis, prophylactic antibiotic therapy is an accepted principle. The infection is usually by Gram negative bacteria (of colonic origin), and the antibiotic chosen should be effective against such organisms, and also capable of penetrating pancreatic tissue. The antibiotic of choice is imipenem-cilastatin administered IV in a dose of 500mg three times a day, and continued for 2 weeks.
- **Nutrition:** In uncomplicated AP, after abdominal distension has settled, oral feeding in the form of clear liquids should be started usually by the third day, and increased gradually. The problem is more complex in patients with severe AP in whom oral feeding may be contraindicated for several days. Total parenteral nutrition (TPN) is the standard practice in such cases. The aim should be to provide approximately 2,000 calories/day, 60% from glucose, and 20% each from proteins and fats.

  Currently, *early enteral nutrition* is employed in preference to TPN. This is achieved by placing a feeding tube endoscopically or under fluoroscopic guidance in the third portion of the duodenum. Enteral nutrition is more physiological, prevents gut mucosal atrophy, and is free from the side effects of TPN (such as fungemia).
- **Other drugs:** Various pancreatic enzyme inhibitors have not been found beneficial. Proton pump inhibitors are effective in reducing the incidence of stress ulceration and upper GI bleeding, but do not influence the course of acute pancreatitis
- **Endoscopic retrograde cholangiopancreatography (ERCP):** ERCP, performed within 24-72 hours of presentation, is known to reduce morbidity and mortality. It is indicated in cases detected to have common bile duct stones or dilated intrahepatic or extrahepatic ducts on CT abdomen. Its inherent risk is bleeding.
- **Special measures:** Laparotomy is indicated when there is diagnostic uncertainty, and other pathologies (with clear surgical treatment) are possible (e.g., perforated viscous, leaking aneurysm, mesenteric ischemia). The clearest *indication for surgery* in acute pancreatitis is **obstructive choledocholithiasis** in which early intervention dramatically improves survival (if ERCP has been unsuccessful). Other

indications include: (1) Drainage of infected necrotic pancreatic tissue, and (2) Upper abdominal mass, suspected to be pseudocyst (late surgery). The precise type and timing of surgical intervention is difficult and best left to the surgeon's discretion.

## Summary

- ❖ Gallstones and ethanol account for majority of cases of AP. An early and precise diagnosis of gallbladder disease is very rewarding as early decompression of the biliary tract (by ERCP or surgery) vastly improves survival as well as late complications of the disease.
- ❖ The diagnosis of AP can usually be made on clinical grounds and confirmed by estimation of serum amylase and lipase. Imaging studies are valuable, especially CT scan which not only helps in diagnosing and staging pancreatitis, but also provides valuable prognostic information.
- ❖ Most of the patients with AP have a simple, benign and self-limiting course, resolving over 2-4 weeks. They can be managed with simple supportive and symptomatic measures.
- ❖ Severe AP (with necrosis and organ failure) occurs in about 20% of cases. Such patients can have a very complex and prolonged clinical course, and require a great deal of medical and surgical expertise.

# CHAPTER 4

# Neurological Emergencies

## ACUTE CONFUSIONAL STATE

### Definition

Confusion implies *an altered state of consciousness* characterized by inability to sustain a normal level of attention *(attention deficit)* coupled with disordered perception and thinking. It represents the first step in the "disorders of consciousness", which range from confusion through drowsiness and stupor to coma. Synonymous terms include delirium, toxic psychosis, and toxic-metabolic encephalopathy. The key feature is that, in contrast to dementia, *confusional states are short lived and reversible.*

### Etiology

Causes of acute confusion can be divided into four groups: (1) Intracranial diseases, (2) Medication/intoxication, (3) Systemic diseases secondarily affecting brain, and (4) Withdrawal syndromes **(Table 4.1)**.

### Pathophysiology

The exact pathophysiology of most confusional states is not understood. The *key feature of confusion is disturbance of arousal and attention.* These functions are located in: (1) the *reticular core of the brainstem and thalamus* from where this activating system projects into the cortex (responsible for arousal), and (2) *the cortex* itself where the incoming impulses are constantly sorted out and stratified, allowing selected focusing on a stimulus to the exclusion of extraneous stimuli ("Attention"). A disruption of these functions at any level results in an inability to maintain a coherent stream of thought or activity. The result may be inattention or fluctuations of attention, or distraction (so that relevant and unrelated stimuli have equal value).

### Clinical Features

Confusion is most common in the elderly and in the hospitalized patients, usually manifesting as delirium. The condition is usually seen in the setting of surgery, multiple drug therapy, or systemic disease. It is typically marked by clouding of consciousness, inattentiveness, and inability to register immediate

**Table 4.1:** Causes of acute confusional state.

| Intracranial diseases | Drugs/Intoxications* |
|---|---|
| • Vascular<br>• Neoplastic<br>• Infections (meningitis/encephalitis)<br>• Subdural hematoma<br>• Epilepsy<br>• Trauma | • Phenothiazines, benzodiazepines<br>• Sedatives, hypnotics, narcotics<br>• Anticholinergics<br>• Aminophylline<br>• Antidepressants<br>• Antihistamines |
| **Systemic diseases**<br>• Renal failure<br>• Hypoglycemia<br>• Electrolyte disorder<br>• Myocardial infarction<br>• Congestive heart failure<br>• Infections, e.g., pneumonia<br>• Diabetic ketoacidosis<br>• Hypo-or-hyperthyroidism<br>• Non-ketotic hyperosmolar diabetic state<br>• Hypo-or-hyperthermia | • Antihypertensives (methyldopa, clonidine, captopril)<br>• Beta-blockers<br>• Cimetidine, ranitidine<br>• Corticosteroids<br>• Digitalis Quinidine<br>• Isoniazide<br>• Antibiotics (quinolones, penicillin, cephaloporins)<br>• Alcohol intoxication<br>• Lidocaine<br>• Mefloquine<br>• Metoclopramide<br>• Metronidazole |
| **Withdrawal syndromes**<br>• Alcohol withdrawal (delirium tremens)<br>• Barbiturate and non-barbiturate sedative drug withdrawal | Nonsteroidal anti-inflammatory drugs |

*Note: This is not an all-inclusive list of medicines which can cause acute confusional state.

events and recall them a few minutes later. Because of disruption of attention there is *impairment of cognitive functions,* which involve logic, comprehension, judgment, and memory. Since neuronal involvement is diffuse in nature, all aspects of intellectual functions are disordered including orientation in relation to time and place (but usually not to person).

In addition to all the above-mentioned negative features of quiet confusion, delirium may supervene and is marked by autonomic and psychomotor overactivity. The resulting signs and symptoms may include restlessness, anxiety, irrational motor behavior, tremors, diaphoresis, dilated pupils, and sometimes, hallucinations. Rapid fluctuations may occur from day-to-day and even from 1 hour to the next. Symptoms often worsen in the evening because of further reduction in visual and auditory inputs into the reticular system, or addition of sleeping pill *("sun-downing syndrome").*

## Diagnosis

Arriving at a diagnosis of delirium involves two steps. The first step is *to exclude dementia and acute transient psychiatric disorders.* The second step is *to define the cause of confusion/delirium* specially to identify any underlying

**Table 4.2:** Important differences between ACS and acute functional psychosis.

| Features | Acute confusional state | Acute functional psychosis |
|---|---|---|
| Onset | Sudden | Sudden |
| Course | Fluctuating | Stable |
| Consciousness | Clouded | Clear |
| Hallucinations | None or visual | None or auditory |
| Involuntary movements | Common (tremor or asterixis) | Usually absent |
| Systemic disease/drug toxicity | Often present | Usually absent |

**Table 4.3:** Acute confusional state/delirium versus dementia.

| Features | Delirium | Dementia |
|---|---|---|
| Onset | Acute | Slow |
| Course | Fluctuating in character and severity | Stable |
| Duration | Days to weeks | Months to years |
| Attention | Disordered | Usually normal |
| Thinking | Disorganized | Limited |
| Precipitating factor(s) | Often present | Usually absent |

neurological disease or associated systemic illness. The exercise can be, at times, complex.

The process of diagnosis should begin with a thorough history and physical examination including neurological check-up. Suitable laboratory tests and other diagnostic studies should then be planned.

Hallucination can occur in both delirium and schizophrenia but are usually visual in the former and auditory in the latter. There may also be evidence of *"conversion reaction"* and dissociative states in the past. Other important differences between confusion and acute functional psychosis are given at **Table 4.2**.

Every case of ACS/delirium must also be *distinguished from dementia,* since the two conditions carry different prognosis **(Table 4.3)**. Important varieties of dementia syndrome are given at **Table 4.4**. Further discussion of the subject is beyond the scope of this text.

## Investigations

These are planned to establish the cause of confusion, especially to rule out reversible/treatable etiologic factor(s). The laboratory tests should include estimation of hematocrit, white cell count, blood glucose, electrolytes, calcium, and hepatic and renal function studies besides routine X-ray of the chest and an ECG. Additionally, blood and urine cultures, blood gases, ammonia level, and thyroid function studies may be carried out when clinically indicated.

**Table 4.4:** Important varieties of dementia syndrome.

| • **Cortical dementia**<br>➢ Senile dementia of Alzheimer type (SDAT)<br>➢ Multi-infarct dementia<br>➢ Encephalitis | • **Frontal dementia**<br>➢ Subdural hematoma<br>➢ Space occupying lesion<br>➢ Hydrocephalus |
|---|---|
| • **Subcortical dementia**<br>➢ Parkinson's disease<br>➢ Huntington's chorea<br>➢ Multi-infarct dementia<br>➢ Demyelinating diseases<br>➢ Post-traumatic | • **Amnesic dementia**<br>➢ Ischemic encephalopathy<br>➢ Post-traumatic encephalopathy<br>➢ Korsakoff syndrome<br>• **Pseudodementia**<br>➢ Depression<br>➢ Confusional state |

Almost every patient in confusional state needs a computerized tomographic (CT) scan or magnetic resonance imaging (MRI) of the brain, especially when a focal lesion is suspected, or asymmetries are observed on examination of nervous system. In selected cases, EEG may also be desirable. Blood level of the drug may be required when intoxication is suspected. Lumbar puncture is essential when CNS infections are suspected or there is a strong suggestion of subarachnoid hemorrhage even though CT scan is normal (15% cases). As far as possible, lumbar puncture should be done after cranial CT.

## Treatment

Almost all patients presenting with acute confusion will require hospitalization. As a domiciliary measure following steps should be practiced: (1) Treatment of any identifiable and reversible medical disorder, (2) Optimal control of fluid and electrolyte balance, blood volume, urinary output, oxygenation, any infection, and (3) Drug therapy. The first two aspects are not discussed further.

### Drug Therapy

This should preferably be decided in consultation with a psychiatrist. The first principle is to *avoid polypharmacy* and *discontinue all nonessential drugs.* All possibly incriminating drugs **(Table 4.1)** should be withdrawn, and (if absolutely essential) replaced by drugs which do not have psychoactive or anticholinergic properties. Even sedatives and hypnotics should be avoided unless one is treating alcohol or benzodiazepine withdrawal.

The drug of choice for managing severe acute confusion/delirium is haloperidol, but even this should be used only if patient is agitated. The usual dose is 1–2 mg orally or IM two or three times a day. The dosage should be adjusted so as to blunt the agitation permitting nursing care and avoiding exhaustion. The aim should be not to totally suppress agitation since this may require very large doses, which can impair vital functions.

Other drugs should be used with caution. These include chlorpromazine and thioridazine for agitation in general, and diazepam for withdrawal symptoms.

# THE UNCONSCIOUS PATIENT

Normal state of consciousness is dependent upon integrity of the reticular system which is chiefly located in the thalamus and upper brainstem. It receives collateral axons from the main spinothalamic and specific sensory pathways, and projects them to the whole of the cerebral cortex. Interruption of activity in this system results in a state of unconsciousness. Pathophysiologically this may be due to:

- **Metabolic and toxic/infective disorders:** Such disorders impair cerebral functions bilaterally, and are amongst the commonest causes of coma **(Table 4.1)**.
- **Supratentorial mass lesions,** such as massive cerebral infarct, brain abscess, and brain tumor, which secondarily encroach upon deep diencephalic structures. These are common conditions, which result in unconsciousness through the mechanism of herniation of brain tissue (either uncal or central transtentorial) with consequent compression and ischemia of the brainstem structures.
- **Subtentorial lesions** arising from the substance of the brainstem and involving reticular formation directly, e.g., brainstem tumor or infarct. Such diseases are relatively uncommon and virtually untreatable.
- **Psychiatric disorders,** which may resemble coma but are physiologically different.

## Etiology

It may be mentioned right at the beginning that like jaundice, coma is only one manifestation of the whole symptom complex and is not a disease by itself. The syndrome of coma, which may range from drowsiness to deep unconsciousness, may be the result of many conditions **(Box 4.1)**. A general approach to arrive at a correct diagnosis in a case of coma is also shown schematically in **Flowchart 4.1**.

### Evaluation of the Unconsciousness Patient

A correct diagnosis of the cause of coma may be obvious (as in hepatic, diabetic, or uremic coma), or may be reached only after a detailed examination of the patient and relevant investigations. However, priority should be to ensure that all vital functions are stable otherwise appropriate resuscitative measures should be immediately instituted. Any bleeding from site of trauma, if present, should also be quickly controlled. Following systematic approach is recommended:

A detailed history should be obtained from the relations, friends and witnesses accompanying the patient especially regarding: (1) Mode of onset

> Box 4.1: Causes of coma.

- **Metabolic/toxic/infective disorders**
  - Poisonings, especially barbiturate, opium, and alcohol
  - Diabetic coma
  - Hypoglycemia
  - Sepsis
  - Hepatic failure
  - Renal failure
  - Cerebral malaria
  - Sunstroke and heat stroke
  - Encephalitis/meningitis
  - Postictal states
  - Electrolyte imbalance
  - Hypoxia/hypercapnia
- **Supratentorial mass lesions**
  - Cerebral vascular catastrophes
    - Cerebral infarct
    - Cerebral hemorrhage
    - Hypertensive encephalopathy
  - Intracranial space occupying lesions
    - Brain tumor
    - Brain abscess
  - Epidural, subdural, or intracerebral hematoma
- **Subtentorial (brainstem) lesions**
  - Brainstem tumor
  - Brainstem infarct or hemorrhage
  - Cerebellar hemorrhage
- **Psychogenic**
  - Hysteria
  - Malingering

of coma, (2) History of any drug addiction, (3) Any possibility of head injury or foul play, and (4) Any significant past illness. If no clues are available, the circumstances under which the patient was discovered should be enquired and a specific search of the environments as well as the patient's clothes made to locate any letter (possible suicide) or drugs which might have been consumed.

A thorough physical examination should then be conducted especially for any signs of trauma or needle marks on the extremities, any systemic organ disease or metabolic disease. Any peculiar odor of the breath should also be noted. Evidence of meningeal irritation should be sought by passive flexion of the neck and by Kernig and Brudzinski's signs. However its absence, in a patient in *deep* coma, does not rule out meningeal pathology. Funduscopy is also desirable.

An attempt should be made to separate out cases of coma due to conditions listed in group 1 from other pathologic states (**Box 4.1**). This is important because *metabolic/toxic encephalopathies involve the cortex and brainstem diffusely, and do not exhibit abrupt or progressive rostrocaudal dysfunction*

Chapter 4: Neurological Emergencies

**Flowchart 4.1:** Evaluation of unconscious patient.

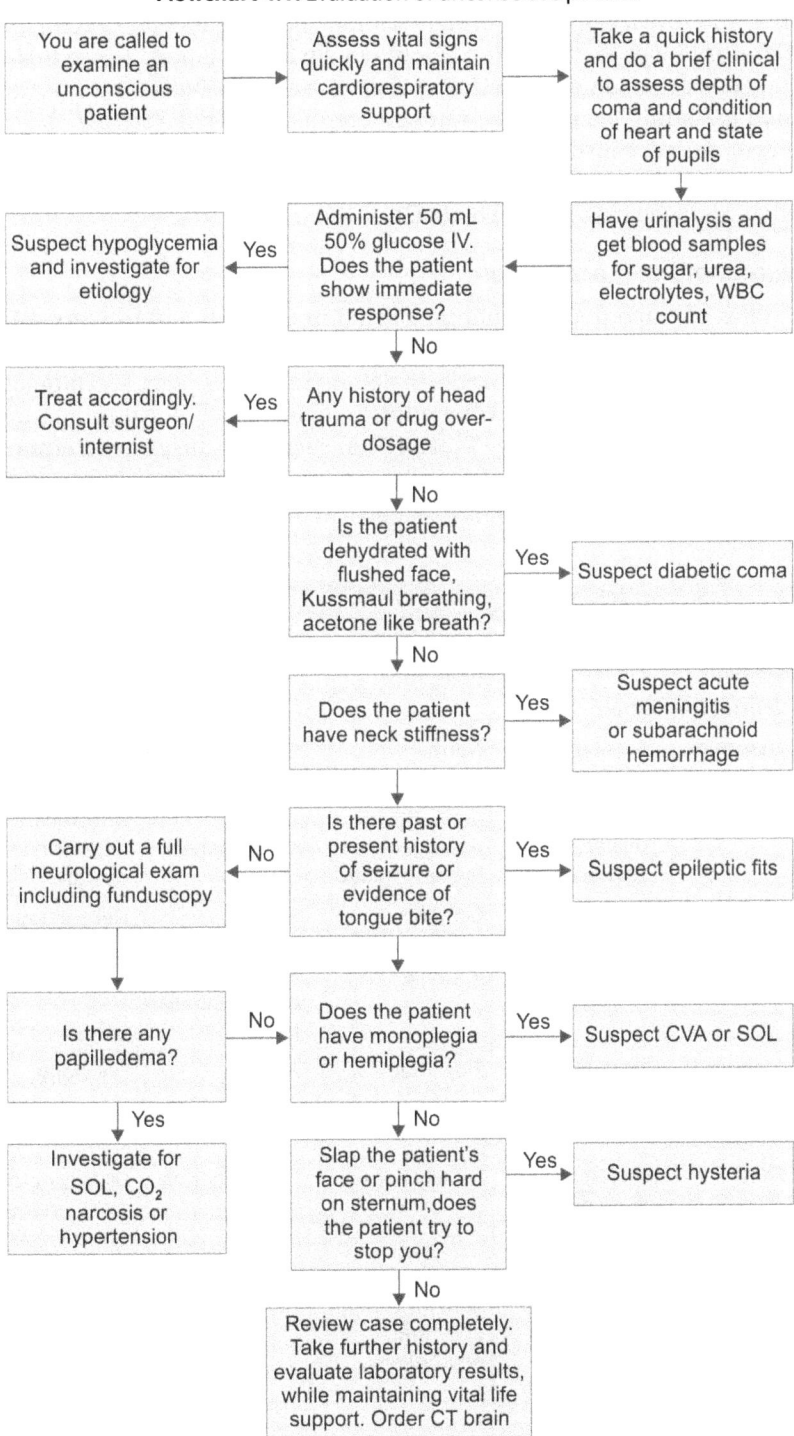

usually seen in neurosurgical setting. The former also have a more gradual onset, and reveal global impairment without any focal lesions. Certain quick laboratory investigations are valuable in such a situation. These include estimation of blood sugar, electrolytes, hepatic and renal functions, and arterial blood gas study. It should be remembered that *altered electrolytes/blood gases and sepsis* constitute important causes of impairment of consciousness, especially in the elderly, in patients who do not have any focal neurological deficit, and who have normal brain CT.

### Neuroanatomic Localization

In states of coma due to conditions listed in Group II and III (**Box 4.1**), a progressive deterioration in nervous system functions tends to occur in a rostrocaudal manner, involving the thalamus, midbrain, pons, and ultimately the medulla, in that order (**"herniation syndromes"**). Neuroanatomic localization of the pathology (**Table 4.5**) in such cases helps in determining the site as well as severity of the disease process. Further, their periodic evaluation helps in determining the course of the disease since such changes

**Table 4.5:** Neuroanatomic syndromes in coma: Salient features.

| Types of herniation | Pupils | Respiration | Eye movements | Motor signs |
|---|---|---|---|---|
| **I. Central Herniation** | | | | |
| a. Thalamic | Small reactive | Normal or Cheyne-Stokes | Usually normal | Usually normal |
| b. Midbrain | Mid or widely dilated, non-reacting | Central neurogenic hyperventilation | Absent ciliospinal reflex | Decorticate or decerebrate posture |
| c. Pontine | Pinpoint, non-reacting | Central neurogenic or irregular | Absent oculocephalic and oculovestibular reflexes | Decerebrate posture |
| d. Medullary | Dilated, fixed (ataxic) | Slow irregular | Absent | Flaccidity |
| **II. Uncal** | | | | |
| a. Early | Ipsilateral pupil dilated but often reactive | Usually normal | Usually normal | Usually normal |
| b. Moderate/advanced | Dilated and usually fixed | Cheyne-Stokes or central neurogenic | HI nerve palsy | Hemiparesis (ipsilateral or contralateral) or decerebrate posture |

often progress in a systematic manner. Following parameters are employed for such assessment:

- **State of consciousness:** This is classified as follows:
  a. *Grade I: Normal* alert wakefulness with intact reflexes, sensory as well as motor.
  b. *Grade II (Drowsiness):* The patient is less aware of his environments, appears disinterested, and his responses to verbal commands are slow and delayed, but appropriate.
  c. *Grade III (Stupor):* Patient can be aroused only by intense stimulation such as loud shouts and deep pressure over the supraorbital notch on both sides. Even this stimulation will evoke, in a stuporous patient, only minor nonverbal reaction of semi-purposeful withdrawal movement. Reflex reactions are usually preserved at this stage.
  d. *Grade IV (Coma):* Patient is unaware of his environments, and even intense painful stimuli evoke either minimum (moderately deep coma) or no response at all (deep coma). All reflex reactions are lost at this stage.

  *Herniation syndromes* result from increased intracranial pressure, and lead to brainstem compression, manifested by arterial hypertension, bradycardia, and respiratory irregularities (Cushing triad). In the initial stages of brainstem compression with only disturbed thalamic functions, there is only confusion, disorientation, and drowsiness. Later, as the midbrain gets involved, drowsiness deepens into stupor and then into coma. As more caudal parts of brainstem get involved, coma deepens, but recognition of the severity of coma is usually not possible at this stage.

- **Pattern of respiration:** In the early thalamic stage, respiration is usually normal but frequent sighing or yawning may occur. As the thalamic dysfunction increases, breathing acquires ***Cheyne-Stokes* character.** Later, with progression into ***midbrain and upper pons,*** Cheyne-Stokes respiration changes to central neurogenic hyperventilation characterized by sustained, deep, rapid and regular hyperpnea. At the *lower pontine and medullary level* compression, **hyperventilation ceases, and gives way to slow respiration, irregular in rate and depth which finally becomes gasping.**

- **Pupillary size and reaction:** The size, equality or inequality of the pupils and their reaction to light provide valuable localizing clues, and should be studied serially, using a strong beam of light.

  At the *thalamic stage,* the pupils are small but react to light. With *early midbrain involvement* the pupils become mid-dilated and nonreactive to light. As damage to the midbrain increases, the pupils become widely dilated and fixed. The *ciliospinal reflex* is also lost at this stage. *Pontine lesion,* usually a hemorrhage, results in very small pupils with minimal reaction to very strong light. Such alterations in pupillary responses generally imply structural brain lesion. *Toxic-metabolic states leave the pupils unaffected with few exceptions* such, as overdose with atropine

(widely dilated and fixed pupils) or opium (pin-point and barely reacting pupils).
- **Eye movements:** Certain eye movements also assist in localizing the site of lesion. Normally, sudden passive turning of the head to one side produces conjugate deviation of the eyes to the opposite side *(doll's eye movements)*. Absence of this *oculocephalic reflex* in a comatose patient implies dysfunction of the pons (where lateral gaze center is located), but does not differentiate between structural and toxic-metabolic pathology.
- **Motor responses:** Presence of local or unilateral paralysis indicates focal structural damage to the brain. This may be detected by alteration of deep reflexes and an extensor planter response on the paralyzed side. However, in the presence of deep coma, planter reflexes lose their significance and may be extensor on both sides.

In the early *thalamic stage* of compression there, may be a generalized increase in tone of all muscles, both flexors and extensors. **Decorticate posture** characterized primarily by fisted upper extremity held in full flexion against the body, occurs with late thalamic and *early midbrain* dysfunction. Later, with *more severe involvement of the midbrain,* **decerebrate state** occurs in which there is extension and adduction of all the four limbs with marked increase in tone. *Pontine-level* dysfunction is invariably associated with extensor posturing. With further deterioration and involvement of *pontomedullary junction,* total flaccidity, and hypotonia result, generally terminal.

A correlation of the observations recorded in respect of the above mentioned five parameters should permit identification and staging of the herniation syndrome in each case of coma. The salient features of these herniation syndromes are summarized in **Table 4.5**.

## *Critical Evaluation of Neurological Signs*

- In a midline *supratentorial mass with rapidly increasing compression* (e.g., diffuse cerebral edema, large subdural or intracerebral hematoma), there is a characteristic rostrocaudal progression of neurological signs starting with features of thalamic dysfunction. Delay in treatment at this stage may convert a recoverable into a nonrecoverable lesion as indicated by appearance of *signs of midbrain involvement,* such as deepening coma, mid-dilated, or widely dilated nonreacting pupils, deep rapid breathing, decerebrate rigidity, and absence of ciliospinal and oculocephalic reflexes.
- When *compression starts from one side* as in laterally placed subdural hematoma, tumor or inflammatory/infective process, the medial portion of the **ipsilateral** temporal lobe (the uncus) is the first to herniate through the tentorial notch. This results in the *uncal herniation syndrome,* characterized by ipsilateral dilated pupil (due to third nerve palsy) and contralateral hemiparesis (due to involvement of ipsilateral pyramidal fibers above the decussation) **(Table 4.5)**. In a few cases with rapidly expanding hemispheric lesions, the other pupil may also dilate in due

course, due to side to side displacement of the brainstem so that the midbrain is grooved by the opposite tentorial edge. Recognition and early treatment of uncal syndrome is most vital since recovery becomes virtually impossible once the opposite pupil dilates. With further increase in compression, the signs mimic those of the central transtentorial herniation.
- In cases with *toxic/metabolic coma,* unlike progressive brain compression, *there is no orderly deterioration in brainstem functions.* In fact, large scale disparities may exist between different parameters (e.g., barely reactive pupils in a patient who intermittently regains consciousness), and deep coma may be present out of proportion to neurological findings. Examination of pupillary reflexes is especially important, since these are preserved in all toxic/metabolic encephalopathies except when due to anoxia or certain drugs, which have specific effects on the pupils (vide supra).

## Investigations

Certain investigations should be done routinely in all cases of coma, and include urine examination, complete blood count, blood urea, sugar and electrolyte estimation, a CXR, and ECG. Non-enhanced CT scan of the brain should be considered when coma is unlikely to be due to toxic/metabolic disorders. *Lumbar puncture, if indicated, should be done preferably after CT brain.* In addition, in all cases suspected of poisoning a gastric lavage should be done and the stomach contents preserved for chemical examination.

## Management

### Emergency Treatment

Patient should be hospitalized as early as possible, and measures instituted to provide a clear airway, stable pulse, blood pressure, and respiration. As already stated, these should take precedence over detailed physical examination and laboratory studies.

### General Measures

- **Posture:** The patient should be nursed on the side (rather than in flat position), to minimize the risk of respiratory complications, and the position changed every few hours to prevent pressure sores. An air mattress or alfa-bed should be used, if the course of illness is likely to be a prolonged one. The bed clothes should be kept dry and free from creases. The limbs should be kept in the optimum position, lightly massaged, and moved through full range frequently, to avoid contractures and deep vein thrombosis. Care should be taken that the patient does not fall from the bed.
- **Nutrition and fluid balance:** As far as possible, nutrition and fluids should be provided every 2-3 hours through a nasogastric tube. Too hot and too

cold fluids must be avoided. The main risk is of aspiration pneumonia in such patients but this can be minimized by: (1) Aspirating the stomach contents before each feed to ensure the correct position of the tube, (2) Elevating the head of the patient during and for a short period after the feed, and (3) Restricting the volume of each feed to 200 mL.

The amount of fluid intake during the first few days should be carefully controlled in all cases where cerebral edema is a factor, especially in acute stroke. There is often a breakdown of blood brain barrier in the damaged area of the brain in such cases which is apt to retain fluid and thus develop cerebral edema. Oral route is to be preferred, but if IV fluid administration is necessary, isotonic saline (0.95%) or *(slightly) hypertonic glucose should be given (not 5.0% glucose which is slightly hypotonic,* isotonic glucose solution being 5.25%). Serum electrolytes should also be monitored.

❖ **Other measures:** Vital functions should be maintained keeping in view that normal autoregulation of blood flow is likely to be lost in the microvasculature in the damaged area especially in cases of ischemic infarction. *Sudden and drastic changes in blood pressure should therefore be avoided,* and hypertension treated only if the blood pressure is >180/110. Episodes of hypotension may be especially dangerous.

Patency of airways and adequate respiration must be ensured. Some patients who may have lost cough reflex and are likely to stay in coma for a long time, may require endotracheal intubation or even tracheostomy for proper removal of secretions. Oxygen therapy is generally beneficial, and some cases with significant respiratory depression may require assisted ventilation. Seizures may occur and are best controlled by phenytoin, since it does not further depress level of consciousness. Neurosurgical consultation should also be considered in suitable cases.

### Specific Measures

*Treatment of increased intracranial pressure (ICP):* Lowering ICP is a vital component of management of comatose patients developing herniation syndromes. This is best reflected by calculating cerebral perfusion pressure (CPP) defined as mean arterial pressure minus ICP. As far as possible, CPP should be maintained >70-80 mm Hg. However, this is possible only in advanced neurological centers. In the absence of ICP monitoring, hyperventilation to a $PaCO_2$ 30-35 mm Hg should be initiated, followed by IV mannitol (0.25-1.0 g/kg). Another measure is use of barbiturates which decrease cerebral metabolism, and thereby reduce cerebral blood flow.

## CEREBROVASCULAR CATASTROPHES (STROKE)

Acute vascular disruption to a specific region of the brain ("stroke") is the second most frequent cause of death world-wide, and constitutes one of the commonest medical emergencies. The term "stroke" originates from biblical reference to being "struck down", implying an acute dramatic neurologic

> **Box 4.2: Classifications of stroke.**
> 
> ☐ **Ischemic stroke**
>   ➢ Transient ischemic attacks (TIA)
>   ➢ Thrombotic stroke (cerebral thrombosis)
>     ♦ Large artery cerebral thrombosis
>     ♦ Lacunar stroke
>   ➢ Embolic stroke (thromboembolism)
>     ♦ Artery-to-artery embolus
>     ♦ Cardio-embolic
> ☐ **Hemorrhagic stroke**
>   ➢ Intracerebral hemorrhage
>   ➢ Subarachnoid hemorrhage

event. The "stroke syndrome" is due either to ischemia or hemorrhage (**Box 4.2**). Ischemia is caused by either blockage of a blood vessel via thrombosis or arterial embolism, or by cerebral hypoperfusion. Hemorrhagic stroke is caused by bleeding of the blood vessels of the brain, either directly into the brain parenchyma (intracerebral hemorrhage) or into the subarachnoid space surrounding brain tissue (subarachnoid hemorrhage). Occasionally, the cerebrovascular (CV) pathology is confined to the cerebral venous system.

## Clinical Evaluation of Stroke

The aim of clinical evaluation should be to determine the *type and magnitude of the stroke*. The history and a careful neurological examination should provide valuable information. A history of recent trauma must always be excluded. Hemorrhagic stroke is often heralded by headache, and generally occurs at a younger age than thrombotic stroke. Presence of hypertension, diabetes mellitus and coronary artery disease reflect underlying atherosclerotic disease and favor vessel thrombosis. On the other hand, atrial fibrillation, valvular heart disease, or recent myocardial infarction will favor cerebral embolism. A *history of recent TIA* can be very significant. Transient neurological deficits occurring in the same vascular territory suggest thrombotic stroke. In contrast, multiple TIAs involving different vascular distributions favor embolic process.

Accurate history of onset and any fluctuations in symptoms is very useful. *A sudden onset of symptoms suggests embolic or hemorrhagic stroke while a progressive or stuttering deficit will favor thrombotic stroke or stroke due to hypoperfusion. Carotid bruit should be looked for and in suspected cases severity of stenosis assessed by Doppler studies. Carotid arteriogram, however, remains the gold standard.*

## Investigations

Besides routine laboratory work up, emergent investigations include blood sugar estimation, an ECG, and non-contrast CT scan of the head. CT brain is very sensitive in detection of hemorrhage, and can reveal valuable information in such cases: (1) Differentiate between ischemic and hemorrhagic stroke (this has important therapeutic implications), (2) Determine the exact location of pathology, presence of prior infarction(s), shift of brain contents, (3) Exclude other pathologies that may mimic stroke (subdural hematoma, tumor, abscess etc.), and (4) Provide important prognostic information since large strokes (involving more than 30% of a hemisphere) are at high risk for hemorrhagic transformation in next 48–72 hours.

However, a *CT scan has certain limitations*. The scan may be normal for up to 48 hours in acute infarction (it cannot differentiate early infarct tissue from normal tissue). It may also be normal in TIAs, in brainstem infarcts, and in many cases of lacunar infarction. These latter conditions are better defined by MRI. In select cases, 4-vessel MRI angiography may be considered to delineate the cerebral arteries in their entire course.

Cardiac assessment is mandatory in every stroke patient, and includes a careful clinical examination, ECG, and an echocardiogram when indicated. Cardiac features to look for include evidence of valvular disease, fresh coronary damage, arrhythmia, or cardiac decompensation.

### *General Principles in Stroke Management*

When consciousness is impaired, proper airway and respiration should be ensured. Oxygen therapy is generally beneficial in such patients. To avoid increase in ICP, head should be elevated to 15–30 degrees, acute flexion or turning of the head avoided, and tracheostomy ties and bandages applied loosely. Fluid balance should be kept slightly below maintenance level using isotonic fluids (5% glucose solution is slightly hypotonic). Lactated Ringer's solution should not be used. Hypotension is dangerous and must be avoided as it may decrease cerebral perfusion in the ischemic region. Electrolytes should be regularly monitored, and hyponatremia avoided as this may worsen cerebral edema.

Any associated disease should be quickly diagnosed and appropriately managed. If hypertension is detected it should be remembered that it may be a physiological response to cerebral ischemia, and that BP often normalizes within 24–48 hours. *Management of persistent hypertension varies in ischemic and hemorrhagic strokes.* In the former, hypertension should be treated only if severe or moderately severe (systolic pressure >190 mm Hg and/or diastolic pressure >110 mm Hg), and *blood pressure reduced gradually over several hours.* In hemorrhagic stroke, on the other hand, severe hypertension should be controlled rapidly (see section on "Hypertensive Crisis").

*Hyperglycemia* is not uncommon in the acute stage of stroke. However, the importance of strict control of blood glucose is not clear. Mild to moderate increase in blood glucose does not per se result in brain injury. Very high levels should be controlled with small doses of soluble insulin administered every 6–8 hours. Aggressive control is not recommended since even transient hypoglycemia is likely to be dangerous.

*Seizures* are a frequent complication of stroke, occur usually within the first few days of the event, are more common with large infarcts, and can be devastating in patients with SAH. The need for prophylactic anticonvulsant therapy should be assessed on patient characteristics, but is almost mandatory in patients with SAH.

*Possible complications* should be kept in mind especially formation of pressure sores, deep venous thrombosis, acute gastric erosions, and aspiration pneumonia in patients on tube feeding. It is easier to prevent bed sores than treat them. Proper positioning of the patient coupled with careful padding, turnings and use of therapeutic beds can be rewarding. Physiotherapy must be instituted early and continued for at least 3–6 months which is the most important period of functional recovery. Therapy with low molecular-weight heparin should be considered in stroke victims likely to be confined to bed for prolonged period. Gastric stress ulcers should be prevented by proton-pump inhibitors and sucralfate. Enteral feeding reduces the risk of acute gastric erosions, and should be instituted early.

# ISCHEMIC STROKE

This is generally due to *cerebral arterial thrombosis or embolism* but can also result from *systemic hypoperfusion* with resultant ischemia and hypoxia *(ischemic-anoxic encephalopathy)*. In the latter condition, regions of the brain (often multiple) with the most marginal vascular supply (i.e., border-zones lying between principal intracerebral arteries) are most often affected. Depending upon the time course of neurologic signs, ischemic stroke may be a transitional episode *(transient ischemic attack)* or a progressing/completed stroke *(thromboembolic stroke)*. In about one-third of all ischemic strokes, there is no obvious explanation/cause, and these are termed as "cryptogenic".

## Transient Ischemic Attacks

Transient ischemic attacks (TIAs) are brief and reversible episodes of focal dysfunction of the brain, without any clinical squeal, and a normal neuroimaging study. The symptoms come suddenly, reach the peak within a few seconds or minutes, and last for an hour or two (always less than 24 hours). TIAs often precede a stroke, and therefore should be properly evaluated.

### Etiology

Transient ischemic attacks result from either an intermittent decrease in perfusion in an area of the brain ("low flow" with inadequate collateral circulation) or from some type of embolization. The latter explains why recurrent TIAs may occur in different parts of the territory supplied by the same major cerebral artery. The emboli may arise from a cardiac source or from platelet-fibrin (atherosclerotic) material in the aortic arch or large arteries in the neck *("artery-to-artery embolus")*. Less common causes include fibromuscular dysplasia or inflammatory disorders involving cerebral arteries.

## Clinical Features

The characteristic feature of TIAs is their *abrupt onset and rapid recovery within minutes or hours.* The specific symptoms will vary according to the arterial territory involved. Carotid arterial system is most often involved and in such cases, possible symptoms include transient hemiparesis, hemisensory loss, monocular blindness, lower facial weakness, aphasia, dysarthria, and visual field loss. Though carotid arteries may be involved at any point in their course, the cervical portion needs careful examination (for intensity of pulsations and/or any bruit) since the pathology here is particularly amenable to specific treatment.

## Management

Most of the patients with TIA can be treated at home. Hospitalization is advisable in patients:
- Presenting within 48 hours of the first attack
- TIAs occurring in a crescendo pattern
- Symptoms persisting for >1 hour
- **Symptomatic carotid stenosis or a known source of emboli exists**

1. **Antiplatelet therapy:** Aspirin in a dose of 75–325 mg daily is the accepted antiplatelet regimen in patients with TIA. It can prevent the stroke, and probably decrease severity even if stroke occurs. *Clopidogrel* is another antiplatelet drug, which may be prescribed (75 mg/day) to patients intolerant to aspirin or to those who have had an ischemic event despite taking aspirin. However, *combination of* **aspirin and Clopidogrel does not** *appear to* **offer greater benefit** *than* **aspirin alone.**
2. **Surgical interventions:** *(a) Carotid endarterectomy:* This procedure is used to remove atherosclerotic plaque from a blocked carotid artery, and has been found useful in preventing future strokes. The procedure is indicated when the vessel has 70-99% blockage, *(b) Carotid angioplasty and stent placement.* This is now widely in use, and has a high degree of technical success with low complication rates. Currently, this non-invasive procedure is increasingly recommended as alternative to carotid endarterectomy.
3. **General measures:** Care must be taken to control comorbid conditions (especially hypertension, diabetes, and hyperlipidemia) as well as life-style aberrations that promote thrombo-occlusive disorders.

## Thrombotic Stroke (Cerebral Thrombosis)

Cerebral thrombosis usually results from atherosclerotic disease especially involving large vessels—the common and internal carotids, vertebrals and Circle of Willis. The occlusion may involve the main artery, but generally one of the principal branches is affected. Less often, thrombosis involves small penetrating arteries resulting in very small cerebral infarcts (lacunar stroke). The clinical picture varies in these two types:

## Lacunar Stroke (Penetrating Artery Disease)

Lacunar infarcts are a form of thrombotic stroke that involve smaller arteries inside the brain, viz., *branches of the circle of Willis, middle cerebral artery, and arteries arising from the distal vertebral and basilar artery.* Any of these penetrating branches can get blocked either by thrombosis at its origin or by marked narrowing of its lumen due to muscular (medial) hypertrophy secondary to chronic hypertension and aging. The narrowed lumen causes distal ischemia resulting in TIAs or infarcts in the territory supplied by the penetrating branches.

The small deep infarcts often cavitate leaving small holes traversed by fine fibrous strands—*"lacunae"/"lacunar infarcts".* Such lacunar infarcts are primarily located in the basal ganglia and pons.

### Clinical features

Lacunar infarcts being small (generally <1 cm$^3$) do not result in significant cerebral edema, and therefore are not associated with symptoms, such as headache, impaired consciousness, or vomiting. On the other hand, because these events occur deep within the brain in the region of the internal capsule where neurons are densely grouped, the neurological deficit is often large (e.g., hemiplegia rather than monoplegia). For the same reason (unlike cortical infarcts), deficits of the face, arm, and leg are typically of equal intensity. Clinically, three well-defined lacunar syndromes can be recognized depending upon the precise location of the lacuna:

1. *Pure motor hemiplegia* due to a lacuna in the internal capsule or pontine base. There are no accompanying important sensory, visual, or cognitive abnormalities.
2. *Pure sensory stroke* resulting in or numbness of the face, arm, and leg on the side opposite to a lacuna in the lateral thalamus or posterior limb of internal capsule.
3. *Ataxic-hemiparesis stroke,* which produces a combination of weakness and ataxia in the arm and/or leg, and occasionally dysarthria, without any sensory loss. The lacunar pathology, in such cases, is in the opposite pons or internal carotid artery.

## Large Artery Cerebral Thrombosis (Cerebral Infarction)

### Clinical features

When one of the large cerebral arteries is occluded, severe, and prolonged ischemia occurs with resultant death of the involved brain tissue. Since, thrombotic occlusion commonly occurs as a gradual process, the symptoms and signs that follow usually develop slowly (compared to embolism or hemorrhage). Thrombosis commonly occurs at night, and a patient who awakens in the morning with a new deficit has probably had a thrombotic stroke.

Since, thrombolytic therapy is being increasingly employed in the acute treatment of thrombotic stroke, the goal should be to determine the exact time of onset of symptoms as the current recommended window of opportunity

> Box 4.3: Common clinical manifestations of stroke syndrome according to vascular supply.

- Anterior cerebral artery
  - Weakness of contralateral extremity (lower limb >upper limb)
  - Bowel and bladder incontinence
  - Altered mentation
- Middle cerebral artery
  - Contralateral hemiparesis (upper limb > lower limb)
  - Contralateral sensory deficits
  - Dysphasia (if dominant hemisphere involved)
- Posterior cerebral artery
  - Contralateral visual field defects
  - Cortical blindness
  - Altered mentation
- Vertebrobasilar arteries
  - Acute vertigo
  - Dysarthria
  - Dysphagia
  - Nystagmus
  - Contralateral superficial sensory deficits (pain and temperature)

for fibrinolytic therapy is 3 hours. Patients who awake with symptoms are considered to have had onset at the time they were last "normal" neurologically (when they went to sleep).

The type of neurologic deficit in each case depends upon the anatomical location of the lesion and the possible vessel(s) involved. Consequently, a variety of "ischemic stroke syndromes" with distinctive patterns may occur **(Box 4.3 and Fig. 4.1)**. Their detailed description is beyond the scope of this text. However, it may be added that when a large artery is involved and occlusion occurs rather rapidly, varying degree of cerebral edema is an invariable accompaniment. This may manifest as impairment in consciousness **(from drowsiness to deep coma), headache, vomiting, hiccup, pupillary abnormalities, and occasionally, disturbed** cardiac and respiratory functions.

*Management*

It is important to realize that occlusion of a cerebral artery does not necessarily indicate immediate complete infarction of the related territory. While certain neurons in the center of the ischemic tissue exposed to extreme deprivation of nutrients die within minutes, *there is a large portion of the affected territory, which may not be functioning (as revealed by neurological deficit) but is still not irreversibly damaged, and can therefore be salvaged.* These are regions of hypoperfusion but preserved oxygen metabolism in which neural damage continues for several hours after the acute episode *("therapeutic window for reperfusion in ischemic infarcts")*. This is the basis of the use of fibrinolytic agents in these cases.

# Chapter 4: Neurological Emergencies

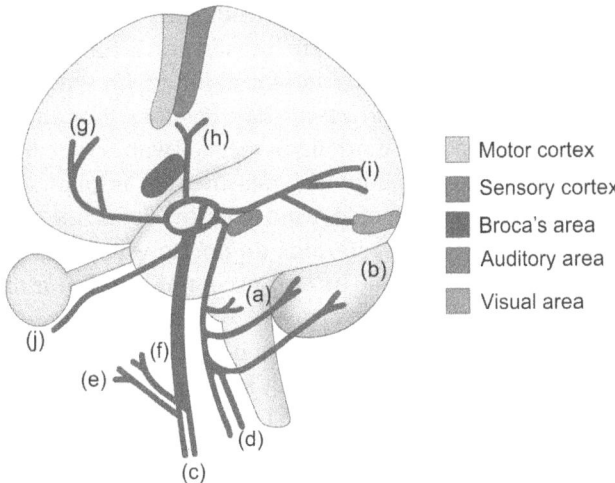

**Fig. 4.1:** Schematic diagram of the arteries supplying the brain. (a) Brainstem; (b) Cerebellum; (c) 2 common carotids; (d) 2 vertebral arteries forming single basilar; (e) 2 external carotids; (f) 2 internal carotids; (g) Anterior cerebrals; (h) Middle cerebrals; (i) Posterior cerebrals and (j) Ophthalmics.

- **Thrombolysis:** Intravenous thrombolysis with tissue plasminogen activator (tPA) is now an accepted and effective treatment in reducing the neurological deficit in proven thrombotic infarction, after CT has excluded intracranial hemorrhage or a multilobar infarction. The standard dosage is 0.9 mg/kg (maximum of 90 mg) of which 10% is given as a bolus over 1 minute and the remainder over 1 hour. The *limiting factor is that thrombolytic therapy must be administered within 4.5 hours after onset of ischemic stroke (or last-known normal state).* Later administration has not been found effective or safe.

  The treatment is *contraindicated in the presence of hypertension* (systolic and/or diastolic pressure >190 and 110 mm Hg, respectively). Other contraindications include: (1) Myocardial infarction in the previous 3 months, (2) Patients with recent hemorrhage or at increased risk of bleeding, (3) Any major surgery in the previous 14 days, and (4) Patients on oral anticoagulants, or with a platelet count <100,000/mm$^3$. It is also essential to fully discuss with the patient and the relatives the potential risks and benefits of tPA therapy.

  It is to be understood that thrombolysis does not improve chances of survival. Benefit is mostly in respect of degree of recovery, and living without disability. Benefit is greater the earlier it is used. The intervention carries a small risk of intracranial hemorrhage, and there is no way to predict who may develop it.

- **Mechanical thrombectomy:** This may be **considered** in **cases** with a **major stroke** due to **occlusion** of the **middle cerebral artery** that **presents within 24 hours** regardless of prior tPA administration. **This intervention must be done only in** specialized stroke centers with experienced staff.

- **Decongestive measures:** Local cerebral edema is the most common cause of neurological deterioration, in such cases, and is directly related to the severity of ischemic brain injury and the rapidity with which it develops. It is *maximal between third and seventh day after the stroke,* and accounts for much of the morbidity and mortality associated with acute cerebrovascular catastrophes. Available therapeutic measures are as follows:
  - *Corticosteroids:* Though often used in brain edema due to brain tumor and other mass lesions, steroids do not appear to have any role in cerebral ischemic events. The only exception possibly is the presence of *extensive vasogenic edema* in cases with massive cerebral infarction and intracerebral hemorrhage (which may behave like a mass lesion). In such cases, these agents probably benefit by their anti-inflammatory and membrane-stabilizing effects by inhibiting release of arachidonic acid products. Dexamethasone is usually prescribed, 8 mg IV initially, followed by 12–16 mg daily in divided doses for 5–7 days.
  - *Diuretics:* Loop diuretics (e.g., furosemide) help to reduce brain edema chiefly by inducing brisk diuresis that reduces intravascular volume. Furosemide 40–60 mg should be given initially IV followed by oral therapy in a dose of 40–80 mg daily for 7–10 days with a close watch on electrolyte levels and fluid intake-output.
  - *Hyperosmolar solutions:* These work as osmotic (and dehydrating) agents and thus help reduce ICP. There is little evidence, however, of any lasting benefit. Mannitol 20% is commonly used in a dose of l g/kg within 1 hour followed by 0.3 g/kg every 6–8 hours for 5–7 days. Prolonged/excessive therapy may worsen the situation.
- **Control of hypertension:** Transient and mild to moderate rise in blood pressure is common in acute stroke, and reflects a compensatory response to maintain cerebral perfusion in the face of acute cerebral ischemia. Also, during acute phase of cerebral ischemia, there is loss of cerebral autoregulation, and lowering of blood pressure may further compromise ischemic areas. Blood pressure reduction should, therefore, be done *only when systolic pressure exceeds 200 mm Hg, and that too only gradually over several hours.*

## Embolic Stroke (Cerebral Embolism)

### Etiology

Embolic stroke refers to the blockage of an artery by an arterial thrombus (from atheromatous plaques in the cervical arteries or from thrombi in the heart). The former usually result in TIAs and the latter in bigger embolic infarcts. Cardiac conditions, which may give rise to such emboli include atrial fibrillation and paroxysmal atrial fibrillation, mitral stenosis, mitral prolapse, bacterial endocarditis, artificial heart valves, atrial myxoma, and mural thrombosis in cases of myocardial infarction and cardiomyopathy. Uncommon causes include air or fat embolism, and paradoxical embolism when deep leg vein thrombi reach the brain through a right-to-left intracardiac shunt *(paradoxical embolus)*.

### Clinical Features

The onset of cardio-embolic stroke is abrupt and symptoms usually are maximal at start. Embolic stroke occurs more often when the patient is awake and active rather than during sleep which is usual for thrombotic stroke. However, since there is no intrinsic disease of the blood vessels, emboli are less adherent to the vessel wall, and hence more *likely to fragment and move distally than clots due to thrombosis*. Therefore, rapid neurological improvement may occur.

Because emboli float in the circulation until encountering a vessel with a sufficiently small lumen, most *embolic strokes involve distal small cortical vessels*, usually in the middle cerebral artery territory. Less often, posterior circulation is involved producing isolated posterior cerebral artery syndromes.

### Management

Broad principles of management of embolic stroke are the same as for thrombotic infarction. The chief difference is in respect of anticoagulation. Ideally, all cases of cardioembolic stroke should be *heparinized at the earliest (after CT has excluded cerebral hemorrhage)* to reduce the risk of re-embolism. However, when embolism is associated with a large infarct or with extensive cerebral edema, it may be safer to delay anticoagulation by 2-3 days (even up to 4-5 days) as such changes indicate a higher risk of bleeding within the infarct. In such cases, a CT should be repeated in 3-5 days, and heparin started only if no hemorrhagic transformation has occurred. For details of anticoagulation, see section on "thrombotic stroke".

*Anticoagulation does not affect the acute course of the disease;* its chief aim is to prevent the risk of recurrent stroke, which is quite high within weeks to months of the initial event. When used, heparin should be followed after 48 hours by oral anticoagulants and heparin discontinued after 5 days allowing 24-48 hours overlap with heparin. The duration of chronic anticoagulation is controversial. It should be continued for more than 6 months (preferably life-long) in patients with cardiogenic cerebral embolism, and for 3-6 months when source of embolus is suspected to be in the large arteries in the neck (shorter period if surgical treatment is instituted earlier). If, for some reason, long term anticoagulation is not possible, aspirin may provide some prophylaxis.

## ■ HEMORRHAGIC STROKE

Hemorrhagic strokes are much less common (20%) as compared to ischemic **strokes** (80%), but carry a higher **mortality. Bleeding may occur within the brain** substance *(intracerebral hemorrhage),* **or in the membranes** surrounding the brain *(subarachnoid hemorrhage)*. **Of the two types, intracerebral hemorrhage (ICH) is more common.**

## Intracerebral Hemorrhage

### Etiology

Intracerebral hemorrhage usually occurs in elderly patients with established *hypertension.* Bleeding occurs primarily in the brain parenchyma, although blood may appear in the cerebrospinal fluid. The most common cause is advancing age and damage to intracerebral arterioles by long standing hypertension. Occasionally, ICH is due to arteriovenous malformation, bleeding diathesis, thrombolytic therapy, anticoagulation, trauma, angiopathy, or drug abuse.

### Clinical Features

The onset of intracerebral hemorrhage is abrupt and symptoms progress within a few minutes to a few hours. The leak probably occurs from micro-aneurysms on small perforating vessels which develop in hypertensive patients. The most common site for hypertensive ICH is basal ganglia followed by pons, thalamus, cerebellum, and cerebral white matter. The extravasated blood can extend into the ventricular system or subarachnoid space resulting in signs of meningeal irritation. Headache and vomiting are common, and seizures are more frequent than in ischemic stroke. However, no specific signs or symptoms reliably distinguish between ICH and ischemic stroke.

Neurological features vary according to the site and extent of hemorrhage. While small intracranial bleed may produce only focal symptoms, a large hematoma often results in features of mass effect of hematoma with displacement and compression of adjacent brain tissue resulting in decreased level of consciousness. Deep coma usually indicates a very large hemorrhage and suggests a grave prognosis. *Hemorrhagic stroke can have any one of the three classical neurological presentations:*

1. *Hemiplegia,* purely motor or sometimes combined with sensory impairment. This is usually due to involvement of thalamus or basal ganglia. Thalamic hemorrhage commonly produces hemi-anesthesia more prominent than hemiplegia, along with impaired upward gaze.
2. *Quadriparesis* of sudden onset when hemorrhage is in the region of the pons. Such patients usually develop coma along with mid-position eyes, and pinpoint pupils.
3. *Ataxia* associated with cerebellar abnormalities, with absent or mild hemiparesis, are characteristic of cerebellar hemorrhage. A quick diagnosis of hypertensive cerebellar hemorrhage is very important since fatal brainstem compression may occur rapidly. Emergency surgical decompression can be lifesaving in such cases.

**Primary ICH** often occurs suddenly, more often during physical activity, with impairment of consciousness in majority of cases. The *outcome is relatively* *good,* the hematoma is located in the subcortical white matter, intermediate in supratentorial hematomas, and almost uniformly grave in posterior fossa hemorrhage (brainstem compression).

## Management

The *general principles of management of ICH* are conservative and supportive. Appropriate care of the airway, breathing and circulation is of primary concern. Decongestive measures are indicated only in patients with evidence of increased intracranial pressure (such as mass effect, midline shift, or herniation on CT). Hypertension should be controlled *rapidly* (by intravenous medication) if the systolic pressure is >200 mm Hg, and gradually when it is around 180 mm Hg.

**Surgical intervention** should be considered in all cases of ICH early in the course of the disease, since the compressive effects of hematoma (including life-threatening herniation syndromes) may be reversible only in the initial stage. *Decompression is helpful* when a large superficial cortical hematoma is exerting mass effect. More urgent surgery is indicated in posterior fossa hemorrhage especially if the hematoma is more than 3 cm in diameter, or has ruptured into the third ventricle. Spontaneous unpredictable deterioration is common in such cases, while early surgical evacuation may lead to substantial recovery in neurological deficit.

## Subarachnoid Hemorrhage

### Etiology

Subarachnoid hemorrhage (SAH) is usually due to rupture of a saccular or berry aneurysm (80%) or arteriovenous malformation (AVM). Other causes include trauma, bleeding from other types of aneurysms (atherosclerotic, mycotic), or as a consequence of blood dyscrasia and anticoagulation. Most of the intracranial aneurysms (IA) are located in the anterior circulation, usually at the base of the brain at the bifurcation of arteries of the circle of Willis. In the posterior circulation, berry aneurysms are usually located at the junction of the vertebral artery and posterior inferior cerebellar artery, and bifurcation of basilar artery. In about a quarter of cases, multiple IA (two or three) may be found.

### Pathology

Intracranial arteries are prone to aneurysm formation as they lack external elastic lamina, and adventitia is very thin. Further, in the saccular or berry aneurysm, tunica media is either very thin or absent, and internal elastic lamina is absent or fragmented. Consequently, the wall of IA is generally composed of only intima and adventitia. Rupture commonly occurs during stress or in association with activities that increase the blood pressure.

### Clinical Features

The mean age of presentation of aneurysmal SAH is 55 years (usual age 45–60 years), and the risk for **women is somewhat greater than in** men. Classically, SAH is **characterized by acute onset of severe headache (often described as the *"worst headache of life"*. The headache usually develops during exertion, may be generalized or localized to neck/occipital region, and may be accompanied by vomiting, transitory weakness, or loss of consciousness.** In a few cases, prodromal episodes of severe headache lasting for hours *(thunderclap headaches)* may occur days or weeks before index SAH. Such symptoms usually represent minor leaks into the wall of the aneurysm or into the subarachnoid space *("warning leak")*, and are often misdiagnosed as migraine, tension-type headache, viral infections, etc. It is important to remember that *a first episode of acute severe headache should not be dismissed as migraine or tension-type headache.* Consciousness is usually impaired following the headache, the depth and duration of coma depending on the site and extent of the hemorrhage. Some cases may have *seizure* at onset.

**Clinical signs** *are a mix of increased intracranial pressure and meningeal irritation.* The former is due to rapid entry of "extra fluid" into the closed cranial cavity, and may manifest as restlessness, confusion, and diminished level of consciousness. Meningeal irritation is indicated by neck stiffness and Kernig and Brudzinski signs (unless the patient is in deep coma). However, since meningeal irritation is caused by the breakdown of blood products within the subarachnoid space, *neck stiffness may not develop until several hours after the hemorrhage.* In some cases, circulation of this bloody cerebrospinal fluid down the spinal axis produces severe low back pain ("lumbosciatica syndrome") which may overshadow the head or neck pain.

**Focal neurological deficit** is absent except when hemorrhage tears into the brain substance, or cerebral ischaemia/infarction occurs due to vasospasm in the vessel adjoining the clotted blood. This usually manifests as cranial nerve dysfunction or motor weakness. *Funduscopy* may be completely normal or reveal some papilledema with venous congestion and unilateral or bilateral retinal or subhyaloid hemorrhages.

The clinical course of SAH is uncertain, but the most important predictor of the outcome is the patient's clinical condition on arrival at the hospital. Depending upon the level of consciousness and extent of neurological deficits, *severity of SAH can be graded* as given at **Table 4.6**.

Another grading system of subarachnoid bleeds is based on patient's condition on presentation **(Table 4.7)** as defined by the World Federation of Neurological Surgeons:

### Diagnosis

The *symptom-triad of sudden onset headache, vomiting, and impairment of consciousness is highly suggestive of SAH.* Difficulty may arise in patients who are febrile, or have prominent focal neurological signs. Differentiation will be required from bacterial meningitis and intracranial space occupying lesion.

**Table 4.6:** Clinical grading of SAH.

| Grades | Severity of SAH |
|---|---|
| Grade 1 | Asymptomatic or only mild headache/neck rigidity |
| Grade 2 | Increasing headache, neck rigidity, cranial nerve palsy; no focal deficit |
| Grade 3 | Confusion, drowsiness, mild focal deficit ± |
| Grade 4 | Stupor, motor deficit, even early decerebrate rigidity |
| Grade 5 | Deep coma, decerebrate rigidity |

**Table 4.7:** Grading of SAH (World Federation of Neurological Surgeons).

| Grades | Glasgow Coma Score |
|---|---|
| I | 15 |
| II | 14 or 13 without motor deficit |
| III | 14 or 13 with motor deficit |
| IV | 12–7 with or without deficit |
| V | 6–3 with or without deficit |

**Table 4.8:** Severity/Grades of SAH on CT scan.

| Grades | CT findings |
|---|---|
| I | Normal (no blood visualized) |
| II | A diffuse deposition or thin layer with all vertical layers of blood < 1 mm thick |
| III | Localized clots and/or vertical layers of blood 1 mm or greater in thickness |
| IV | Diffuse or no subarachnoid blood, but with intracerebral or intravascular clots |

The first diagnostic study should be a *non-contrast CT scan of the brain,* which is 98% accurate within the first 12 hours (CT sensitivity decreases over time and may be <50% after 7–10 days).

Lumbar puncture should be performed only if CT is negative but the suspicion of SAH remains high. Cerebrospinal fluid (CSF) examination is also required if there is the least suspicion of meningitis, but only after CT has excluded SAH. Spinal fluid showing xanthochromia is diagnostic. However, it takes 12 hours after the bleeding for spinal fluid to become xanthochromic, and it will remain xanthochromic for about 2 weeks. Blood in CSF may be due either to SAH or traumatic lumbar puncture. The standard method of decreasing red cell count in successive tubes to identify traumatic lumbar puncture is questionable. If the diagnosis is still in doubt angiography may be indicated.

CT scan of the brain in SAH also helps in grading the pathology and assessing overall prognosis (Fisher scale, **Table 4.8**). MRI study is more useful during subacute or chronic phase of illness when CT findings may have reverted to normal; *during the acute stage, MRI is less sensitive than CT study.*

**Localization of aneurysm(s):** *Angiography* is the gold standard in imaging cerebral aneurysms. Better results may be available with two new techniques—*CT angiography* (CTA) and *magnetic resonance angiography* (MRA). CTA is easier to perform in critically ill patients, and has sensitivity between 70-100%. The advantage of MRA is that it can detect very small lesions (even 2-3 mm) in diameter, and is especially useful in detecting thrombus in the aneurysmal sac.

## Management

The general principles of management especially with regard to unconscious state and brain edema, if present, are the same as in "thrombotic infarction". *Specific management of SAH is aimed to: (i) Tide the patient over the immediate crisis, (ii) Prevent cerebral artery vasospasm, and (iii) Avoid recurrence of bleeding.*

- **Immediate measures:** Complete bed rest in a quiet room should be advised for the first few days, and unnecessary manipulation of the patient avoided. Only mild sedation is advised to control restlessness since deeper sedation may interfere with periodic neurological assessment.
- **Special measures**
  - *Hypertension:* Elevated blood pressure must be controlled quickly and kept within safe limits until the aneurysm has been secured. Too drastic reduction in blood pressure may interfere with cerebral perfusion pressure.
  - *Seizures:* These are not uncommon and increase the risk of rebleeding after SAH. Prophylactic use of anticonvulsants is, therefore, recommended in all cases of SAH. Most commonly used drug is phenytoin (loading dose 15 mg/kg administered over 1-2 hours) followed by 300 mg/day.
  - *Vasospasm:* Cerebral artery vasospasm is a frequent complication of SAH, and can result in high morbidity and mortality rates. It usually involves arteries at the base of the brain (anterior, middle, or posterior cerebral arteries) where blood collects after SAH. Cerebral vasospasm develops between 4 and 14 days after the bleed, and is maximal about 7 days. Clinically, vasospasm results in delayed cerebral ischemia with consequent increase in cerebral edema and a focal neurological deficit depending upon the artery involved.

There are no specific agents to control or even ameliorate the vasospasm. Nimodipine (Nimotop) 60 mg every 4-6 hours is recommended usually for 2-3 weeks. Hemodynamic augmentation by IV fluids (hypervolemia, hemodilution, and induced hypertension—triple "H" therapy) has been suggested. Mean arterial pressure should be maintained around 110 mm Hg.

**Prevention of aneurysmal rebleeding:** Aneurysmal rebleeding may be secondary to hypertension or aneurysmal clot fibrinolysis, the risk being maximal within a few days of the initial episode. Early intervention (within

2-3 days of the hemorrhage) is, therefore, strongly recommended. The procedures available are craniotomy and clipping of the base of the aneurysm or *interventional endovascular coiling*.

## Summary

- Stroke syndromes constitute one of the most common emergencies in medical practice. It is a dreaded disease not only on account of the initial high mortality but more so because of its frequent crippling sequel.
- Strokes are classically divided into ischemic and hemorrhagic. The former can be due to thrombosis, embolism, or hypoperfusion. Hemorrhagic stroke may be intracerebral or subarachnoid.
- A history of TIAs is important, because it is a powerful warning sign of impending stroke.
- CT brain is the most valuable investigation in the diagnosis and treatment of stroke patients.
- Hypertension is often recorded in patients with ischemic strokes. It is important to realize that it may be only an adaptive response of cerebral autoregulation, and should not be over-treated.
- Anticoagulation is of unproven value in the acute management of ischemic stroke; its main role is to prevent recurrences in patients with cardio-embolic stroke.
- Fibrinolytic therapy in "selected" cases of thrombotic stroke improves quality of life after survival in some patients. It has no effect on survival rates.

## HYPERTENSIVE ENCEPHALOPATHY

Hypertensive encephalopathy (HE) is an acute neurological dysfunction induced by acute rise in blood pressure *(hypertensive crisis)*. **The exact levels at which encephalopathy may develop varies according to previous blood pressure status.**

**In** chronic hypertension, **because** of **structural** thickening of the **arterioles, encephalopathy usually occurs** with **severe and sustained elevation** of **blood** pressure. However, in patients previously normotensive, severe encephalopathy may occur even with relatively little hypertension, e.g., in cases of eclampsia or in children with acute glomerulonephritis.

The *mechanism of hypertensive encephalopathy* is not understood. In normotensive subjects, cerebral autoregulation maintains a relatively constant cerebral blood flow at a mean arterial pressure (MAP) in the range of 60-90 mm Hg. In chronically hypertensive patients, autoregulation is altered and shifted upward to a higher MAP to maintain effective cerebral blood flow. An acute rise in blood pressure in such cases possibly induces cerebral arterial spasm resulting in cerebral ischemia.

## Clinical Features

Symptoms and signs are a *mix of diffuse cerebral dysfunction (due to cerebral edema) and focal neurological damage*. The former include severe headache, nausea, vomiting, and altered mental status ranging from lethargy and confusion to coma. Focal findings include seizures, cranial nerve palsies, blindness, aphasia, and a varying degree of paralysis of one or more limbs.

*A characteristic feature of HE is clearing of the altered sensorium within hours of control of blood pressure,* followed by rapid recovery in neurological deficits. However, if uncontrolled severe hypertension persists, hypertensive encephalopathy may progress into ischemic or hemorrhagic stroke.

## Diagnosis

In the acute phase, differentiation from ischemic or hemorrhagic stroke may be virtually impossible. It must also be distinguished from other disorders associated with alteration in mental status in which elevated blood pressure may be a coincidental finding (such as hypoglycemia, meningitis, encephalitis, subarachnoid hemorrhage). Routine blood sampling, ECG, chest X-ray, arterial blood gas analysis, and cranial CT scan are required. Diagnosis depends essentially on normal brain scans and a quick clinical recovery (during the next 24-48 hours) following rapid and effective lowering of blood pressure.

## Management

The goal of treatment in HE should be to lower the blood pressure rapidly (within 2-6 hours), taking care to avoid excessive blood pressure reduction, which may induce ischemic events (stroke or coronary ischemia). It is usually safe to reduce MAP by 25% and lower the diastolic blood pressure to 100-110 mm Hg. Additionally, cerebral edema should be taken care of, and, if the patient is comatose, general measures instituted as described in the section on "The Unconscious Patient". The patient should be hospitalized but antihypertensive medication must be started immediately (without waiting for actual hospitalization or results of laboratory tests).

- ❖ **Pharmacological therapy:** *Parenteral antihypertensive agents are usually* required the drug of choice being IV sodium nitroprusside (an arteriolar and venous dilator). Initial dose is 0.25-0.5 mcg/kg/min with a maximum of 8-10 mcg/kg/min. The drug acts within seconds and the duration of action is only 2-5 minutes. Alternative drugs include nicardipine and labetalol (for further details see section on "Hypertensive Crisis").
  *Oral hypotensive drugs:* Because of milder and slower onset of action these drugs have limited role in the management of HE. However, when there is no rapid access to parenteral medication, and as a first aid measure, sublingual Captopril 25 mg can substantially lower the blood pressure within 10-30 minutes in many patients.

❖ **Measures to reduce cerebral edema:** Because of various factors stated above, a certain degree of cerebral edema is usual in patients with HE. The drug of choice in this setting is furosemide which also helps to control the BP. Corticosteroids are contraindicated.

# CEREBRAL VENOUS THROMBOSIS

## Etiopathogenesis

Thrombosis of the cerebral veins and sinuses occurs most commonly as a *complication of pregnancy in the peripartal period,* at any rate in India and other developing countries. While the exact mechanism is not known, it is probably related to a hypercoagulable state and stasis that occur during pregnancy. Occasionally, cerebral venous thrombosis (CVT) may be encountered in *states of marked toxemia* (e.g., untreated and severe typhoid fever) and severe malnutrition, or as an extension of infection *from a neighboring septic focus,* which may be in the ear, nose and throat, or over the face or scalp. Uncommon causes include polycythemia, inflammatory bowel disease, collagen vascular disease (like lupus), sickle cell disease, nephrotic syndrome, protracted use of oral contraceptives, malignancy, and cyanotic congenital heart disease.

In cerebral venous sinus thrombosis blood clots usually form in the veins of the brain and the venous sinuses. This results is cerebral edema (both vasogenic and cytotoxic), and small petechial hemorrhages. Thrombosis of the sinuses with consequent decreased reabsorption of cerebrospinal fluid accounts for increase in intracranial pressure.

## Clinical Features

The most common symptom of CVT is headache, which may worsen over a period of several days. Seizures can occur especially in peripartal cases, are usually unilateral, but may be generalized. Additionally, there may be fever and some degree of neck stiffness. The neurological deficit depends upon the part of the cerebral venous system occluded. When sinus thrombosis occurs in the peripartal period, *superior sagittal sinus is generally involved resulting in paraplegia.* Hemiplegia results if only cortical veins are affected.

**Other early features may include decreased level of consciousness** and **papilledema. Occasionally,** *coma supervenes especially if thrombosis involves deep venous system.* **Two distinctive syndromes** have also been **recognized with** CVT *viz.* pseudotumor cerebri (which mimics brain tumor) and cavernous sinus thrombosis.

*The clinical course and prognosis* are variable. It is grave in cases in which deep venous system is involved and when deep coma develops. In others, it is generally better than cerebral arterial thrombosis. In such cases, if the patient survives the acute stage, functional recovery is fairly satisfactory and usually better than seen after ischemic cerebral infarction.

## Diagnosis

The diagnosis is usually obvious from the clinical background of the case. In fact, CVT can occur in all clinical states known to be associated with calf and pelvic vein thrombosis, and should be suspected when appropriate neurological features develop in such a setting.

Some degree of leukocytosis and raised ESR are not uncommon, but are nonspecific. Likewise, *CSF may be normal* or show only a slight nonspecific increase in proteins. However, in view of increased intracranial pressure in many of these cases, *lumbar puncture should be avoided.* The diagnosis is confirmed by CT scanning with radiocontrast in the venous phase. MRI venography is equally informative but has the additional advantage of detecting damage to the brain as a result of the increased pressure on the obstructed veins.

## Management

There is no specific treatment of CVT. Antibiotics are indicated only in cases of secondary- CVT when there is associated calf or pelvic vein thrombosis, or there is evidence of infection in gynecological or urinary tract. *Anticoagulants* have been recommended to restrict thrombus extension once CT has confirmed the pathology to be confined to the venous system. Treatment should be started with heparin or low molecular weight heparin and followed by oral anticoagulation provided there are no contraindications. The duration of anticoagulant treatment depends upon the underlying cause of the condition. In peripartal cases three months are regarded as sufficient. If the condition was unprovoked and there are no clear causes, anticoagulation for 6-12 months is recommended. If there is a severe underlying thrombosis disorder, anticoagulation may need to be continued indefinitely. Patients with pathology in the cortical regions are prone to convulsions, and should receive prophylactic *anticonvulsant therapy.*

Some degree of cerebral edema is invariable, and therefore cerebral decongestants should be used as described in the section on "Thrombotic Stroke".

## ACUTE BACTERIAL (PYOGENIC) MENINGITIS

### Etiopathogenesis

Acute bacterial meningitis (ABM) is an acute infection of the central nervous system (CNS) that causes an intense inflammation in the subarachnoid space. The pathology is not confined to pia-arachnoid, and is invariably associated with infection and inflammation within the brain with its consequences of cerebral edema, and blockage of CSF pathway.

The *pathogenic organisms vary according to the age group.* In neonates, the common causes are Group B streptococcus, *Listeria,* and *Escherichia coli.*

Older children usually have *Neisseria meningitides, Streptococcus pneumoniae,* and *H. influenza* as infecting organisms. On the other hand, in adults (18–50 years), *N. meningitides* and *Streptococcus pneumoniae* together account for more than three-fourths of the cases; whereas in elderly subjects (>50 years), *S. pneumoniae*, gram-negative bacilli, and *Listeria monocytogenes* are the dominant pathogens.

Most bacteria enter CSF as a result of colonization of the nasopharynx or through hematogenous spread. Bacterial meningitis may also occur by direct invasion across the protective meninges which may be disrupted by trauma/surgery (e.g., secondary to shunt or CSF leak), or by spread of infection from parameningeal infective focus, such as sinusitis and otitis media. Rarely ABM may result from rupture of a brain abscess into ventricles or subarachnoid space.

## Clinical Features

Acute bacterial meningitis can start as a sudden acute illness characterized by marked toxemia, meningeal symptoms, and impaired sensorium ranging from drowsiness to coma *("fulminant cases")*. This may be preceded by a day or two of premonitory symptoms, such as fever, upper respiratory tract infection, headache, and vomiting. More often, however, the onset is subacute and features of CNS involvement develop over several (2–7) days. In general, the symptoms and signs can be ascribed to: (1) *Febrile illness* (e.g., fever, lethargy, anorexia), (2) *Meningeal inflammation* (e.g., nausea, vomiting, photophobia, stiffness of neck to flexion but not to lateral rotation), and (3) *Encephalopathy* (e.g. headache, altered sensorium, and seizures). When suspected, *the two strongest indicators of ABM are a change in mental status coupled with features of meningismus.*

The classical sign of ABM is involuntary rigidity of the neck muscles resulting from meningeal irritation. *Kernig and/or Brudzinski sign* are often positive. The former comprises pain or resistance in extending the knee in a supine patient with the hip flexed at 90 degree. Brudzinski sign is involuntary hip and knee flexion on bending the neck forwards. However, features of meningeal irritation may be minimal or absent at extremes of ages, or in comatose patients who do not respond to pain.

Additional problems may develop in the early stage of the illness. The brain tissue may swell, and *intracranial pressure may increase* with herniation through the skull base. This may be noticed by a decreasing level of consciousness, loss of **pupillary light reflex, and abnormal posturing (see section on "The Unconscious Patient"). *Hydrocephalus* is a possibility, and *seizures* may occur.**

*Cranial nerve palsies* may occur due to inflammation of the nerves as they traverse the meninges. The nerves most affected are those arising from the brainstem. Additionally, 6th nerve palsy may occur as a result of increased intracranial pressure, while 3rd nerve palsy will indicate brain herniation.

## Diagnosis

The disease may need to be differentiated from subarachnoid **hemorrhage,** other types of meningitis, and meningeal reaction (meningismus) sometimes associated with acute infections like enteric fever, pneumonia, septicemia, mastoiditis, cervical adenitis, and peritonsillar abscess.

A clinical diagnosis of the *type of ABM is* often difficult, if not impossible. However, certain features do correlate with a particular infection. For example, *presence of skin rash* (especially purpuric), large ecchymosis, circulatory collapse and occurrence of the disease in small epidemics, strongly favor meningococcal meningitis. *Seizures and focal neurologic deficits* are more common in pneumococcal meningitis compared to either meningococcal or *H. influenzae* meningitis. Associated infection in the ear, nose, or throat also suggests pneumococcal meningitis. Both meningococcal and pneumococcal infections occur mostly in adults though the former is not uncommon in children. The commonest cause of ABM in children is *H. influenzae,* and this usually follows upper respiratory tract infection.

While attention to clinical details will be helpful, a *conclusive diagnosis of meningitis can be made only by study of spinal fluid.* Ordinarily, lumbar puncture (LP) is a safe procedure and can be done without waiting for cranial CT except in patients with coma, papilledema, or focal neurologic findings. In such cases, a CT scan of the brain should be obtained (before LP) to exclude possible mass lesions or cerebral edema, but *treatment must be started without waiting for results of imaging,* since instituting antibiotic therapy rarely changes the cellular and biochemical pattern of CSF in the first 2-4 hours.

The salient features of CSF in common types of meningitis are given at **Table 4.9**. These findings may, however, be modified to a varying degree by antibiotic therapy administered more than a few hours ago. In pyogenic meningitis, however, such a therapy results more often in negative cultures,

| Types of meningitis | Pressure (mg%) | Proteins (mg%) | Glucose | Cells/cmm | Cell type |
|---|---|---|---|---|---|
| Tubercular | ↑↑ | >100 | ↓ (mild to moderate) | 100–500 | Lymphos* |
| Pyogenic | ↑↑↑ | >100 | ↓↓ | 200–400 | PMN† |
| Viral (aseptic) | Normal or ↑ | <100 | Normal | 100–700 | Lymphos* |

**Table 4.9:** Cytobiochemical CSF findings in various types of meningitis.

**Note:** When assessing CSF sugar, simultaneous blood sugar estimation is essential (patient should not be receiving glucose infusion). Concentration of CSF glucose is normally above 40% of that in blood. In ABM it is much lower, and a ratio (CSF glucose to serum glucose) of 0.4 or less is highly suggestive of bacterial meningitis.

*Instead of lymphocytes, polymorphs may predominate in the early phase.

†Instead of polymorphs (PMN), lymphocytes may predominate when the total cell count is not very high.

leaving the other characteristics largely unaffected. Nevertheless, in some cases, there may be a genuine difficulty in differentiating between viral and bacterial meningitis. In such cases, if the patient is not seriously ill, specific therapy should be withheld for 12 hours, after which a repeat CSF examination will usually reveal a correct diagnosis in nearly all patients.

It is always desirable to obtain bacterial culture of the CSF, which is likely to be positive in up to 75% of cases of ABM. While waiting for culture report, a rapid working diagnosis of the causative organism can be made by: (i) *Gram stain of the sedimented CSF,* and (ii) *Measurement of bacterial antigen in CSF by latex fixation* to determine the presence of a specific capsular polysaccharide associated with *H. influenzae, Pneumococcus,* and *Meningococcus*. This test is of special value in partially treated cases when CSF Gram stain and culture results may be negative. However, the test is of only limited value in meningitis due to gram-negative bacilli. Furthermore, a negative test does not rule out ABM.

Other useful investigations include white cell count, blood cultures, and X-ray chest. *Neuroimaging should be considered in the presence of following clinical features:*

- Seizures (focal or generalized) that are recurrent or occur after the 3 days of treatment
- Focal seizures at any point in the illness
- Prolonged or secondary fever
- Rapidly enlarging head circumference (in children)
- Focal neurological deficits
- Prolonged depression of consciousness, or other signs of increased intracranial pressure.

## Management

Acute bacterial meningitis is a grave medical emergency, and despite significant advances in intensive care management and introduction of new antibiotics, it **continues to be associated with a significant morbidity and mortality. Any patient with suspected ABM should, therefore, be hospitalized.**

### Specific Measures

- **Antibiotics:** Antimicrobial therapy in full doses should be initiated rapidly since a close correlation exists between the time from onset of symptoms to administration of antibiotics and the prognosis, both short and long term. The goal should be to administer antibiotics IV *within 30 minutes* after a patient with ABM has sought treatment. While choosing an antibiotic regimen care should be taken to select only bactericidal drugs (and not bacteriostatic drugs). Following factors affect the bactericidal activity of an antibiotic in CSF:
    - *CSF penetration:* Only those antibiotics should be used which cross blood-brain barrier adequately **(Table 4.10)**.

**Table 4.10:** CSF penetration of various chemotherapeutic agents.

| Satisfactory, even with normal meninges | Satisfactory with only inflamed meninges | Poor or no penetration (even with inflamed meninges) |
|---|---|---|
| Sulfonamides | Penicillin G | Streptomycin |
| Chloramphenicol | Ampicillin | Kanamycin |
| Trimethoprim | Carbenicillin | Gentamicin |
| Sulfamethoxazole | Methicillin | Erythromycin |
| Isoniazid | Tetracycline | |
| Rifampicin | Vancomycin | Polymyxin |
| Ethambutol | Cephalosporins | Tobramycin |
| Pyrazinamide | (3rd generation) | |

- *CSF concentration:* Large doses of antibiotics are required since infected CSF decreases antibiotic activity partly because of its low pH (e.g., aminoglycosides), and partly due to high CSF protein content which reduces the concentration of active free drugs, such as beta-lactams (especially cephalosporins), which are highly protein-bound.

### Empiric Treatment

The choice of antibiotic(s) should be guided by knowledge of the possible pathogen. Gram stain of CSF and measurement of bacterial antigen in CSF by latex fixation are measures for quick identification of causative organism, in many cases of bacterial meningitis. However, when these results are negative or there is delay in CSF examination, empiric therapy should be started on the basis of patient's age, health status, and expected state of meninges **(Table 4.10)**. The therapy should be modified as soon as organisms can be identified or results of CSF culture and antibiotic sensitivity become available. Although CSF penetration of vancomycin is not optimal, it is given empirically in conjunction with ceftriaxone due to reported rates of *Streptococcus pneumoniae* resistance to third generation cephalosporins. Vancomycin should be continued until MICs have resulted. When strep pneumonia is likely to be the causative agent, the patient should receive a one-time dose of dexamethasone prior to or with the initial antibiotic dose. The use of dexamethasone decreases CSF inflammation and has been shown to decrease neurologic sequelae of bacterial meningitis **(Table 4.11)**.

In immunocompromised patients or in whom bacterial meningitis is associated with head trauma, neurosurgery, CSF shunt or CSF rhinorrhea, antibiotic choice should include coverage of pseudomonas and MRSA until cultures show a definitive organism.

### Specific Antibiotic Therapy

Once the pathogenic organism is identified, antimicrobial regimens should be modified to provide highly active but narrow coverage against organism's

| Table 4.11: Empiric treatment of acute bacterial meningitis. ||||
| Patient group | Likely pathogens | Antibiotic regimen | Alternative regimen |
| --- | --- | --- | --- |
| Neonates | Group B strep, E. coli Listeria | Ampicillin + ceftriaxone + vancomycin | Chloramphenicol+ gentamicin |
| 3 months–18 years | H. influenzae, S. pneumoniae N. meningitidis | Cefotaxime or ceftriaxone | Meropenem |
| 18–50 years | N. meningitidis H. influenzae S. pneumoniae | Ceftriaxone + vancomycin | Meropenem |
| Over 50 years | S. pneumoniae Gram (-)bacilli Listeria | Ampicillin+ ceftriaxone + vancomycin | Ampicillin + fluoroquinolone |

| Table 4.12: Optimal antibiotic dosage regimens in bacterial meningitis.* |||
| Pathogen | Drug of choice | Alternative regimens |
| --- | --- | --- |
| S. pneumoniae | Ceftriaxone/cefotaxime + vancomycin | Penicillin, meropenem |
| N. meningitidis | Penicillin G/ampicillin | Cefotaxime, Chloramphenicol |
| Listeria | Ampicillin + gentamicin | Ampicillin + fluoroquinolones |
| H. influenzae | Ceftriaxone/cefotaxime | Chloramphenicol |

**Note:** There should be an interval of at least half an hour between ampicillin and chloramphenicol administration.

isolated (**Table 4.12**). The aim should be to achieve effective bactericidal CSF concentration, and therefore optimal systemic doses of antibiotics must be administered.

**Duration of antibiotic therapy:** Antibiotic therapy for bacterial meningitis should be continued IV for 10 days except in cases of meningitis due to gram-negative bacilli or *Listeria* in whom longer period of treatment for 2–3 weeks may be required. It is essential that throughout this period, the antibiotics are continued in full dosage since the meningeal inflammation, and hence the penetration of most of the antimicrobial agents into the meninges, declines rapidly and progressively as the patient improves. Oral or IM therapy is not reliable and in fact early switch over to these modes of administration of antibiotics may account for occasional treatment failures. *Repeat LP should not be done if clinical recovery is satisfactory.* It is warranted only in cases of meningitis caused by Gram- **negative** bacilli, when therapeutic response is inadequate, or when complications arise.

## General and Symptomatic Measures

If the patient's consciousness is impaired, general principles of management described under "The Unconscious Patient" should be followed. **Cerebral** edema of varying severity is nearly always present, and should be treated with 20% mannitol as described in the section on "Cerebral Thrombosis". **Seizures** of various types often complicate acute meningitis and should be suppressed by phenytoin.

### Complications

- ❖ Hyperpyrexia
- ❖ Peripheral circulatory failure. This may be due to severe toxemia or result from adrenal apoplexy (Waterhouse Frederickson syndrome) especially in cases of meningococcal meningitis.

### Summary

- ❖ The causative organism in ABM usually varies according to age of the patient. Majority of cases of ABM are due to Group B streptococci in neonates, *H. influenzae* and *N. meningitides* in children and young adults, and *Streptococcus pneumoniae, and N. meningitides* in adults/ older patients.
- ❖ Spinal fluid should be examined and cultured in all cases of suspected meningitis. Gram stain and latex fixation test for bacterial antigen are useful in quick identification of the causative pathogen.
- ❖ Because of high morbidity and mortality, antibiotic therapy should not be delayed on account of diagnostic testing. *The first dose of antibiotic must be given as soon as ABM is suspected on clinical grounds,* preferably within 30 minutes of patient reaching the hospital.
- ❖ Antibiotics must be given IV and continued in full dosage for 10–14 days or longer according to etiology.

## TUBERCULAR MENINGITIS

Tubercular infection of the meninges (TBM) usually has a subacute clinical course, and hence is not a medical emergency in the strict sense. However, more often than not, the exact diagnosis is delayed until the patient develops impairment of consciousness and various paralytic features, and at this stage, the patient's condition often warrants emergency management. The disease has become quite uncommon in the past few decades since the introduction of isoniazid and rifampicin which are not only highly potent antitubercular drugs but, more importantly, freely cross the blood-brain barrier.

### Pathology

Tubercular infection of the meninges is invariably secondary to tuberculosis elsewhere in the body, the pathogenic organism (*Mycobacterium tuberculosis*) *reaching the brain via bloodstream.* The pathology usually begins with seeding of the meninges or subpial brain by tubercle bacilli. A caseating lesion develops, which discharges bacilli into the subarachnoid space resulting in meningeal inflammation in the brain and spinal cord. The pathology is confined mostly to the basal areas of the brain involving leptomeninges, though the cerebral cortex is always inflamed. The exudate is most marked in the interpeduncular fossa but spreads in all directions. It involves cranially the optic chiasma and anterior cerebral vessels, extends laterally into the Sylvian fissures encircling middle cerebral artery and its penetrating branches, and caudally into the cerebellomedullary cisterns where the dense exudate may block the foramina of Luschka thereby resulting in hydrocephalus.

An important component of pathology is vasculopathy. Blood vessels of all types (arteries, capillaries, veins) are involved. The brunt is maximal on the arteries, and the lesions include periarteritis, fibrinoid necrosis, panarteritis, and luminal occlusion of both small and medium sized cerebral arteries. These vascular changes compromise cerebral perfusion and may result in various types of ischemic insult.

## Clinical Features

The clinical spectrum can be wide varying from silent or asymptomatic cases to fulminant disease. Three distinct stages can be recognized:

**Stage I:** Cases presenting purely as meningitis.

**Stage II:** Cases with apparent meningitis + definite neurological deficit but alert consciousness.

**Stage III:** Cases with the triad of meningeal features, paralysis, and impaired consciousness. Often there is an overlap between different stages.

**The disease usually starts as a flu-like illness with rather severe headache to which** features such as apathy and irritability are soon added. Diagnosis, at this stage, requires a high index of suspicion since many cases may neither have fever nor features, of meningeal involvement. The headache becomes persistent and more troublesome, pyrexia develops or continues, and mental confusion and gastrointestinal features like anorexia and vomiting supervene. **Convulsions** are not uncommon, at this stage, especially in infants and children. Within a few days, classical features of meningitis develop in the form of photophobia, neck stiffness, and positive Kernig sign. As the disease progresses consciousness is increasingly impaired, **paralytic features** (especially ocular palsies) supervene, and papilledema may be seen (more often than in pyogenic meningitis). *Sometimes the dominant presentation comprises a stroke syndrome often associated with cranial nerve palsies.*

## Diagnosis

Tubercular infection of the meninges can be suspected on the basis of history, physical examination and an X-ray of the chest, but a firm diagnosis rests on examination of spinal fluid. The fluid is clear, under increased pressure* and may form a "cobweb" on standing (of course, not diagnostic of TBM). The cellular reaction is predominantly lymphocytic (count usually <500 cells/mm$^3$) with a modest increase in protein content (usually < 200 mg %). However, the characteristic change is a reduction in glucose level to nearly half the blood value or less (around 30 mg%).

Such typical CSF changes are, however, present in only about three-fourth of the cases. In others, CSF picture may resemble that of aseptic meningitis, encephalitis, acute bacterial meningitis, or may be modified by findings of spinal block. Rarely, CSF may be normal initially but another LP done after 48 hours provides diagnostic information. Neuroimaging studies, such as *CT scan or MRI* of the brain can be helpful but are not diagnostic.

## Management

Successful management depends on the stage of the disease treatment is started. Chances of recovery are remote once coma has set in.

### Specific Measures

- **Antitubercular therapy:** Treatment should be started with four first line drugs comprising isoniazid (INH), rifampicin, pyrazinamide, and ethambutol. All the four drugs cross the blood-brain barrier freely (especially the first two). If drug resistance is a possibility, treatment should be suitably modified. If fluoroquinolones are added, their epileptogenic potential should be kept in mind.
  This intensive treatment should be continued for three months, after which only INH and rifampicin should be continued for another 12 months. Pyridoxine 40 mg may be added once or twice a week to prevent INH related neuropathy.
- **Intrathecal therapy:** Since the discovery of INH, intrathecal streptomycin therapy has become obsolete. Likewise, there is no role of intrathecal administration of corticosteroids except when spinal block is suspected.
- **Corticosteroids:** Steroid therapy is often added to antitubercular regimen soon after a firm diagnosis of TBM is established. The aim is to reduce cerebral edema, decrease inflammatory exudates (with the hope that it will check formation of adhesions and blocks), and to lessen vasculopathy. Treatment is usually started with injection dexamethasone 4 mg 3 or 4 times a day IV for about a week and then continued as oral prednisolone 20-40 mg daily for 2-3 months.

### General Measures

These are generally similar to those described under "Pyogenic Meningitis", but will need to be continued for a longer period because of the protracted course of the disease. For the same reason, the diet should be high in calories, rich in proteins, and supplemented with adequate vitamins.

## Complications
❖ Hydrocephalus
❖ Multiple cranial nerve palsies
❖ Paralytic features resembling stroke syndromes

## Summary
❖ TBM is now a fairly uncommon disease. It involves predominantly the leptomeninges, but vasculopathy and cerebral cortical inflammation are also important in its pathogenesis.
❖ Features of meningitis are common to all cases of TBM; neurological deficits and impairment of consciousness worsen prognosis.
❖ Spinal fluid examination is central to the diagnosis of TBM. Imaging studies are helpful in patients responding poorly to treatment, and in detection of complications.
❖ Standard treatment comprises 4-drug therapy; INH and rifampicin are most important because of their free access to CSF. Corticosteroids are helpful in reducing cerebral edema and inflammatory exudates.

# ASEPTIC MENINGITIS

## Etiology
Aseptic meningitis refers to meningitis without a bacterial or fungal cause. By definition, the Gram stain or culture of CSF is negative. Aseptic meningitis, sometimes used interchangeably with viral meningitis, is usually caused by enterovirus or herpes simplex virus (HSV). Nonviral causes of aseptic meningitis include medications, such as nonsteroidal anti-inflammatory drugs (NSAIDs), antibiotics, IVIG, as well as hematologic malignancies.

The most common viral cause of meningitis in the summer months is enterovirus. The most common cause of viral meningitis year-round is HSV2. Other viral etiologies of meningitis include EBV, CMV, and West Nile Virus.

## Clinical Features
Patients with aseptic meningitis present with low-acuity symptoms, such as cough/cold, mild headache. The most notable feature of aseptic meningitis is the presence of normal cognitive function, which differentiates it from encephalitis. Of note, meningitis due to West Nile Virus causes characteristic back pains, myalgias, and Parkinsonism, which, in addition to CSF findings, can be diagnostic.

Mollaret's Syndrome is benign recurrent lymphocytic meningitis, lasting 2-5 days, recurring multiple times in a month.

## Diagnosis
The diagnosis of aseptic meningitis is made by a sterile CSF Gram stain. PCR may be used to identify enterovirus, HSV, EBV, or other viral causes of

meningitis. West Nile virus must be diagnosed by CSF IgM antibodies; it will not appear positive on a PCR test.

### Management

In general, aseptic meningitis is treated with supportive cares and resolves on its own. In cases where the etiology of aseptic meningitis is a medication, removal of the offending agent should be curative.

## ACUTE VIRAL ENCEPHALITIS

### Etiology

Viral encephalitis is an inflammation of the brain parenchyma caused by a viral infection. In some cases, meninges (meningoencephalitis) and brainstem or spinal cord may also be **involved. Direct infection of neurons accounts** for majority of cases. Many types of viruses can involve the nervous system.

**Some of** these are associated with specific disease syndromes (e.g., poliomyelitis, **rabies**) while **others** result in **aseptic meningitis with or** without mild encephalitis (e.g., virus of lymphocytic choriomeningitis, mumps virus, the enterovirus group (including Coxsackie virus and echo viruses), and Epstein-Barr virus of infectious mononucleosis). Furthermore, some viruses cause a wide spectrum of clinical disorders (e.g., herpes-viruses) with acute encephalitis as the most serious clinical manifestation. The description that follows is confined to acute viral encephalitis with special reference to herpes simplex encephalitis which is the only type of viral infection of the brain for which a specific antiviral therapy is available. It is important to understand the difference between viral meningitis and viral encephalitis. The clinical presentation is more severe in the latter, and more aggressive therapeutic regiments are indicated in viral encephalitis.

### Clinical Features

The onset is acute or sub-acute with nonspecific (flu-like) symptoms, such as fever, headache. Alterations in mental state soon set in and may range from confusion and delirium to frank coma. Other common features include behavioral and speech disturbance, focal or generalized seizures, cranial nerve palsies, and neurological deficits, sometimes focal but usually diffuse. Meningeal involvement is frequent and can be detected by positive Kernig or Brudzinski sign. The acute phase of illness lasts from a few days to a week, and runs a variable course. It may be a short-lived benign illness or a fulminant one leading to pronounced impairment of cerebral functions. The recovery can be quick or gradual with improvement continuing over a period of weeks to months. However, the disease carries a significant mortality if diagnosis and treatment are delayed.

*Herpes simplex virus* predominantly infects temporal lobe, initially unilaterally and then bitemporally as the illness progresses. The resulting acute focal encephalitis leads to aphasia, anosmia, temporal lobe seizures, and focal neurologic deficits. The course can be progressive and devastating unless interrupted (successfully) by specific and prompt treatment.

## Diagnosis

Several conditions characterized by acute high fever and impaired sensorium need to be differentiated. These include typhoid fever, pneumonia, acute meningitis, sepsis, heat stroke and cerebral malaria. Clinical details are important in differential diagnosis. Whenever acute encephalitis is suspected, distinction between generalized and focal neurological findings is vital. *Focal neurological features coupled with pleocytosis (lymphocytic) and elevated CSF protein in a patient with features of encephalitis in the absence of identifiable pathogens should be considered to be due to herpes simplex virus until proved otherwise.*

## Investigations

Routine laboratory testing should be done as in any emergency, and include estimation of CBC, glucose, liver and renal functions, and electrolytes. Lumbar puncture should be performed after obtaining an emergent CT brain. Encephalitis is suggested by moderate pleocytosis (50-500 lymphocytes), elevated proteins, and normal glucose. A few cases may, however, show completely normal CSF. Cultures of CSF for isolation of virus, and serological studies for detection of antibodies in the serum or CSF are too insensitive, and the results are too long delayed to be clinically useful. More useful investigations include electroencephalogram (EEG) and MRI of the brain.

In herpes simplex encephalitis, EEG may reveal focal changes, such as periodic lateralizing epileptiform discharges, focal temporal spikes, or slow waves. MRI will help exclude many other diseases, which mimic acute encephalitis, and may also help in specific diagnosis of herpes simplex encephalitis by revealing temporal lobe localization. The combination of clinical, CSF, EEG, and radioimaging studies often provide enough evidence of herpes simplex encephalitis to justify prompt institution of antiviral chemotherapy. Additional confirmatory evidence can be obtained by polymerase chain reaction (PCR) in the CSF, which is a rapid and sensitive and specific test for early diagnosis of HSV infection.

## Management

### General Measures

These include proper control of fluid and electrolytes, and pyrexia. If the patient is lethargic or comatose, general principles of management as described in the section on "The Unconscious Patient" should be observed. Seizures frequently occur and should be controlled with phenytoin. A major threat to life comes from cerebral edema, which should be managed with decongestive therapy (see section on "Thrombotic Stroke"). Corticosteroids are contraindicated (risk of enhancing spread of virus within the brain).

### Specific Measures

Specific therapy for HSV encephalitis comprises treatment with acyclovir, 10 mg/kg intravenously every 8 hours for 10 days or more. The drug is generally free of toxicity, but dosage should be adjusted for renal impairment. The results are particularly encouraging if therapy is instituted early (within four days of the onset of disease) and the patient's consciousness is not deeply impaired. Acyclovir is also effective in patients with Epstein-Barr virus, and Varicella-Zoster virus encephalitis.

## SEIZURES

### Etiology

A seizure is a transient disturbance of cerebral function resulting from abnormal paroxysmal neuronal discharge in the brain. Convulsive seizures may **result from cerebral** or **extracerebral conditions (Table 4.13). However, in majority** of **cases, seizures are apparently idiopathic though these may be related to microscopic lesions resulting from trauma at** birth **or later in life, or to scars** resulting from infective, degenerative, or vascular disorders of the brain.

### Pathophysiology

**The pathophysiology** of seizures is not fully **understood at** the neuronal level. However, it is generally agreed that both excitatory (acetylcholine) and inhibitory (gamma aminobutyric acid—GABA) neurotransmitters exert significant effect resulting in "electrical overactivity" and "electrical

**Table 4.13:** Common causes of seizures.

| Cerebral | Metabolic |
|---|---|
| • Epilepsy<br>• Stroke syndrome<br>• Intracranial space occupying lesion<br>• Encephalopathy<br>• Meningitis<br>• Eclampsia | • Hypo- or hyper<br>• Hypo- or hypernatremia<br>• Hypocalcemia<br>• Hyperpyrexia |
| Infections | Drug/substance related |
| • Malaria<br>• Cysticercosis<br>• Toxoplasmosis | • Lidocaine<br>• Theophylline<br>• Alcohol withdrawal<br>• Cocaine<br>• Isoniazid<br>• Lead poisoning |

underactivity", respectively. For an individual to be conscious, their relative normal functioning is essential in at least one cortical hemisphere and reticular activating system. *Continuous seizure activity (with or without convulsions) for more than 30-60 minutes often results in permanent neuronal injury,* either directly or through rapid depletion of vital metabolic substrates, such as oxygen and glucose, or calcium influx into neurons.

## Classification

Epileptic seizures can take a varied form, and are best classified as follows:
- **Generalized seizures:** These include:
  - Tonic-clonic (grand mal) seizures
  - Absence (petit mal) seizures
  - Myoclonic seizure
  - Atonic seizures (epileptic drop attacks)
- **Partial seizures** which may be of the *"simple partial"* or *"complex partial"* type.

## Clinical Features

Epileptic seizures can have a varied and sometimes baffling presentation. A common characteristic is occurrence of chronic and recurrent seizures, each with a stereotype clinical pattern, and quick recovery. Their detailed description is beyond the scope of this text. *Acute medical problems arise only in "tonic-clonic" type of epileptic seizures (and sometimes in "complex partial" seizures) which is often associated with loss of consciousness.* Further discussion is therefore confined only to this type.

The diagnosis of "tonic-clonic" (grand mal) epilepsy is often easy if the patient is seen in an actual fit. However, more often than not, an attack of grand mal is already over by the time the doctor actually arrives, and in such cases, the diagnosis depends upon obtaining careful details from eyewitness of the event. Grand mal seizures are characterized by sudden loss of consciousness associated with generalized rigidity in which the patient may fall to the ground, if standing (tonic phase). This phase is very brief (usually less than a minute) and is followed by a clonic phase characterized by jerky movements of the body. This may last for 2-4 minutes and is in turn followed by a phase of flaccid coma which may last for several minutes. During the seizure, the patient may bite the tongue or lips, may become incontinent, and sustain injury. Immediately after the attack the patient may recover consciousness, drift into sleep, or develop features of *"postictal automatism".*

*Pseudo-seizures* imply both hysterical conversion reaction and malingering attack. Of the two, hysterical fits are most common, occur more often in women, without any aura (but may be preceded by a period of emotional stress), and are of longer duration (usually stretching over several minutes or even hours). The attack superficially resembles grand mal seizure, but there is often no tonic phase, clonic movements are asynchronous and bizarre, tend to increase, if restrained, and there may be accompanying groans and cries. Consciousness may be retained in the presence of bilateral jerking. Pupillary responses, and tendon and plantar reflexes are normal during and immediately after convulsion. Absence of history of tongue bite, incontinence, or of patient sustaining any injury during such a fit will also favor a diagnosis of hysterical fit. The differentiation is important if unneeded and prolonged anticonvulsive treatment is to be avoided in these cases. An EEG and MRI of brain can be of help in establishing correct diagnosis.

## Management

During the actual epileptic fit when the patient is unconscious, following measures should be instituted:
- Turn the head of the patient to one side so as to prevent aspiration
- Loosen all clothes around the chest and the neck
- Do not try to open the mouth with a tongue depressor or any other device since this may damage the gums or tongue, and also possibly dislodge loose teeth, which the patient may aspirate
- Patient should be placed in such a position that he does not injure himself by striking against hard or sharp pointed objects
- **No attempt should be made to feed the patient during the fit.**

**Recurrence of fits** should be controlled by maintenance therapy with anticonvulsants, such as phenytoin, phenobarbital, valproate and carbamazepine. The dosage of these drugs, their half-life and the optimal frequency of administration are given at **Table 4.14**. Phenytoin is the drug prescribed most often but the choice should depend upon the age and sex of the patient as well as physician preference. Antiepileptic drugs are **most effective** and have the **least adverse effects** when they are used as **monotherapy.** Many other drugs including gabapentin, lamotrigine, topiramate, and levetiracetam are available for control of epileptic seizures. Their precise usage is best left to the specialist.

Finally, all cases of convulsive seizures must be thoroughly investigated to discover the etiological factor which, if found, should be appropriately treated.

**Table 4.14:** Pharmacokinetics of commonly used anticonvulsant drugs.

| Name of drug | Average oral dose (mg/kg/day) | Half-life (hours) | Frequency of administration (per day) | Peak cone after single oral dose (hours) |
|---|---|---|---|---|
| Phenytoin | 5–7 | 20–24* | Once | 2–6 |
| Phenobarbital | 3–5 | 20–120 | Once | 6–18 |
| Carbamazepine | 10–20 | 10–20 | 2–3 times | 2–6 |
| Sodium valproate | 30–60 | 8±2 | 2–3 times | 1–2 |

*Highly variable: may range from 8 to 72 hours.

# STATUS EPILEPTICUS

## Definition

The International League against Epilepsy has defined status epilepticus (SE) as "a seizure that persists for a sufficient duration of time, or repeated frequently enough that recovery (of consciousness) between attacks does not occur. The definition of duration of convulsive SE is controversial, but generally duration of 5 minutes is accepted as the guiding criterion. There can be essentially as many types of status as there are types of epileptic seizures. It can be classified as:

- **Generalized convulsive** (tonic-clonic) **SE.** This is the most dangerous type of SE.
- **Nonconvulsive SE** is a state of electromechanical dissociation where the epileptiform discharges evident on EEG are not accompanied by clinical manifestations, such as motor symptoms or coma. Two categories of nonconvulsive SE are recognized: absence status and complex partial seizures.

In this section, discussion is confined to generalized (tonic-clonic) SE since it is the most common type of SE, and also because it constitutes a medical emergency.

## Pathophysiology

Several physiological changes may occur during convulsive stage from excitotoxic neuronal injury (possibly related to calcium influx into neurons, or rapid depletion of vital substrates, such as oxygen and glucose), and secondary effects of systemic complications. The latter include hypoxia, lactic acidosis, aspiration pneumonia, rhabdomyolysis, and hyperkalemia. In addition, marked hyperactivity of autonomic nervous system occurs which may result in tachycardia, hyperpyrexia, neurogenic pulmonary edema, and cardiac arrhythmias. Status lasting more than 60 minutes is especially likely to lead to irreversible brain damage and cardiovascular collapse.

**Precipitating factors:** Status epilepticus may be precipitated (in an epileptic patient) by sudden stoppage of anticonvulsants, change in antiepileptic drug or dosage, and withdrawal or over-indulgence in alcohol. Occasionally, the very first attack of epilepsy may be an episode of SE. This may result from any severe infection, electrolyte disturbances (especially hyponatremia), hypoglycemia, or an underlying intracranial pathology, such as space occupying lesion, vascular stroke, cerebral tumor, and intracranial infection.

## Management

### General Measures

Initial management should comprise maintaining adequate ventilation and circulation. Electrolyte and fluid balance should also be adequately monitored keeping in view the increased fluid requirement in such cases because of excessive muscular activity and frequently associated pyrexia. Blood glucose level should be determined immediately and hypoglycemia excluded. Hypoxia may not be clinically manifest and oxygen supplementation is recommended in all patients in SE.

## *Specific Measures*

Status epilepticus is a medical emergency and warrants immediate attention especially since longer a seizure continues the more difficult it is to stop it. In case there is no past history of seizures and immediate blood sugar estimation is not practical, 25-50 mL of 50 % dextrose should be given IV to rule out hypoglycemia as a cause of seizure activity. If seizures continue following steps are suggested.

- ❖ **Anticonvulsants:** Antiepileptic drugs (AEDs) used in SE can be broadly divided into first and second line drugs. The former include benzodiazepines - lorazepam, diazepam, and midazolam. The second line AED is phenytoin. Treatment may be started with any drug most familiar to the physician.

  Intravenous lorazepam and diazepam have shown similar benefits but the safety profile is slightly better with the former. Usual dose of lorazepam is 0.1 mg/kg, for diazepam 0.2 mg/kg, and midazolam 0.05-0.2 mg/kg. **Any of the three drugs may be used and administered as a bolus at the rate of 2 mg/min. The issue with** all these drugs is respiratory and possibly also, hemodynamic compromise that is possible during bolus injection. Intravenous benzodiazepines should, therefore, be administered cautiously, preferably in a set up where emergency intubation is possible. In prehospital setting intramuscular diazepam can also be effective.

  Phenytoin can be given IV as a bolus in a dose of 15-20 mg/kg at the rate of 50 mg/min followed by a maintenance dose of 4-6 mg/kg/day orally for long-term seizure control. The bolus dose is given diluted in 100 mL *normal saline* over 20-30 minutes (not glucose containing infusions in which phenytoin precipitates). Therapeutic level is achieved within 10-20 minutes after starting the infusion. Side effects include hypotension and arrhythmias, and therefore, the drug should be administered under electrocardiographic control and with a close watch on blood pressure. IV phenytoin is contraindicated in patients with heart block or severe myocardial disease. Phenytoin should not be given IM since it is poorly absorbed.

  As soon as SE is controlled, oral therapy should be started for the long-term management of the disease. Treatment is usually started with any one of the three drugs (phenytoin, carbamazepine, and valproate) depending upon individual characteristics of the patient.

- ❖ **Treatment of underlying cause** after the acute phase is over an attempt should be made to uncover any organic lesion which may be the cause of epilepsy. This is, however, found in only a minority of cases but when discovered, should receive appropriate attention including surgical intervention, if required.

## Complications

- ❖ Sudden death (always a possibility in SE)
- ❖ Hyperpyrexia
- ❖ Dehydration and peripheral circulatory failure
- ❖ Aspiration pneumonia
- ❖ Hypoxia, acidosis, hyperkalemia, and renal failure

# ACUTE HEADACHE

## Etiology

The causes of headache are legion. Though brain parenchyma itself is insensitive to pain, many cranial tissues are pain-sensitive and can result in headache. These include scalp and its arteries, head and neck musculature, venous sinuses, duramater, dural and intracerebral arteries, certain cranial nerves (V, VII, IX, and X), and second and third cervical nerves. Headache can be broadly classified into three main groups **(Table 4.15)** according to the mechanism by which the pain is produced:

1. Vascular headaches which include headaches caused by abnormal reaction of the cerebral arteries, with a tendency toward dilatation
2. Muscle contraction headaches produced by persistent contraction of the muscles of the head, neck and face, and
3. Organic headaches resulting from increased intracranial pressure and inflammation/traction on pain sensitive cranial tissues **(Table 4.15)**.

## Diagnosis

A schematic approach for arriving at a precise diagnosis in a case of acute severe headache is given in the accompanying "**Flowchart 4.2**". Of utmost importance is a thorough clinical history with details of onset of headache, its location and severity, time course of episode, previous headaches, associated symptoms, and precipitating factors. Differentiation should be made between first onset/onset of new type and recurrent headaches. *Acute first-onset*

**Table 4.15:** Etiological classification of headache.

| Vascular headaches | Muscle contraction headaches | Organic headaches |
|---|---|---|
| • Migraine<br>　➤ Classic (with aura)<br>　➤ Common (without aura)<br>• Hemiplegia<br>• Ophthalmic<br>• Complicated<br>• Cluster (histamine)<br>• Hypertensive | • Tension headache<br>• Cervical osteoarthritis<br>• Chronic myositis | • Stroke (brain edema)<br>　➤ SAH<br>• Infections<br>• Mass lesions including subdural hematoma<br>• Arteritis<br>• Cranial neuralgias<br>• Diseases of eye, ear, nose, throat and teeth |

headache should always be taken seriously, and raise suspicion of serious organic causes, such as acute meningitis, SAH, stroke, or arteritis. An acute headache that is accompanied by fever and neck stiffness suggests acute meningitis. A "thunderclap headache", sudden and severe, and often described as 'the worst headache of my life', is usually the result of SAH. However, in so-called warning leaks of SAH, the headache may resemble any other severe, acute, or atypical head pain.

*Chronic/recurrent headaches* are much more frequent, and in general, benign. Such headaches include all forms of vascular and tension headaches, cranial neuralgias, and headache due to diseases of the eye, ear, nose, throat, and teeth. Misuse of analgesics or anti-migraine drugs itself may result in chronic headaches—**"analgesic headaches".** Caffeine-containing beverages, often consumed for relief, further worsen such headaches. A chronic headache with recent change in symptoms, or a recent headache with progressive course, often worse in the morning, or associated with a personality change and/or seizure, should raise strong suspicion of intracranial space occupying pathology.

## Investigations

Few laboratory tests are required in patients with prolonged, recurrent headaches, and normal physical examination including ophthalmic and ENT examination. When systemic disorders are suspected, several investigations may be called for including complete blood count, blood sugar, renal and liver function tests, and CXR. CSF should be examined, if there is the least suspicion of meningitis. Indications for **CT/MRI of the brain** are as follows:

- Recent acute onset headache
- "Aura" symptoms always affecting the same side of the body, and either very brief (<5 minutes) or unusually prolonged (>60 minutes)
- Sudden change in the character of the headache or a substantial increase in attack frequency
- Onset above age 50 years
- Headache associated with high fever or abnormal neurological examination.

## Physical Examination

Neurological profile is normal in most types of headache. Presence of meningeal signs, such as Kernig and/or Brudzinski sign is of great value, and (in a case with acute sudden headache), strongly suggests SAH or acute meningitis. Focal neurological deficit especially when associated with papilledema suggest intracranial mass lesion. *Physical findings which suggest a serious cause of headache include:* (a) Altered consciousness, (b) Fever and neck stiffness, (c) Evolving or persistent neurological deficit, (d) Papilledema, (e) Tender temporal artery, and (f) Macrocephaly.

**Flowchart 4.2:** Evaluation of acute severe headache.

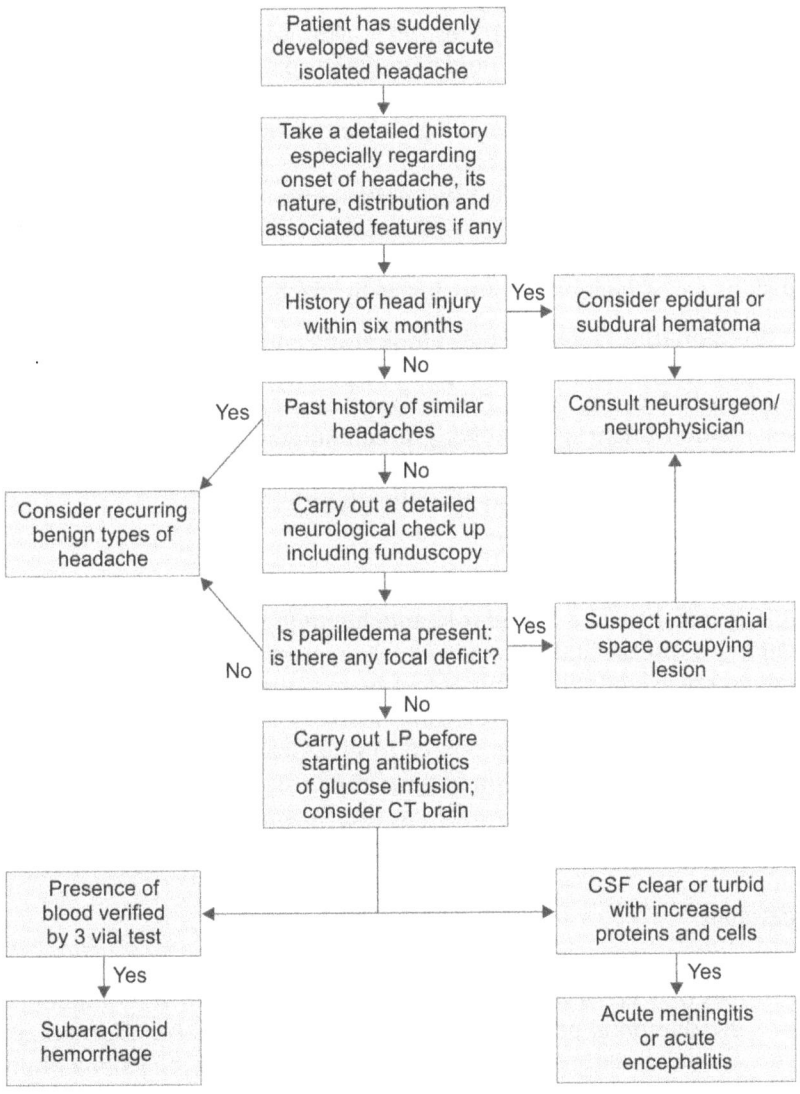

Further discussion is confined to migraine and cluster headache which are the two most common types of headache.

# MIGRAINE

Migraine is the most important cause of (recurrent) acute severe headaches, and can be of two types—migraine with aura *(classic migraine)* and without aura *(common migraine)*. The latter (migraine without aura) is the more *common* type and accounts for about 80% of migraine cases.

## Clinical Features

Migraine without aura is characterized by a throbbing or pulsating headache, which is generally unilateral, and of moderate or severe intensity. Headache attacks last 4–72 hours (unless successfully terminated), and are invariably associated with nausea or vomiting. Other common associated features are photophobia and phonophobia.

Patients of migraine with aura experience transient neurologic symptoms prior to acute headache. The most common aura is visual-scotomas and scintillations. Sometimes, the aura is in the form of dysphasia. As the aura subsides, vasodilatation follows causing headache.

**Precipitating factors** include physical and emotional stress, certain foods, such as chocolates containing phenethylamine, wine, and monosodium glutamate (a flavoring agent). Other triggers can be fasting, oral contraceptives, menstruation, bright lights (working on computers continuously for prolonged periods, or watching television for long periods especially fast moving colored pictures), and vasodilators, such as nitroglycerine.

## Pathophysiology

Initially considered a vascular headache, migraine is now thought to be primarily a disease of the brain in which an electrical discharge in the brain leads to release of neurogenic inflammatory mediators. These mediators activate trigeminal nerve, the main sensory nerve supplying the head and face. Pain appears to be related to sensitization of perivascular nerve terminals leading to activation of the central trigeminal system. As a result, a self-sustaining process develops causing further pain, inflammation, and sensitization of central trigeminal neurons.

## Treatment

- ❖ **Acute attack:**
    - NSAIDs given in high dose remain the first line of treatment. The fundamental principal of symptomatic therapy (to abort an acute attack) is early intervention. Naproxen in a dose of 500 mg orally is quite effective, and is preferred because of its quick absorption and safety profile. An exceptionally severe attack may require intramuscular NSAID, e.g., diclofenac acid. To counter gastric hypomotility (which often accompanies migraine) and improve its absorption, naproxen should be combined with domeperidon 10 mg orally.
    - *Triptans:* In cases with disabling attack of migraine, triptans are the preferred first line of treatment. Triptans have a high affinity for serotonin-1 receptors, and are available in several forms - as tablets, nasal spray, and as injection. The nasal spray acts fastest, followed by injection and tablets. Oral medication is effective only after 30–90 minutes. It is not advisable to take more than two SC

injections or three 100 mg tablets in a day to prevent *"sumatriptan misuse headache".* Triptans are contraindicated in patients with hypertension and coronary, cerebral, or peripheral vascular disease. Triptans *should be used very cautiously in patients receiving selective serotonin reuptake inhibitors (SSRIs) because of risk of potentially fatal "serotonin syndrome".*

- *Ergots:* Since ergot medications are less effective than triptans, and also because of risk of causing coronary ischemia, these are now seldom used. However, if at all ergot medications are to be used, dihydroergotamine (DHE) should be preferred over ergotamine since it is a less powerful arterial vasoconstrictor. It is given IV 1 mg in normal saline over 5 minutes, following an IV antiemetic.

❖ **Recurrences:** This is a situation in which the headache is relieved initially but returns within 24 hours. Early treatment with a high-dose triptan and concomitant administration of an NSAID reduces rates of recurrence of migraine.

❖ **Prolonged attacks (status migraine):** Prolonged attacks of migraine lasting over 72 hours, and sometimes for days can lead to development of painful cutaneous swelling (a sterile inflammation), in the distribution of the trigeminal nerve. Such patients complain that brushing hair is painful, and their glasses are uncomfortable. Best medication, in such cases, is dexamethasone 16 mg IV. Alternatives include valproic acid, ketorolac, and DHE.

❖ **Preventive measures:** Such measures are required when migraine attacks occur 2-3 times or more often per week, but conventional drugs are only partially successful. In these cases, a search should be made for comorbidities associated with migraine, such as depression, panic attacks, anxiety disorder, and epilepsy. Amitriptyline and SSRIs can be useful in such cases. Other drugs to be considered are beta-blockers, flunarizine, valproate, and gabapentin. Once a drug or a combination of drugs has been found to help, it should be continued for several months, and then tapered off. Life-style modifications are also helpful.

# CLUSTER HEADACHE

Cluster headache is a syndrome of distinct attacks of severe headache marked by striking circadian periodicity. Cluster headache is also defined as a *trigeminal autonomic cephalgia.* The typical age of onset is usually 20-40 years, and it is four times more common in men than in women.

The attack is characterized by extremely severe pain occurring in the distribution of trigeminal nerve, more commonly in the temporal and periorbital regions. The headache begins more rapidly than migraine and the episodes are often nocturnal making patients sleep deprived. Attacks occur one to three times daily, often at nearly the same time. During the active cluster period, each attack develops and increases over 15-20 minutes, and may last up to 3 hours. These patients with the *episodic form* have at least two cluster periods of 1 week to several months with remission for at least 1 month.

Some patients experience *chronic cluster headaches* without remission. These patients have at least one cluster period lasting at least 1 year with either no remission or very brief remissions lasting less than a fortnight. Triggers for cluster headache include vasodilators (e.g., alcohol, nitroglycerine) and histamine. In fact nitroglycerine challenge (sublingually) can be diagnostic, producing a typical headache in 30-60 minutes.

Cluster headache is often associated with typical autonomic symptoms, which may include ipsilateral ptosis, lacrimation, miosis, conjunctival injection, rhinorrhea, eyelid edema, and forehead and facial swelling.

### Diagnosis

The unique pattern and combination of symptoms usually make the diagnosis of cluster headache fairly easy, yet other headache disorders with similar or overlapping features need to be differentiated. Neuroimaging is not useful in the diagnosis of cluster headache but is of value in differentiating other forms of severe, acute onset headaches such as intracranial bleed.

### Treatment

Standard treatment for acute attack (abortive therapy) of cluster headache is supplemental oxygen at 8-10 L/min for 15 minutes. Complete pain relief is observed in three-fourths of the cases. Sumatriptan 6 mg subcutaneously is also effective and provides complete relief in over 90% of cases at 15 minutes. Intranasal sumatriptan has a faster onset of action. The drug is contraindicated in patients with known cardiovascular disease. Other drugs used for treatment of acute attack of cluster headache are dihydrergotamine, ergotamine, somatostatin, and intranasal lidocaine, but their efficacy is not proven. Cluster headache is typically resistant to indomethacin.

Prophylactic treatment should be instituted simultaneously with abortive therapy and continued for 2 weeks past the last attack. The most commonly used drug is verapamil in a dose of 240 mg/day. In resistant cases corticosteroids (prednisolone 60-80 mg/day tapered over 2 weeks), and ergotamine 2 mg at bed time or twice daily may be tried.

For chronic cluster headache, verapamil or lithium may be used. Deep brain stimulation is also an option for such cases.

## ACUTE VERTIGO

Vertigo is a feeling of motion when there is no motion, or an exaggerated sensation of motion in response to certain bodily movement. Its severity varies from a spinning sensation and unsteadiness to patient falling suddenly forward or backward. *Vertigo results from some disturbance of vestibular system or its connections with the brainstem.* Vertiginous feeling may be more or less continuous, though more often it comes in attacks lasting from a few minutes to several hours.

## Etiology

Vertigo may be either *peripheral or central in origin*. The former *(vestibular vertigo)* accounts for majority of cases, and comprises conditions, such as Meniere's disease, labyrinthitis, vestibular neuronitis, cervical vertigo, acoustic neuroma, and benign paroxysmal postural vertigo. *Central vertigo* can result from any pathology involving the medulla and cerebellum, such as stroke syndromes, tumor and inflammatory diseases. Sometimes, vertigo occurs from certain physiological causes as in motion sickness, hyperventilation, and standing at a height much above the surrounding environment.

## Clinical Features

Symptoms depend upon the precise type and cause of vertigo. *In peripheral type,* vertigo is usually sudden in onset and occurs in discrete episodes lasting seconds, minutes, or hours. Often mild and transitory, peripheral vertigo can be so severe that the patient is unable to stand or walk, and may fall down. Such patients usually have associated symptoms, such as nausea, vomiting, sweating, prostration, and gait ataxia. The most important sign is *nystagmus,* usually of horizontal type with a rotatory component, and with its Fast phase Opposite to the *Side* of Zesion *(FOSL).* Associated hearing loss and tinnitus provide strong evidence of peripheral vertigo, usually of otologic origin.

*Vertigo due to central lesions,* on the other hand, usually starts gradually as a sensation of dizziness, and then becomes progressively more severe and disabling. Nausea and vomiting are uncommon. Nystagmus is less common, and when present it is not rotational. With progression of vertigo, other features of brainstem dysfunction manifest, such as dysarthria, dysphagia, and sensory abnormalities.

## Diagnosis

As a first step, it should be decided if the vertigo is of peripheral or central origin. A thorough history and physical examination are of great help. Of the two types, peripheral vertigo is much more common. Salient differentiating features of important causes of peripheral vertigo are given below (very briefly):

❖ **Cervical vertigo:** This is usually seen in elderly people and is precipitated by neck movements especially hyperextension *("cathedral ceiling syndrome").* It is generally associated with degenerative disease of cervical spine which impairs functioning of proprioceptive receptors located in the facets of the cervical spine. Prolonged abnormal positioning of the neck such as in watching television lying down in bed, is an important predisposing factor.

- **Benign paroxysmal vertigo:** This type of vertigo is generally triggered by a *"change" in the position of the head* (also called *"positional vertigo"*); actual position of the head is not important. Symptoms usually develop a few seconds after head movement, subside rapidly, and often occur in clusters that last several days. Such episodes are usually benign but can sometimes be due to vertebrobasilar insufficiency.
- **Migrainous vertigo:** Migraine and vertigo sometimes occur together and may be temporally related to each other. Uncommonly however, vertigo may be the sole symptom and may last for several hours. The point to remember is that it is episodic and not associated with tinnitus. A background history of migraine in the patient or family members is usually available.
- **Labyrinthitis:** Vertigo usually starts acutely in these cases, is usually moderate/severe in intensity, and often lasts for several days. Accompanying tinnitus and hearing loss are common. Recovery may take several weeks. The exact cause of labyrinthitis is not clear, but it may be viral or bacterial in origin. Clinically, labyrinthitis may resemble *vestibular neuronitis,* but the latter is not accompanied by any hearing loss or tinnitus.
- **Meniere's syndrome:** This is characterized by brief episodic vertigo, not related to position or movement of the head or neck. Each episode may last from a few minutes to several hours. Such attacks are however, recurrent, wax and wane, and may in the long run be associated with tinnitus and hearing loss. The underlying pathology is believed to be distension of the endolymphatic sac of the inner ear.

## Investigations

Whenever the nature and cause of vertigo is obscure, a detailed history, physical examination, and routine laboratory tests including blood sugar, CBC, and liver and kidney function tests should be done. Special investigations are called for when vertigo is recurrent or a suspicion exists for a neurological disorder. These include otologic evaluation and MRI of brain.

## Management

This should aim initially at control of the distressing symptom by intramuscular anticholinergic/antihistamine preparations, such as promethazine *(Phenergan)* or prochlorperazine *(Stemetil)*. After the acute attack is over, vestibular suppressants (e.g., benzodiazepines, meclizine) should be continued orally for a few days.

In every case, after the acute attack is over, cause of vertigo should be determined and treated appropriately.

# CHAPTER 5

# Renal Emergencies

## INTRODUCTION

The kidneys normally serve a number of important functions, which include:
- Fluid and electrolyte balance,
- Acid-base equilibrium,
- Removal of metabolic waste,
- Regulation of blood pressure,
- Vitamin D metabolism, and
- Synthesis of erythropoietin.

Of these, the first three have a vital role in preserving the *"milieu interior"*. Any serious disturbance in these functions can result in life-threatening emergencies.

## CLINICAL FLUID, ELECTROLYTE, AND ACID-BASE ABNORMALITIES

Disorders of electrolytes and acid-base are common in all types of medical emergencies. Usually minor and of little clinical import, these may sometimes be complex and life-threatening. The aim here is to provide the practicing physicians simple guidelines for their proper interpretation and management. Their diagnosis and principles of treatment based on laboratory values comprise the *"science"* of electrolyte and acid-base physiology. However, the actual treatment, especially replacement therapies, must take into account the entire clinical setting, and constitute the *"art"* of medicine.

### Electrolyte Abnormalities

Though all the electrolytes present in body fluids and cells are required for maintaining a normal *milieu interior*, it is the sodium, potassium, and calcium that are most important.

## SODIUM ABNORMALITIES

### Hypernatremia

A relatively uncommon condition, hypernatremia (serum sodium >150 mEq/L) is usually due to a *deficit in total body water (TBW);* sodium excess being an uncommon cause. In both states, serum osmolality increases resulting in increased thirst and augmented secretion of antidiuretic hormone (ADH), which in turn stimulate water reabsorption (in the kidneys) to restore sodium equilibrium.

### Etiology

Hypernatremia can be due to: **(1) pure or predominant water deficit** due to diminished intake or excessive loss of water as in GI disorders, increased insensible loss (burns, tachypnea, and hyperthermia), excessive use of diuretics, and diabetes insipidus, and **(2) sodium overload** due to improper fluid management in critically ill patients, or excessive sodium bicarbonate administration during cardiopulmonary resuscitation.

### Clinical Features

Sustained hypernatremia usually occurs in patients who lack access to free water or are unable to respond to thirst by drinking water (e.g., young children and physically or neurologically impaired patients). Consequently, central nervous system dysfunction results causing mental confusion, lethargy, stupor, and even seizures. *Hypovolemia* is invariable and commonly manifests as orthostatic hypotension, absence of tears during crying, dry mucous membranes, and decreased skin turgor.

### Treatment

The treatment usually revolves around correction of the cause of the fluid loss, and replacement of water and electrolytes as required. Water constitutes about 60% of body weight, of which about two-thirds is intracellular fluid and the remainder extracellular. TBW deficit can be calculated as follows:

Total body water (TBW) deficit = Normal TBW − Current TBW
Normal TBW = 0.6 × body weight in kg

$$\text{Current TBW} = \frac{\text{Normal serum sodium} \times \text{TBW}}{\text{Estimated serum sodium}}$$

In mildly symptomatic patients *without hypotension* 1–2 L of fluid may be administered over 24 hours IV (as D5W) or orally if patient does not have nausea or vomiting. In more severe cases with dehydration and orthostatic hypotension, TBW deficit should be calculated and $V_i$ of the calculated water deficit replaced in first 24 hours. The remainder should be administered gradually over next 24–48 hours, keeping a serial record of serum sodium levels. *Sodium correction must be done slowly* (about 2 mEq/L/hour) especially if hypernatremia is of long standing, to avoid complications such as cerebral edema and even convulsions.

## Hyponatremia

### Definition and Etiology

Hyponatremia is the most common electrolyte abnormality observed in clinical practice, especially in hospitalized patients. Though normal serum

[Na⁺] ranges between 136 and 145 mEq/L, a decrease in values up to 130 mEq/L is common and usually asymptomatic. *Most of the cases of hyponatremia are due to water imbalance (not sodium imbalance).*

From clinical point of view, hyponatremia is considered severe when serum [Na⁺] is 120 mEq/L or less, *moderate/moderately severe* between 121 and 130 mEq/L and mild between 130 and 135 mEq/L. The cause of hyponatremia varies depending upon whether the patient is hypovolemic, normovolemic, or hypervolemic.

- ❖ **Hypovolemic hyponatremia:** Sodium deficiency in these cases is due to *excessive sodium loss either in urine or through other sources.* The former include diuretic therapy, mineralocorticoid deficiency (e.g., Addison's disease, hypopituitarism), and salt-losing nephropathy. Excessive loss through nonrenal sources occurs in conditions such as diarrhea, vomiting, hot humid weather, and severe burns.
- ❖ **Normovolemic hyponatremia:** This is a heterogeneous group including conditions such as hypothyroidism, renal failure patients with excessive fluid intake, psychogenic polydipsia, postoperative hyponatremia, and the *syndrome of inappropriate secretion of ADH* **(SIADH),** which itself may be due to diverse clinical states (such as acute neurological disorders, malignancy, pulmonary diseases, and certain drugs (e.g., carbamazepine, chlorpropamide, amitriptyline), and in conditions associated with stress (emotional, physical, and surgical). Plasma urea and creatinine are invariably normal indicating that the glomerular filtration rate (GFR) is normal. Diagnosis of SIADH is suggested if the urine osmolality exceeds serum osmolality and the urine [Na⁺] level is more than 40 mEq/L (implying that the urine is inappropriately concentrated).
- ❖ **Hypervolemic hyponatremia:** This is seen in states characterized by *edema* such as congestive cardiac failure, nephrotic syndrome, hepatic cirrhosis, and advanced renal disease. Renal hemodynamics is disturbed in such cases so that total extracellular water is increased (hypervolemia). Such patients have more water than [Na⁺].

### Clinical Features

Symptoms of hyponatremia depend upon the *degree and speed with which sodium level declines.* Mild hyponatremia is usually asymptomatic; overt symptoms of hyponatremia are seen only in patients with moderate or moderately severe [Na⁺] deficiency (125 mEq/L or less). Besides nausea and vomiting, these patients may have headache, and lethargy. *The critical level for hyponatremia is <120 mEq/L, especially if it develops rapidly.* Such patients can have altered sensorium, muscle twitches, irritability, and even seizures, coma and respiratory arrest.

### Treatment

Isotonic saline or lactated Ringer's solution is used in cases of *hypovolemic hyponatremia.* The rate and volume of fluid replacement will be determined by the clinical status.

In patients with *normovolemic hyponatremia* who are *asymptomatic*, sodium level should be corrected by fluid restriction to about 1,000–1,500 mL/day, and oral supplementation by 10–15 g common salt. In some patients with SIADH who cannot follow water restriction or when effect of fluid restriction is inadequate, demeclocycline (300–600 mg twice daily) may prove beneficial by inhibiting the action of ADH at distal tubular level. However, if serum sodium is <120 in asymptomatic patients, normal saline infusion along with furosemide may be used.

Treatment of *hyponatremia in hypervolemic patients* (cirrhosis, heart failure, etc.) depends on the underlying disease. Specific treatment for *symptomatic severe hyponatremia* comprises IV administration of hypertonic saline (3%). This should be done only in intensive care units, when serum sodium is <120 on two closely spaced estimations, and the patient has seizures. The amount of [Na$^+$] required is determined by multiplying the calculated [Na$^+$] deficit in plasma (mEq/L) by TBW (60% of body weight). For example, if a 50 kg patient has a [Na$^+$] level of 112 and is seizing, his immediate [Na$^+$] requirement will be (120 – 112) × (50 × 0.6) = 8 × 30 = 240 mEq.

The calculated amount of hypertonic saline should be infused slowly so as to increase plasma [Na$^+$] by no more than 1–1.5 mEq/L/hour in acute cases and 0.5–1.0 mEq/L/hour in chronic cases. As a general rule plasma [Na$^+$] should not be increased by more than 12 mEq/L over first 24 hours since a rapid increase can cause neurological damage. Infusion should be discontinued when [Na$^+$] level reaches 120 mEq/L. Further correction of hyponatremia should be done slowly by fluid restriction and oral [Na$^+$] supplementation.

## POTASSIUM ABNORMALITIES

Normal serum [K$^+$] level is maintained between 3.5 and 5.5 mEq/L, but this constitutes only about 2% of the total body potassium, which is about 160 mEq/L. Most of the [K$^+$] (approximately 98%) is inside the cells, and intracellular [K$^+$] concentration is about 40 times that in extracellular fluid (ECF). However, serum [K$^+$] is important because even a small variation in its level can be life-threatening.

Ordinarily, extracellular and intracellular changes occur in the same direction, and therefore alteration in serum [K$^+$] level is a good measure of change in total body potassium. The only exception to this rule is the [K$^+$]-alterations in acid-base imbalance. In metabolic acidosis excess [H$^+$] ions migrate into the cells, displacing potassium into the serum, resulting in hyperkalemia. The reverse occurs in metabolic alkalosis.

*Potassium plays an important role in nerve-muscle function, cell membrane activity and acid-base balance.* An average daily diet contains about 40–100 mEq potassium most of which is excreted in urine (40–80 mEq/day).

## Hypokalemia

Hypokalemia, defined as serum potassium below 3.5 mEq/L is the most frequent electrolyte disturbance. Body potassium is regulated by *aldosterone*, which facilitates potassium excretion in urine in distal renal tubules. Healthy subjects lose only minimal amount of potassium (5–15 mEq/day). Hypokalemia may result from a decrease in total body stores of potassium as after diuretic use, from increased gastrointestinal (GI) or renal losses, or in the setting of alcohol, malnutrition, or decreased intake. Various causes of hypokalemia are listed at **Box. 5.1**. In our country (and other developing countries), the most common cause of hypokalemia is GI loss due to infective diarrhea.

### Clinical Features

The most common feature of hypokalemia is *impaired neuromuscular conduction*. Milder cases may be asymptomatic or have only fatigue, muscle weakness, and cramping. Increasing hypokalemia may be associated with constipation, abdominal distension (ileus), hyporeflexia, hypercapnia, lethal arrhythmias, and tetany. Extreme cases may develop almost total paralysis. The severity of symptoms is also related to how quickly the hypokalemia develops.

### Diagnosis

Whenever a significant alteration in [K⁺] level is observed, the value should be rechecked before initiating treatment. The cause of hypokalemia is often obvious from the history. *ECG changes develop when potassium level is below 2.7, and can rapidly progress to serious arrhythmias* (**Box 5.2**).

### Treatment

The cause of hypokalemia should be identified and corrected as best as possible. When replacement therapy is planned, following points should be kept in mind.

---

**Box 5.1: Important causes of hypokalemia.**

- **Decreased availability:**
  - *Deficient intake:* Malnutrition, alcoholism, prolonged IV therapy with fluids lacking potassium
  - *Reduced absorption:* Malabsorption, small bowel-bypass.
- **Increased loss:**
  - *Extra renal (gastrointestinal):* Vomiting, diarrhea, fistulae, villous adenoma, Zollinger-Ellison syndrome
  - *Renal:* Diuretics, glucocorticoid excess (exogenous therapy, Cushing syndrome), hypomagnesemia, renal tubular acidosis, metabolic alkalosis, aldosteronism
- **[K⁺] shift into cells:** Drug-induced (insulin, Beta-2 agonists), familial periodic paralysis, thyrotoxicosis, metabolic alkalosis

> **Box 5.2: ECG changes in hypokalemia.**
> 
> - Decreased T-wave amplitude
> - T-wave inversion
> - ST-segment depression prominent LP wave
> - Prolongation of QT interval
> - Ventricular tachycardia Torsade's de pointes

- ❖ On average, a decrease of 0.3 mEq/L in serum potassium is associated with a 100 mEq deficit in total body stores.
- ❖ During acute replacement therapy most of the potassium rapidly enters the cells so that administration of 100-200 mEq results in increase in plasma [K⁺] concentration by about 1 mEq/L.
- ❖ Intravenous potassium replacement therapy should be started only when adequate urine output is ensured.
- ❖ Intravenous potassium should not be given in glucose-containing solution as this may stimulate insulin release and result in worsening hypokalemia through shifts of potassium into the cells.
- ❖ Magnesium values should be checked and corrected (if low) especially in resistant cases of hypokalemia.

In patients with hypokalemia who are *asymptomatic or mildly symptomatic*, potassium depletion can be treated by oral replacement using potassium chloride (20-40 mEq every 4-6 hours). Oral therapy is preferred provided the patient can tolerate it. Higher doses carry risk of esophageal and gastric irritation.

In *moderately symptomatic patients* (but without cardiac arrhythmias), one-half of the estimated potassium deficit should be replaced over the first 18-24 hours, and the remaining over next 24 hours. Even in these cases oral route is preferable. *In severely symptomatic patients with serum potassium below 2.5,* IV therapy is indicated. When infusing through a peripheral vein, potassium concentration should not exceed 20 mEq/L to avoid pain at infusion site and sclerosis of the veins. Administering potassium at 20 mEq/hour is expected to increase potassium by 0.25 mEq/hour.

The rate of infusion should not exceed 20 mEq/hour (or more than 200 mEq/day) except in cases of myocardial infarction with significant ventricular arrhythmia, in patients with paralysis of respiratory muscles, or when there is evidence of large continuing loss of [K⁺] in urine. In such cases the rate of initial [K⁺] infusion can be doubled. Potassium infusion should always be given in **intensive care unit** under close ECG monitoring and with hourly estimations of serum [K⁺]. **Potassium should never be administered through a central venous catheter** because local hyperkalemia may result in arrhythmias, heart block, and asystole.

## Hyperkalemia

This is one of the most serious electrolyte disturbances, and may be life-threatening. The plasma [K⁺] is usually 5.0 mEq/L or more.

| Table 5.1: Important causes of hyperkalemia. | |
|---|---|
| **Increased exogenous potassium load** | • Potassium supplements (oral or IV) (especially with impaired renal function)<br>• Stored blood (>10 days old)<br>• Potassium penicillin |
| **Increased potassium release from cells**<br>($K^+$ released from cells) | • Cell destruction (burns, crush injuries)<br>• Rhabdomyolysis<br>• Severe intravascular hemolysis<br>• Tumor lysis<br>• Succinyl choline |
| **Renal disorders**<br>• Decreased GFR<br>• Tubular disorders (Decreased $K^+$ excretion) | • Acute and chronic renal failure<br>• Analgesic nephropathy<br>• Obstructive uropathy<br>• Interstitial nephritis<br>• Chronic pyelonephritis |
| **Hypoaldosteronism**<br>• Primary<br>• Secondary | • Addison disease, adrenogenital syndrome<br>• Hyporeninemic (type IV), renal tubular acidosis<br>• Drug-induced (NSAIDs, ACE inhibitors, aldosterone antagonists, heparin, cyclosporine) |
| **Transcellular shifts**<br>($K^+$ shift from intracellular to extracellular space) | • Acidosis<br>• Hyperosmolar diuresis<br>• Acute digitalis over dosage<br>• Insulin deficiency<br>• Hyperkalemic periodic paralysis<br>• Succinylcholine exercise |
| **Spurious** | • Hemolysis blood sample<br>• Thrombocytosis and leukocytosis with release of potassium (plasma potassium will be normal). Repeated fist clenching during drawing blood sample resulting in release of potassium from forearm muscles |

## Etiology

Important causes of hyperkalemia are listed at **Table 5.1**. *Excess potassium is mainly eliminated by the kidneys.* Accordingly, the most frequent cause is decreased renal excretion. Hyperkalemia can also occur with transmembrane shift of intracellular potassium as seen in metabolic acidosis.

*Severe hyperkalemia* can sometimes develop rapidly with massive tissue damage (e.g., accidents, military casualties). Such cases often have associated acidosis and acute renal insufficiency, and plasma [$K^+$] can increase by as much as 2–3 mEq/L in a day.

## Clinical Features

Hyperkalemia can interfere with normal neuromuscular functions and may result in nonspecific symptoms comprising muscular weakness (including muscles of respiration), fatigue, paresthesias, and palpitation. Occasionally diarrhea and abdominal distension may occur.

Cardiac abnormalities constitute an important feature of hyperkalemia, and these are often well *reflected in ECG*. The earliest change is *peaking of T-waves,* usually seen with [K⁺] levels between 6.0 and 7.0 mEq/L. With progressive increase in plasma [K⁺], *PR and QRS become prolonged, and complete heart block* may develop. Terminally, *ventricular fibrillation/standstill* may occur. However, ECG may be normal in many cases of hyperkalemia.

## Diagnosis

When significantly high, potassium level should be confirmed by a second analysis, preferably by measuring plasma potassium level to exclude spurious causes. In all cases renal and cardiac status as well as current medication should be reviewed. Hyperkalemia is commonly associated with metabolic acidosis, and a venous blood gas may be helpful in guiding treatment.

## Treatment

Several measures are available to control hyperkalemia. The precise therapy in a given case is determined by *degree of hyperkalemia* which is *graded as mild, moderate, or severe,* with [K⁺] levels 6.0 mEq/L or less, 6.0–8.0 mEq/L, and >8.0 mEq/L, respectively.

Mild hyperkalemia usually calls for slow correction coupled with elimination of the underlying cause (such as use of [K⁺]-sparing diuretics and ACE inhibitors). Volume depletion and acidosis should be corrected and loop diuretics administered to increase [K⁺] excretion. In all cases diet should be modified avoiding [K⁺]-rich items (fruit juices, etc.). *More severe or progressive hyperkalemia,* especially when associated with cardiac arrhythmias and conduction defects in ECG, warrants *aggressive therapy*. Following drugs/measures are available in such cases.

- ❖ **Calcium gluconate:** Calcium antagonizes the effect of potassium on cardiac membrane potential and is the first line drug to be used whenever potassium level is >7.0 or when ECG changes are present. Both calcium gluconate and calcium chloride are available as 10% solution, but calcium chloride has three times as much calcium available as calcium gluconate, and is more irritating, if it extravasates. Calcium gluconate is therefore preferred; 10 mL of 10% solution is given as IV push over 1 minute and may be repeated at 2–5 minute intervals up to three doses, preferably under continuous ECG monitoring. If calcium chloride is used only one ampule should be given over 5 minutes. Calcium acts within minutes and its effect lasts for about an hour. It *restores membrane excitability but does not lower plasma potassium level.*

ote

> (1) Calcium should be used with extreme caution in patients receiving digitalis since calcium potentiates the myocardial toxicity of digoxin. (2) Calcium and HCO₃ should be administered separately through different IV lines, or sequentially with good flushing, if there is a single line.

- **Insulin and hypertonic glucose infusion:** Ten units of regular insulin may be given along with 500 mL of D10W administered rapidly over 30 minutes. The infusion also improves hyperkalemia by simple dilution of plasma [K⁺], which may be lowered by 1-2 mEq/L within 30-60 minutes. If fluid overload is a problem, 50 mL of D50W may be given through a central line. *Hypertonic glucose provokes insulin release with consequent shift of [K⁺] into the cells.* In hyperglycemic patients only insulin is required. Insulin lowers serum potassium level by 1-3 mEq/L within minutes and the effect usually persists for 4-5 hours.
- **Sodium bicarbonate:** Infusion of $NaHCO_3$ alone has a variable effect and should not be used as a monotherapy. However, it potentiates the potassium-lowering effect of insulin. Two ampules of $NaHCO_3$ (100 mEq) should be administered IV within 2-5 minutes in cases with severe hyperkalemia and metabolic acidosis. This therapy is effective within 20-40 minutes and the effect lasts for 4-5 hours.
- **Potassium elimination:** This can be achieved by: (1) using a *sodium-potassium exchange resin*, (2) *hemodialysis*, which is usually required for patients with renal failure and severe hyperkalemia, and (3) *loop diuretics* used in conjunction with saline infusions (useful only in patients with good urine output and modest hyperkalemia).

## ■ CALCIUM ABNORMALITIES

Normal serum/plasma calcium varies between 9.0 and 10.5 mg/dL. Of this ionized calcium comprises 4.7-5.3 (about 50% of total calcium), and it is this component that is necessary for muscle contraction and nerve function. Calcium value is closely related to serum albumin concentration, and decreases by about 1 mg for every 1 g fall in albumin. In fact *hypoalbuminemia is the most common cause of low serum calcium* observed in clinical practice.

In normal subjects serum calcium level is tightly regulated by **parathyroid hormone** through: (1) increase in bone resorption, (2) decrease in renal excretion of calcium, and (3) activation of vitamin D, which increases reabsorption of calcium from the gut. It is to be noted that despite alterations in serum calcium values observed frequently in clinical practice, emergency situations are uncommon.

### Hypocalcemia

*Etiology*

Hypocalcemia is defined as ionized calcium less than 4.4 mg/dL. Many conditions can result in hypocalcemia (**Table 5.2**), the most common being *renal failure in which decreased production of active vitamin D3* (1,25 dihydroxyvitamin $D_3$) and hyperphosphatemia play an important role. However, only a few of these clinical conditions are associated with an acute decrease in serum calcium (**hypocalcemic crisis**). These include damage

| **Table 5.2:** Important causes of hypocalcemia. | |
|---|---|
| **Decreased intake/absorption**<br>• Nutritional deficiency<br>• Malabsorption<br>• Small bowel bypass<br>• Vitamin D deficit<br>  ➢ Anticonvulsants<br>  ➢ Glucocorticoids<br>  ➢ Chronic renal failure | **Increased loss**<br>• Diuretic therapy<br>• Alcoholism<br>• Chronic kidney disease |
| | **Multifactorial**<br>Sepsis<br>Pancreatitis<br>Magnesium deficiency |
| **Endocrinal disorders**<br>• Hypoparathyroidism<br>• Pseudohypoparathyroidism<br>• Familial hypocalcemia | **Physiological**<br>• Hypoalbuminemia<br>• Hyperphosphatemia |

**Box 5.3: Clinical manifestations of hypocalcemia.**

- **Central nervous system**
  - Seizures
  - Confusion, hallucinations, psychosis, extrapyramidal disorders, dysarthria, papilledema
- **Cardiovascular**
  - Decreased myocardial contractility
  - Decreased vascular tone
  - Arrhythmias
  - Prolonged QTc

to parathyroid glands during surgery, acute pancreatitis, intestinal fistula, transfusion of large amount of citrated blood, and marked alkalosis.

### Clinical Features (Box 5.3)

It is to be noted that the rapidity of fall in calcium level is as important as actual degree of hypocalcemia. Basically, hypocalcemia facilitates the transmission of impulses across the myoneural junction resulting in increased neuromuscular excitability which may clinically manifest as tetany. Early symptoms include paresthesia, muscle cramps and carpopedal spasms. More *severe cases* can develop seizures, laryngeal stridor, dysarthria, and cardiac arrhythmias. In cases with *protracted hypocalcemia,* cerebral symptoms may supervene including depression or psychosis, confusion and drowsiness. Papilledema occurs sometimes and is a source of confusion with intracranial space occupying lesion.

### Diagnosis

Hypocalcemia is diagnosed when serum $Ca^{++}$ is <9.0 mg/dL (in true hypocalcemia the ionized calcium level is also low, i.e., <4.7 mg/dL). However, serious symptoms of hypocalcemia (tetany, arrhythmias, and seizures) manifest only when calcium level falls below 7.5 mg% (except in alkalosis). In respiratory alkalosis, total serum calcium may be normal but ionized fraction is decreased. ECG shows prolongation of QTc.

## Treatment

**Asymptomatic hypocalcemia** rarely progresses to a life-threatening situation. Oral calcium supplements (1–2 g elemental calcium) are useful but because of the rampant vitamin D deficiency, it is more important to provide vitamin D-3 supplements. Note should be made of even mild symptoms due to hypocalcemia because of the potential for significant problems should hypocalcemia worsen.

**Symptomatic (severe) hypocalcemia** should be treated with IV 10% calcium gluconate, 10–20 mL (containing 93 mg elemental calcium per 10 mL ampule). Intravenous calcium should be administered slowly to avoid serious cardiac complications (20 mL over 10–20 minutes). The effect of such bolus injection is short lived, and therefore it should be followed by an infusion of 0.5–1.5 mg/kg/hour of elemental calcium in dextrose or saline for 4–6 hours (up to a maximum of 2.0 g). Because of the risk of serious cardiac arrhythmias (especially in patients on digitalis therapy), calcium infusions should be administered only in intensive care units, with frequent monitoring of calcium level (every 6–8 hours) so as to maintain serum calcium between 7.5 and 8.5 mg/dL.

In the presence of *hypomagnesemia* (serum magnesium <1 mg/dL), symptoms may remain refractory until serum magnesium is also corrected. Patients with renal disease or hypoparathyroidism may have simultaneously *hyperphosphatemia* (serum phosphate >6.0 mg/dL). Such cases should not be treated with supplemental calcium to avoid risk of metastatic calcification; rather, treatment should focus on eliminating phosphate by using insulin and glucose to shift phosphate into cells. Volume expansion may also be useful.

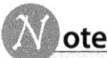ote

> When hypocalcemic symptoms are due to respiratory alkalosis (e.g., psychogenic hyperventilation), rebreathing from a paper bag or infusion of 1/2 to 1 L of normal saline will ameliorate symptoms.

## Hypercalcemia

Hypercalcemia is defined as serum calcium more than 11.0 mg/dL. As with hypocalcemia, the rate at which calcium increases is important in assessing the symptoms of hypercalcemia. Though many conditions can result in hypercalcemia **(Table 5.3)**, about 90% cases are due to **primary hyperparathyroidism** or **malignancy.** The differentiation is important from therapeutic point of view as prednisolone is useful in patients with hypercalcemia mediated by mechanisms other than parathyroid excess.

**Table 5.3:** Causes of hypercalcemia.

| Endocrine disorders | Increased intake or absorption |
|---|---|
| • Hyperparathyroidism<br>• Acromegaly<br>• Adrenal insufficiency<br>• Pheochromocytoma | • Vitamin D excess<br>• Milk-alkali syndrome |
| **Neoplastic diseases** | **Miscellaneous causes** |
| • Malignancy anywhere (especially lung, kidney, ovary)<br>• Multiple myeloma<br>• Immobilization | • Chronic granulomatous diseases (calcitriol production)<br>• Thiazide diuretics<br>• Paget's disease<br>• Familial<br>• Lithium therapy<br>• Lymphoma |

**Table 5.4:** Clinical manifestations of hypercalcemia.

| Renal | Cardiovascular |
|---|---|
| Natriuresis, hypovolemia Impaired renal concentrating ability polyuria, polydipsia, renal lithiasis, nephrocalcinosis, renal failure | Increased myocardial contractility, increased vascular tone shortened QTc |
| **Gastrointestinal** | **Central nervous system** |
| Ileus, constipation, anorexia, vomiting, peptic ulcer disease, pancreatitis | Lethargy, fatigue, depression, confusion, psychosis, coma |

## Clinical Features (Table 5.4)

There is *poor correlation between the elevated serum calcium level and severity of symptoms*. Clinical manifestations of hypercalcemia are mostly mild and nonspecific.

With mild or moderate hypercalcemia, *gastrointestinal symptoms* are common (anorexia, nausea, vomiting, and constipation). Some cases may also develop *impairment of renal function* and present with polyuria and polydipsia simulating diabetes insipidus. Renal colic and hematuria may result from nephrolithiasis. More severe degree of hypercalcemia often results in hypertension, cardiac arrhythmias, and neuromuscular symptoms such as lethargy, muscular hypotonia, flaccid paralysis, stupor, or even coma. Chronic cases develop calcium metastases in various organs with terminal renal failure.

## Diagnosis

Serum calcium level is increased (usually above 12.0 mg/dL), but should be *correlated with serum albumin level*. Highest calcium values (>15 mg/dL) generally occur in malignancy. There may be associated hypercalciuria (urinary calcium >20 mg/day) and hypophosphatemia. The electrocardiogram reveals a shortened QTc. Radiological examination can reveal evidence of trabecular bone disease, and chest radiograph may disclose malignancy or granulomatous lesion. The diagnosis between hyperparathyroidism and malignancy is confirmed by study of: (1) parathyroid hormone (PTH)

### Box 5.4: Treatment of severe hypercalcemia.

- **Acute treatment**
  - Restore intravascular volume rapidly by isotonic saline infusion
  - Then administer furosemide 20–40 mg every 4–6 hours to increase $Ca^{++}$ excretion. Without adequate saline infusion, diuretics can actually worsen hypercalcemia
  - Follow urinary magnesium and potassium losses and replace as warranted
  - Dialysis with low or no calcium dialysate (in emergency situations).
- **Pharmacological measures**
  - *Hypercalcemia associated with hyperparathyroidism:*
    - Bisphosphonates
    - Vitamin D and vitamin D analogues
    - Calcitriol
  - *For hypercalcemia of malignancy*
    - Bisphosphonates
    - Gallium nitrate
    - Calcitonin
    - Other drugs (corticosteroids, plicamycin).

which is elevated in hyperparathyroidism, and (2) PTH-related protein, which is increased in neoplastic diseases (along with level of PTH).

### Treatment

Though there is no specific cut off value, serum ionized calcium greater than 6.5 mEq/L warrants emergency treatment, even if asymptomatic. Specific therapy may be instituted, if a precipitating cause is identified. In the meanwhile, however, **renal excretion of $Ca^{++}$ should be promoted by volume expansion and saline diuresis (Box 5.4)**. It is to be remembered that most patients with severe hypercalcemia are profoundly volume depleted, and initial treatment should be directed toward volume replacement with isotonic saline until the patient is normovolemic. This will increase glomerular filtration rate and thereby promote diuresis. Once extracellular volume has been normalized, further urinary excretion of calcium should be promoted by loop diuretics.

Such acute treatment of hypercalcemia is usually successful, and serum calcium concentration can be lowered by 3–6 mg/dL within 24–48 hours in most patients. Long-term pharmacologic measures may be required in some patients.

ote

(1) Renal and cardiovascular status should be assessed prior to rapid administration of saline, (2) Fluid overload should be avoided. Ideally, central venous pressure should be monitored and kept 10–14 cm $H_2O$.

## Clinical Acid-base Disorders

The terminology and some concepts of acid-base disorders need to be recapitulated:
- Normal acid-base values are: **pH:** 7.40 ± 0.04; **PaCO$_2$:** 40.0 ± 4.0 mm Hg; and **HCO$_3$:** 24.0 ± 2 mEq/L
- **"Acidosis"** (pH <7.36) results from accumulation of acid [H⁺] or elimination of [HCO$_3$], while **"alkalosis"** (pH >7.44) is due to excessive addition of base or elimination of acid
- **Metabolic processes** primarily affect bicarbonate concentration, and **respiratory processes** primarily affect PaCO$_2$
- These primary disturbances are *accompanied by compensatory changes (ventilatory or renal)* in an attempt to maintain pH as near normal as possible (7.40). The former (ventilatory) involves rapid elimination of CO$_2$ by lungs, while the latter (renal) is through increasing HCO$_3$ level by either increased tubular reabsorption or generation of new bicarbonate. If the compensation is adequate, it is *simple acid-base disorder,* if not, it is a *mixed acid-base disorder.* Mixed disorders are difficult to interpret in general clinical practice.

### *Pathophysiology*

The pH is normally maintained within a very narrow range by means of a precise balance between acid [H⁺] production and excretion. Acid is produced in two forms: **(1) volatile component, i.e., carbonic acid (H$_2$CO$_3$)**, which principally results from carbon dioxide produced during metabolism, and **(2) nonvolatile acids, such as sulfuric, phosphoric, and uric acids.** The primary organs, which remove this acid load and maintain the constancy of pH are the lungs and kidneys. The lungs rapidly eliminate carbon dioxide maintaining a PaCO$_2$ of 40 mm Hg, while kidneys excrete the bulk of nonvolatile (fixed) acid load. The renal response to changes in pH is slower than the ventilatory response, and may take 24–48 hours. Any imbalance between the excretion and rate of production of CO$_2$ results in respiratory acid-base disturbance. Similar alterations in the rate of production and excretion of fixed acids results in metabolic acidosis or alkalosis.

**Buffers:** These are substances that oppose changes in free [H⁺]. The *buffer system has two components:* (1) carbonic acid system (CO$_2$/HCO$_3$); and (2) noncarbonic buffer system comprising hemoglobin and protein buffers. Of these the former is more important clinically since its components are readily measurable, and also because determination of CO$_2$ and HCO$_3$ allows differentiation between metabolic or respiratory origin of the problem under consideration.

**Compensations:** Whenever the primary disturbance alters the blood pH, compensatory (adaptive) responses set in to bring the pH towards normal. These compensations work differently when pH is threatened by metabolic or respiratory disorders (**Table 5.5**).

**Table 5.5:** Primary and compensatory responses in acid-base disorders.

| Disorder | Primary abnormality | Compensation | pH | PaCO$_2$ | HCO$_3$ |
|---|---|---|---|---|---|
| Metabolic acidosis | HCO$_3$ | PaCO$_2$ | <7.35 | <40 | <22 |
| Metabolic alkalosis | HCO$_3$ | PaCO$_2$ | >7.45 | >40 | >28 |
| Respiratory acidosis | (PaCO$_2$) | HCO$_3$ | <7.35 | >45 | >24 |
| Respiratory alkalosis | (PaCO$_2$) | HCO$_3$ | >7.45 | <35 | <24 |

- **Metabolic acidosis** *(decrease in HCO$_3$)*. The respiratory center in medulla responds to metabolically induced lowering of pH by hyperventilation, so CO$_2$ is washed out and pH is restored toward normal. This **compensatory response** is directly proportional to the degree of metabolic acidosis. Simply stated (in compensated metabolic acidosis) *PaCO$_2$ decreases by 1.0 mm Hg for each 1 mEq fall in bicarbonate* **(RULE 1)**. However, PaCO$_2$ rarely falls below 20 mm Hg. For example, with bicarbonate 10 mEq/L, PaCO$_2$ should decrease by "base deficit" × 1.0, i.e., (24 − 10) × 1.0 = approximately 14 mm Hg. Therefore, the predicted PaCO$_2$ is 40 − 14 = 26 mm Hg. If the measured PaCO$_2$ is more than 26, in the face of this severe acidosis, it implies **a mixed disturbance** (i.e., mixed metabolic acidosis and respiratory alkalosis).

  Maximum compensation usually occurs at pH 7.1; if blood pH further decreases, there is no more increase in ventilatory compensation possibly due to muscle fatigue and depression of respiratory center.

- **Metabolic alkalosis** *(increase in HCO$_3$)*: Change in bicarbonate and PaCO$_2$ is opposite to that seen in metabolic acidosis. Therefore, as a *primary change* bicarbonate increases, and *compensation* (adaptation) leads to increase in PaCO$_2$. In simple terms, *PaCO$_2$ increases by 0.7 mm Hg for every 1 mEq rise in bicarbonate* **(RULE 2)**. This compensatory response in PaCO$_2$ is, however, seldom >50–55 mm Hg.

- **Respiratory acidosis** *(increase in PaCO$_2$)*: This is reflected *primarily* in increase in PaCO$_2$. As *compensation* sets in, bicarbonate increases in a linear and predictable manner so that *for every 10 mm Hg increase in PaCO$_2$ above 40, bicarbonate increases by 1 mEq/L in* **acute** *respiratory acidosis* **(RULE 3)** and *4 mEq/L in* **chronic** *respiratory acidosis* **(RULE 4)**.

- **Respiratory alkalosis** *(decrease in PaCO$_2$)*: This is due to hyperventilation resulting in a decrease in PaCO$_2$. Compensation/adaptation results by decrease in bicarbonate due to increased renal excretion and reduced generation. Here again the alteration in bicarbonate is proportional to change in PaCO$_2$ so that *for every 10 mm Hg decrease in PaCO$_2$ below 40, bicarbonate decreases by 2 mEq/L in* **acute** *respiratory alkalosis* **(RULE 5)** *(seldom <18 mEq/L), and 5 mEq/L in* **chronic** *cases* **(RULE 6)** but usually not below 14 mEq/L.

**Adverse consequences:** Severe acidosis (pH <7.20) and severe alkalosis (pH >7.60), irrespective of the type or the cause, can per se result in serious

**Table 5.6:** Important adverse effects of severe acidosis.

| | |
|---|---|
| Cardiovascular | • Impaired cardiac contractility<br>• Increased pulmonary vascular resistance<br>• Decreased cardiac output and blood pressure<br>• Increased risk of ventricular arrhythmia |
| Metabolic | • Hyperkalemia<br>• Insulin resistance<br>• Increased metabolic demands |
| Miscellaneous | • Hyperventilation<br>• Impaired brain metabolism<br>• Progressive coma |

**Table 5.7:** Important adverse effects of severe alkalosis.

| | |
|---|---|
| Cardiovascular | • Arteriolar vasoconstriction<br>• Decreased coronary flow; increased risk of supraventricular and ventricular arrhythmias |
| Metabolic | • Hypokalemia<br>• Increased anaerobic glycolysis<br>• Decreased ionized calcium fraction |
| Miscellaneous | • Hypoventilation resulting in hypercapnia and Hypoxemia<br>• Decrease in cerebral blood flow<br>• Tetany, seizures<br>• Lethargy, delirium and stupor |

hemodynamic and metabolic consequences **(Tables 5.6 and 5.7)**. Of these, the effects on the cardiovascular system can be particularly deleterious.

## METABOLIC ACIDOSIS

### Etiopathogenesis

Many pathologic states can result in metabolic acidosis **(Table 5.8)**. Three mechanisms are involved:
1. *Bicarbonate depletion* as in diarrhea and proximal renal tubular acidosis
2. *Retention of acid metabolites* such as sulfuric and phosphoric acids (as in uremia)
3. *Overproduction of metabolic acids,* e.g., betahydroxybutyric acid and acetoacetic acid in diabetic ketoacidosis, and lactic acid in cardiac arrest and acute circulatory failure.

The cause of metabolic acidosis is usually obvious from the clinical setting. As far as laboratory studies are concerned, it is useful to determine the **anion-gap** and then classify these cases into two categories— *increased anion-gap group and normal anion-gap group*. However, this discussion is beyond the scope of this text.

**Table 5.8:** Causes of metabolic acidosis.

| Normal anion-gap | Increased anion-gap |
|---|---|
| **Gastrointestinal disorders**<br>• Diarrhea<br>• Fistula (pancreatic)<br>• Ileal loop | **Exogenous**<br>• Poisoning (salicylates, methanol, ethylene glycol, paraldehyde)<br>• Hyperalimentation |
| **Renal (Loss of $HCO_3$)**<br>• Renal tubular acidosis<br>• Potassium sparing diuretics<br>• Carbonic anhydrase inhibitors<br>• Hypoaldosteronism | **Endogenous**<br>• Ketoacidosis<br>• Lactic acidosis<br>• Renal failure |

**Table 5.9:** Diagnostic features and symptoms of various acid-base disturbances.

| Acid-base disturbance | Diagnostic feature | Chief symptom | Other symptoms |
|---|---|---|---|
| **Metabolic acidosis** | ↓pH and ↓$HCO_3$ | Hyperventilation | pH <7.35 |
| **Metabolic alkalosis** | ↑pH and ↑$HCO_3$ | Tetany (in severe cases) | See **Table 5.5** |
| **Respiratory acidosis** | ↓pH and ↑$PaCO_2$ | Confusion (when $PaCO_2$ >70) | Symptoms of underlying disease |
| **Respiratory alkalosis** | ↑pH and ↓$PaCO_2$ | Related to hypocalcemia | Cerebral and cardiac ischemia (in severe cases) |

## Diagnosis and Clinical Features

See **Table 5.9**.

## Treatment

The treatment of metabolic acidosis depends upon the acuteness and severity of acidosis as well as on the nature of the underlying disorder. Specific therapy is not required in mild cases ($HCO_3$ >15 mEq/L) or when metabolic acidosis is associated with chronic renal failure unless it is severe. Likewise, in acute acidosis due to overproduction of metabolic acids as in diabetic ketoacidosis and lactic acidosis, effective treatment of the primary disorder will rapidly result in conversion of accumulated acids into bicarbonate with consequent improvement in metabolic acidosis.

When metabolic acidosis is significant ($HCO_3$ <15 mEq/L) but slow in onset, oral treatment with sodium bicarbonate may be all that is required. The usual dose is 1 g sodium bicarbonate 2–4 times daily, the exact dose depending upon the response in bicarbonate levels which should be frequently monitored. In acute severe metabolic acidosis, however, parenteral bicarbonate therapy becomes mandatory. In such cases base (bicarbonate) deficit is calculated as follows:

Total body $HCO_3$ deficit = $HCO_3$ (base) deficit × total body water

Where:

a. Base deficit = Desired $HCO_3$ − Actual HCO

b. Total body water = Body weight × 0.6

For example, if in a patient weighing 60 kg, plasma $HCO_3$ is 10 and it is planned to increase it to 18, bicarbonate deficit is 18 − 10 = 8 mEq/L, and TBW will be 60 × 0.6 = 36 L. The total bicarbonate deficit therefore, is 36 × 8 = 288 mEq. One half of this can be given IV over 10 minutes as 7.5% sodium bicarbonate solution (50 mL contains 90 mEq bicarbonate), and the remaining half replaced subsequently according to pH measurements. In practice it may be safer to restrict initial replacement to no more than 100 mEq since overzealous treatment can result in severe hypernatremia, hyperosmolar state, and in tetany (in patients with renal failure or hypocalcemia). The only exception would be cases with extreme and protracted acidosis (pH <7.1). In such cases larger doses (even equal to total calculated bicarbonate deficit) may be given in keeping with the clinical condition of the patient and the physician's expertise.

## METABOLIC ALKALOSIS

This is a state characterized by *increase in pH and plasma bicarbonate associated with a compensatory increase in $PaCO_2$*.

### Etiology (Box 5.5)

Metabolic alkalosis usually results from loss of fixed acids from the gastrointestinal tract or kidneys, and is nearly always associated with hypokalemia. Occasionally, it is the result of excessive alkali administration (bicarbonate or its precursors—citrate, lactate, and acetate). The causes of metabolic alkalosis can be divided into two groups according to whether it

---

**Box 5.5: Causes of metabolic alkalosis.**

- **Chloride sensitive** (urinary chloride <10 mEq/L)
  - *Gastrointestinal*
    - Vomiting/nasogastric suctioning
    - Some cases of diarrhea
    - Excessive alkali intake (milk-alkali syndrome)
  - *Renal*
    - Diuretics
    - Post-hypercapnic alkalosis
    - Severe potassium depletion
- **Chloride resistant** (urinary chloride >10 mEq/L)
  - *Excessive mineralocorticoids*
    - Adrenal over activity (e.g., Cushing syndrome, Conn's syndrome)
    - Exogenous steroid administration

is **chloride-sensitive or chloride-resistant.** Of the two, the former is much more common and is often associated with hypochloremia and hypokalemia.

## Clinical Features

While metabolic alkalosis is a common finding in seriously ill patients, it has few signs and symptoms, and the clinical picture is usually dominated by the underlying disease state. Severe alkalosis can, however, per se result in a variety of symptoms and signs **(Table 5.6)** with ECG changes resembling those of hypokalemia. In the presence of hepatic failure, encephalopathy may be worsened due to increase in ammonia levels.

## Diagnosis

Metabolic alkalosis is diagnosed by an increase in pH along with increase in bicarbonate. Respiratory compensation is in the form of hypoventilation, but is only modest and $PaCO_2$ is seldom >50–55 mm Hg. As a general rule $PaCO_2$ increases by an average of 0.7 mm Hg for every 1 mEq rise in bicarbonate. For example, if a patient in metabolic alkalosis has a $HCO_3$ of 38, the $PaCO_2$ should be - $PaCO_2$ + (increase in bicarbonate × 0.7) = 40 + (38 - 24) - 0.7 = ~50 mm Hg. If the measured $PaCO_2$ is less than 50 it implies a component of respiratory alkalosis.

The cause of metabolic alkalosis is usually obvious from the clinical setting. When in doubt, it is useful to determine urine chloride content.

## Treatment

Mild or moderate cases of metabolic alkalosis (plasma bicarbonate up to 30 mEq/L) seldom require specific treatment. Nasogastric drainage should be stopped, if possible, exogenous administration of bicarbonate and other alkalis discontinued, use of diuretics curtailed, and salt restriction relaxed.

In more severe cases treatment involves replacing extracellular fluid volume deficit (group 1 cases) with isotonic NaCl solution, and potassium. The provision of chloride results in increased [Na$^+$] reabsorption and enhanced $HCO_3$ excretion in proximal tubule. Since less [Na$^+$] is now presented to distal tubule, alkalosis begins to resolve as less [FT] is secreted and less $HCO_3$ is generated. These adjustments, however, occur slowly and may take 3–4 days to improve metabolic alkalosis.

*In chloride-resistant metabolic alkalosis,* treatment of the underlying disease often resolves alkalosis. These cases generally have large [K$^+$] depletion (500 mEq or even more), and [K$^+$] replacement invariably corrects alkalosis. Aldosterone antagonists (e.g., spironolactone) or acetazolamide may also prove useful in such cases by increasing renal excretion of bicarbonate.

## RESPIRATORY ACIDOSIS

This is an acidotic state in which decrease in pH is associated with increase in $PaCO_2$ and a compensatory increase in bicarbonate level.

### Etiology

Respiratory acidosis results from retention of $CO_2$ secondary to decreased alveolar ventilation. Any disease state which results in hypoventilation, if sufficiently prolonged, can lead to respiratory acidosis, e.g., chronic obstructive pulmonary disease (COPD), pneumonia, pneumothorax, flail chest, congestive heart failure, myopathy, pathological obesity, upper abdominal surgery limiting diaphragmatic excursion, respiratory depressants (narcotics or other drug overdose), etc.

### Diagnosis

As $PaCO_2$ concentration rises above 40 mm Hg, $HCO_3$ level tends to increase. Initially (in acute cases), this compensation is rather poor (only 1 mEq/L increase for every 10 mm rises in $PaCO_2$). However, as respiratory acidosis becomes stable (after 6-12 hours of respiratory failure) the renal synthesis and retention of $HCO_3$ is stimulated. Accordingly, bicarbonate increases substantially (4 mEq/L for every 10 mm Hg rise in $PaCO_2$), and electrical balance is maintained by renal excretion of chloride. Acidosis, therefore, is less marked—pH decreases by only 0.03 for every 10 mm increase in $PaCO_2$.

### Clinical Features

*See* **Table 5.9**.

## RESPIRATORY ALKALOSIS

It is a frequent problem in seriously ill patients and is often iatrogenic. The salient feature is hyperventilation. Various causes of respiratory alkalosis are given at **Box. 5.6**.

### Diagnosis and Clinical Features

Laboratory diagnosis of respiratory alkalosis comes from *an increase in pH coupled with a decrease in $PaCO_2$*

Compensation occurs by a decrease in $HCO_3$, which (like in cases of respiratory acidosis) is much more in chronic than in acute cases (5-6 mEq/L and 2 mEq/L, respectively for every 10 mm Hg decrease in $PaCO_2$).

The clinical picture in acute cases can be characteristic and is related to *decrease in ionized calcium without any significant alteration in total calcium.*

> **Box 5.6: Causes of respiratory alkalosis.**
>
> ❑ **Central**
>   ➢ Anxiety, pain
>   ➢ Hyperventilation syndrome
>   ➢ Cerebral diseases (e.g., head injury, tumors, encephalitis)
>   ➢ Fever, septicemia, salicylate intoxication
> ❑ **Peripheral**
>   ➢ Pulmonary diseases (e.g., embolism, pneumonia, asthma)
>   ➢ Congestive heart failure, pulmonary edema
>   ➢ High altitude hypoxemia
> ❑ **Miscellaneous**
>   ➢ Hepatic insufficiency
>   ➢ Pregnancy
>   ➢ Excessive mechanical ventilation

## Treatment

The main principle of treatment is to *identify the underlying cause of respiratory alkalosis,* and manage it as best as possible. Proper use of ventilator and correction of any existing potassium deficit are important. In iatrogenic hyperventilation, reassurance, sedation, and "rebreathing" into a paper bag will relieve the symptoms.

## Summary

Proper interpretation of arterial blood gas (ABG) report requires not only values of pH, $PaCO_2$, and $HCO_3$, but also knowledge of patient's past health, medication, and present clinical status. Furthermore, since production and removal of $[H^+]$ ions may change rapidly with treatment or even spontaneously, frequent measurements are often required. Many systems are defined for analyzing ABG. **One system for stepwise analysis of ABG based on findings of three variables (pH, $PaCO_2$, and $HCO_3$) is as follows:**

Step 1: Look at pH (1st variable):
   a. Below 7.35 is acidosis
   b. Above 7.45 is alkalosis
   c. Values between 7.35 and 7.45 imply no acid-base disorder, or a compensated disorder, or a mixed disorder.

Step 2: Look at $PaCO_2$ and $HCO_3$ to find the variable responsible/main disturbance — respiratory or metabolic (2nd variable). For example, if acidosis is associated with increased $PaCO_2$ (>45), it is mostly respiratory; if it is associated with a decrease in $HCO_3$, and then a major component of acidosis is metabolic.

Step 3: Study the 3rd variable (which may be $PaCO_2$ or $HCO_3$, depending upon observation of Step 2). Finally, keeping in view the clinical status of the patient, calculate the predicted value of this 3rd variable according to Rules 1 to 6 (described above) whichever is applicable, and compare it with the measured value. If the calculated and the measured values are near identical, acid-base disturbance is fully compensated, otherwise it is a partially compensated or a mixed acid-base disorder.

### Examples

- A 60 kg patient in septic shock has pH 7.10, $PaCO_2$ 20 mm Hg, and $HCO_3$ 5.0 mEq/L. He has acidosis (↑pH) and it is primarily metabolic (↑$HCO_3$). The predicted fall in $PaCO_2 = ↓HCO_3 \times 1.0$ (Rule 1) = $(24 - 5.0) \times 1.0 - 19.0 \times 1.0 = 19$ mm Hg, and therefore the predicted $PaCO_2$ is $40 - 19 = 21$, which is about the same as measured $PaCO_2$. Metabolic acidosis in this case is therefore, already fully compensated.
- A patient with septicemia, and on ventilator, has a pH of 7.49 with a $PaCO_2$ 30 mm Hg and $HCO_3$ 26 mEq/L. He has chronic respiratory alkalosis (↓pH with ↑$PaCO_2$); his $PaCO_2$ is less by $(40 - 30) = 10$ and his bicarbonate should be $(24 - 5) = 19$ (bicarbonate decreases by 5 mEq/L for every 10 fall in $PaCO_2$ (Rule 6). Since the measured bicarbonate is 26, it represents associated metabolic alkalosis.
- A patient of COPD develops postoperative shock and has a pH of 7.22, $PaCO_2$ 75 mm Hg and $HCO_3$ 26. He has chronic respiratory acidosis (*↓pH* with ↑$PaCO_2$) and should have a compensatory increase in bicarbonate by 14 mEq/L (4 mEq/L increase for every 10 mm increase in $PaCO_2$ over 40). His bicarbonate should therefore be 38 mEq/L. However, his measured bicarbonate is only 26, leaving a deficit of 12 mEq/L. This is the metabolic component of acidosis.

## ACUTE RENAL FAILURE

### Definition

Acute renal failure (ARF), also called *"acute kidney injury"* is a rapidly progressive loss of renal functions, generally characterized by oliguria developing within hours to weeks, and usually presents as oliguria (urine output <15 mL/hour or <400 mL/day in adults). *The best marker of ARF is serum creatinine level* but it usually lags behind oliguria or anuria. Various stages of ARF are shown in **Table 5.10**.

### Etiology

The etiology of ARF varies with rapidity of the process, and whether it develops in *ambulatory or hospital setting*. In the former, renal failure usually develops

**Table 5.10:** Staging criteria of acute renal failure.

| ARF stage | Serum creatinine | Urine output |
|---|---|---|
| 1 | Increased by 1.5–2.0 times baseline | <15 mL/hour or <0.5 mL/kg/hour for 6 hours |
| 2 | Increased between 2 and 3 times baseline | <15 mL/hour or <0.5 mL/kg/hour for 24 hours |
| 3 | Increased by >3 times baseline or to >4 mg/dL | <0.3 mL/kg/hour for 24 hours |

in a **subacute or chronic** manner, most often in patients with poorly controlled hypertension and/or diabetes mellitus. **Acutely developing renal failure** in such patients is usually due to glomerulonephritis, vasculitis, and obstructive nephropathy. On the other hand, when ARF develops in hospitalized patients, it is usually associated with shock (low cardiac output states), or administration of nephrotoxic drugs, surgery, trauma, or sepsis.

Acute renal failure can be classified into three groups depending upon the anatomic site of pathology: **(1) prerenal, (2) postrenal, and (3) intrarenal.** *Parenchymal/intrarenal causes are usually considered after the other two are excluded.*

### Prerenal Failure

This is the most common type of ARF and results from decreased renal perfusion with decrease in GFR. It can be due to:

- **Decrease in intravascular volume:** Hypovolemia may be due to gastrointestinal fluid losses, massive hemorrhage, dehydration, excessive diuresis, or when large amount of fluids are sequestrated in the extravascular space as in burns, pancreatitis, and trauma.
- **Change in vascular resistance:** Alterations in vascular resistance may occur at the systemic level (sepsis, anaphylaxis, after-load reducing drugs, anesthesia), *or selectively involve afferent or efferent renal arterioles.* The latter include angiotensin-converting enzyme (ACE) inhibitors and angiotensin receptor blockers (ARB), NSAIDs, epinephrine, high-dose dopamine, norepinephrine, and anesthetic agents.
- **Low cardiac output:** The result is renal hypoperfusion and decreased GFR. This is characteristically seen in cardiogenic shock, but can also occur in cases with congestive heart failure, pulmonary embolism, and cardiac tamponade. It is important to remember that *all patients on positive pressure ventilation have decreased venous return leading to lower cardiac output.*

The kidneys are intrinsically intact in such cases (with normal glomerular and tubular functions). Prerenal azotemia can be quickly reversed with correction of hypovolemia and restoration of renal blood flow. If however, hypoperfusion persists (mean arterial pressure below 60–70 mm Hg) and is protracted (lasting >30 minutes), intrinsic renal injury is likely.

## Postrenal Failure

This is an uncommon cause of ARF and is due to obstruction to urinary outflow from both kidneys **(obstructive uropathy).** The outstanding feature is complete cessation of urine flow which may occur almost abruptly unlike prerenal or intrarenal ARF in which oliguria occurs over a period of hours to days. The normal fall in pressure from kidney to bladder is altered resulting in increased intraluminal pressure in each nephron and consequent decrease in GFR. It is important to remember that to cause azotemia, **the obstruction need not be complete but must be bilateral, or be located at the bladder outlet** as in prostatic enlargement.

## Intrarenal Failure

The *renal injury/pathology can be at the level of (i) tubules, (ii) interstitium, and (iii) small vessels/glomeruli* **(Box 5.7)**.

- ❖ **Tubular disorders:** Acute tubular necrosis (ATN) is the most common cause of intrinsic renal failure and can be due to: (i) *tubular ischemia,* **and** (ii) *toxin exposure.* Predisposing factors, in both types include advanced age, dehydration, associated hypertension, diabetes, and pre-existing renal disease.

   Of the two, *tubular ischemia* is more frequent and results from severe/protracted renal hypoperfusion. It is important to remember that *prolonged periods of hypotension result not only in decreased GFR with consequent ischemic ATN but can also lead to renal parenchymal dysfunction from inadequate renal blood flow.*

   **Nephrotoxin exposure (Box 5.7)** dominates other cases of ATN. Renal failure (usually nonoliguric) typically occurs 7–10 days after exposure. Both exogenous and endogenous nephrotoxins can cause ATN. In the former subgroup, commonly incriminated drugs are *NSAIDs, aminoglycosides, and ACE inhibitors.* NSAIDs block PGE2 formation, and thereby prevent afferent arteriolar vasodilatation resulting in decreased GFR. Likewise, ACE inhibitors alter intrarenal hemodynamics in patients with mild renal dysfunction (serum creatinine >3 mg/dL) or impaired perfusion (e.g., renal artery stenosis). Because of their synergistic effect on intrarenal perfusion, *a combination of the NSAIDs and ACE inhibitors is especially dangerous* in predisposed patients. Aminoglycosides, on the other hand, cause renal insufficiency directly by binding with and damaging cellular proteins in the proximal tubule. Since aminoglycosides can remain in renal tissues for as long as a month, recovery in renal functions may take a long time after stopping the medication.

   Though either tubular ischemia or nephrotoxins can result in necrosis of tubule epithelial cell and ATN, the risk is maximal when both factors operate together. It is also important to remember that the term *"ATN"* and *"intrinsic renal failure" are not interchangeable* since many renal parenchymal disease states (e.g., interstitial nephritis and vasculitis) can cause ARF without tubular cell necrosis.

- **Interstitial nephritis:** This is a common cause of intrinsic renal failure, but often remains unrecognized. Majority of cases are due to an allergic response to a specific drug in which cell-mediated immune reactions prevail over humoral responses. Other causes include infectious diseases and autoimmune disorders (**Box 5.7**). The typical pathology comprises interstitial inflammation along with edema and tubular-cell damage. The most common drugs involved are penicillin, cephalosporin, ciprofloxacin, sulfonamides, thiazides, rifampin, phenytoin, and allopurinol.

  Clinical features are usually nonspecific and comprise fever, rash, and arthralgia. Accompanying oliguria and a rising serum creatinine level often provide early diagnostic clues. An increase in eosinophil count is highly suggestive. Urine findings are generally nonspecific but some degree of proteinuria, white cell casts, and increase in white cells commonly occur. The disease generally carries a good prognosis, but recovery may take weeks to months. Removal of the offending cause and high dose corticosteroid therapy generally prove effective. Some cases may require dialysis for a brief period, but progression to end-stage renal disease is rare.

- **Glomerulonephritis/small vessel vasculitis:** These are common causes of intrinsic ARF in ambulatory patients, and may result from many disorders (**Box 5.7**). Renal involvement is suspected in such cases by the presence of *active urine sediment* containing protein, leucocytes,

---

**Box 5.7: Causes of intrinsic (intrarenal) acute renal failure.**

1. **Tubular (ATN)**
   - *Ischemic:* All causes of prerenal ARF untreated or inadequately treated sepsis
   - *Nephrotoxic*
     - Exogenous:
       a. Drugs: Cisplatin, vancomycin, radiographic contrast agents
       b. Heavy metals: Lead, mercury, arsenic, bismuth, lithium, cadmium
       c. Chemicals: Potassium chlorate, insecticides, organic solvents (e.g., ethylene glycol), acetaminophen
     - Endogenous: Myoglobin (rhabdomyolysis), hemoglobin, porphyrins
2. **Interstitial nephritis drugs:** Antibiotics (penicillin, cephalosporin, sulfonamides, NSAIDs, phenytoin, rifampicin, protein pump inhibitors, allopurinol
   - *Immune-mediated:* Lupus erythematosus, sarcoidosis, transplant rejection
   - *Infective:* Histoplasmosis, leptospirosis
   - *Infiltrative:* Lymphoma, leukemia, sarcoidosis
   - *Intratubular obstruction:* Uric acid, sulfonamides, myeloma proteins
3. **Glomerular/small vessel vasculitis:**
   - *Glomerulonephritis/Vasculitis:* Rapidly progressive polyarteritis, Wegener granulomatosis, hypersensitivity, lupus erythematosus, Goodpasture syndrome
   - *Microvasculature:* Scleroderma, Henoch-Schonlein purpura, toxemia of pregnancy, hemolytic-uremic syndrome, disseminated intravascular coagulation, accelerated hypertension, toxemia of pregnancy

and (characteristic) red blood cell casts. The proteinuria is more severe than in interstitial nephritis, and may be in the nephrotic range. Specific diagnosis is made by study of markers of immune-mediated diseases, serum complement, and hepatitis B surface antigen. Therapy is mainly directed at underlying disease. For renal failure per se, supportive measures are generally sufficient, but some cases may require temporary dialysis.

## Pathophysiology

The term prerenal failure is best considered in the clinical setting of marked hypovolemia and/or shock. Consequently, GFR is reduced to about 50 mL/min or less (normally 125 mL/min) with significant fall in urine output (<400 mL/day) and accumulation of waste products of metabolism **(prerenal azotemia).** Sometimes, however, urine output is not significantly reduced **(nonoliguric ARF)** because the kidneys do not avidly reabsorb water and sodium. These patients have a better prognosis probably because of lesser intensity of renal insult.

The oliguria and azotemia up to this point are often fully reversible on timely correction of the primary disturbance, since renal blood vessels, glomeruli and tubules are intact. With more severe and protracted hypotension and continuing impaired renal perfusion, oliguria and renal failure may persist despite correction of the precipitating factor(s). Marked renal vasoconstriction is present in such cases, and may be perpetuated by angiotensin, produced in response to reduction in blood volume. Consequently, *necrosis and desquamation of tubular lining cells occur at several places along the course of the nephron, and then ATN becomes established.*

## Signs and Symptoms

In the early stage of kidney disease many patients do not feel sick or notice any symptom. When kidney pathology worsens, filtration is affected, waste products of metabolism accumulate, and blood indicators of renal dysfunction (BUN and serum creatinine) start increasing **(azotemia).** Mild azotemia may produce few, if any, symptoms. With continuing renal dysfunction, patient begins to experience certain symptoms, and this stage is termed as **uremia** (renal failure accompanied by noticeable symptoms).

Uremic symptoms can be due to many factors, often working together. However certain symptoms are more closely related to a particular biochemical disturbance.
1. **Increased level of BUN/serum creatinine:** Nausea, vomiting, appetite, bad taste
2. **Increased $K^+$ level:**
   - Muscle weakness/paralysis
   - Cardiac arrhythmias

3. **Hyperphosphatemia:** Pruritus, bone damage, muscle cramps (caused by low levels of calcium which can be associated phosphates).
4. **I synthesis of erythropoietin:** Anemia
5. **Proteinuria and hypoproteinemia:** Edema of feet, face or abdomen, foamy urine

## Diagnosis

Clinical features of ARF usually do not develop until GFR falls to about 10-15% of normal. ARF in its early stages is therefore diagnosed by elevated blood urea nitrogen (BUN) and creatinine. Oliguria is frequent, but not invariable. Physical examination may provide clues to the underlying pathology, as well as indicate the state of hydration. **In all cases of ARF, postrenal obstruction must first be excluded** by appropriate history, physical examination, radioimaging, and if necessary, by catheterization of the bladder.

*Differentiation between prerenal azotemia and ATN is clinically important but may be difficult.* Besides history and physical examination, valuable clues may be provided by **radioimaging of the kidneys (Table 5.11) and study of certain blood and urinary indices.** The latter include study of *serum BUN creatinine ratio* (which is normally about 20:1), and certain urinary indices (especially urine specific gravity and osmolality). Their discussion is beyond the scope of this text.

**Radioimaging:** Abdominal ultrasonography, especially the kidney size, can provide valuable clues to the cause of ARF **(Table 5.11)**. In general, prerenal azotemia is characterized by kidneys of normal size, while small kidneys suggest a more chronic process.

**Other investigations:** Intravenous pyelography **(IVP)** is relatively contraindicated in cases of multiple myeloma, and in patients with impaired renal functions (serum creatinine >3 mg/dL) who may be at risk of developing ARF. **CT scan and MRI** are now replacing IVR. The gravity of renal failure can be assessed by ECG and serum K⁺ level. Other useful laboratory tests include study of hematocrit and serum albumin (both of which are decreased in chronic renal

| Table 5.11: Kidney size in relation to etiology of renal failure. | | |
|---|---|---|
| **Normal size** | **Enlarged** | **Small size** |
| Acute tubular necrosis | Amyloidosis | Chronic renal failure |
| Acute interstitial nephritis | Obstructive uropathy | Hypertensive kidney |
| Acute glomerulonephritis | Interstitial nephritis | Renal artery stenosis |
| Hepatorenal syndrome | | |
| Malignant hypertension | Acute glomerulonephritis | |
| Renal artery stenosis | Renal vein thrombosis | |
| Collagen disorders | | |

disease, and are usually normal in acute azotemia), ABG studies, and (at least one) urine culture with antibiotic sensitivity pattern.

## Management

Hospitalized patients who develop ARF often have multiple risk factors, and more than one specific insult may be involved. On the other hand, in domiciliary practice ARF is seen usually in patients with comorbid conditions and a debilitated state. The prognosis has vastly improved with availability of dialysis and other support technologies.

### *Principles of Management*

Once acute renal failure is established, only supportive therapy is available. Therefore, the best treatment is primary prevention. In a patient with ongoing oliguria, after excluding postrenal causes and eliminating prerenal factors, the primary approach should be to try to reverse oliguria. Correction of hypovolemia, and discontinuation of any nephrotoxic drug(s) are most important measures. The management should also include: (1) *identification and treatment of underlying cause,* (2) *control of fluid and electrolyte imbalance,* (3) *appropriate nutritional support,* and (4) *dialysis,* when required. Furthermore, suitable measures should be taken to prevent/treat various complications **(Table 5.12)**, which may arise during the course of disease/treatment.

*Identification and treatment of underlying cause*

Pre- and postrenal azotemia can be identified to a large extent by clinical details. When obstructive nephropathy is suspected, appropriate investigations (especially radioimaging) will help in identifying the pathology. Cases of intrinsic renal failure due to ATN, glomerular/vascular factors and interstitial pathologies constitute a heterogeneous group, and require a careful review of the history (including details of medication), physical examination, and laboratory data. In selected cases renal biopsy may be required.

**Table 5.12:** Important complications of acute renal failure.

| **Metabolic** | **Gastrointestinal** |
|---|---|
| • Hyponatremia<br>• Hypocalcemia<br>• Hyperphosphatemia | • Nausea/vomiting |
| **Cardiovascular** | **Neurological** |
| • Fluid overload<br>• Hypertension<br>• Pericarditis | • Neuropathy<br>• Confusion<br>• Seizures |
| **Hematologic** | **Infections** |
| • Anemia<br>• Coagulopathy | • Urinary tract<br>• Pneumonia<br>• Sepsis |

## Chapter 5: Renal Emergencies

*Fluid management*

This is one of the cornerstones in the management of ARF oliguric patients often have fluid overload manifested by pedal/presacral edema, engorged jugular veins, hepatomegaly, and pulmonary congestion. Monitoring central venous pressure is of great help.

While estimating volume deficit, note should be taken of all types of fluid loss in the form of urine, vomiting, diarrhea, aspirates, sweating, and an insensible daily loss of 500–1000 mL (0.5 mL/kg/hour). The latter increases by 10% with every 1o rise in body temperature, and varies according to the environmental temperature (as much as 1 L of additional fluid may be lost per day during the hot tropical summer, if the patient is not in air-conditioned environment). On the other hand, about 400 mL of endogenous water is produced daily by average caloric expense in a starving patient. Fluid management will vary according to the stage of the disease.

❖ **Oliguric phase:** At this stage an attempt should be made to convert it into nonoliguric type since it greatly simplifies fluid management, and is associated with a lower mortality. This requires the *fluid status to be optimized.* Unless there are clear signs of fluid overload (vide supra), a **fluid challenge** by rapid infusion of 500–1000 mL normal saline is advised. If oliguria persists, this volume loading should be **followed** by **furosemide infusion** at a rate of 0.2–0.5 mg/kg/hour, which may be increased to 0.8 mg/kg/hour, if required. A loading dose of 20–40 mg is advised at the start. The role of mannitol is suspect. To make precise estimate of urine flow, the output should be recorded every 2 hours initially, with the help of an indwelling catheter.

Such measures are likely to be successful if undertaken within a few hours of the onset of reduction in urine flow. *Persistent oliguria for more than 12–24 hours is ominous,* and usually signifies superadded tubular damage. Renal-dose dopamine infusion (1.5–3.0 mcg/kg/min) may also be tried but usually fails to induce diuresis.

It is to be emphasized that the window of opportunity is often narrow, and therefore these measures should be used early in the course of oliguria. The aim is to prevent tubular damage; once ATN is established, it is not reversible. If oliguria persists despite correction of hypovolemia and furosemide therapy, it can be presumed that tubular damage has supervened. Complete anuria is rare, and urine volume less than 100 mL may continue for several days. Not infrequently, urine output becomes adequate spontaneously or following furosemide, but the quality of urine and renal functions do not improve, and azotemia continues to progress.

Blood urea nitrogen and creatinine concentration increase approximately by 10–25 mg% and 0.5–1.5 mg%, respectively per day during the first few days; the rate of increase is higher in patients with hypercatabolic states.

It is to be noted that during oliguric phase **too much fluid can be as dangerous as too little.** All too often patients of ARF are seen loaded with fluid due to iatrogenic factors such as administration of mannitol and/or large amounts of IV fluids in an attempt to "force" diuresis. Fluid intake in these cases must be drastically reduced, keeping the patients slightly dehydrated so that the body weight falls by about 0.2 kg daily. Many of these cases will ultimately require dialysis (vide infra).

- **Diuretic phase:** If the patient survives the oliguric phase, the kidneys begin to function again. This is manifested by onset of diuresis, clearing of azotemia, and progressive improvement in clinical status. The urine output gradually increases and at times may reach 2-4 L or even more per day. The cause of the diuresis is not clear but is possibly due to tubular dysfunction continuing in the face of recovering GFR. Fluid therapy at this stage is directed to combat dehydration, and fluids should be administered orally as far as possible. When IV supplementation is required, isotonic saline and D5W should be given in a ratio of 1:2. After 2-3 days only 75% of the urine volume should be replaced in an attempt to decrease urine output. In favorable cases, tubular functions improve rapidly and urine specific gravity begins to increase. As the BUN decreases to about 50% of the original high level, full and free intake of food and water should be permitted.

*Control of electrolytes and pH*

- **Sodium:** During the oliguric phase, there is retention of sodium and therefore, sodium intake should be limited to 500 mg/24 hours. A low sodium level at this stage indicates over-hydration *(dilutional hyponatremia)*, and will improve with fluid restriction. Hypernatremia is much less common and when encountered is due to inadequate water intake or excessive administration of IV isotonic saline.
- **Potassium:** Some degree of *hyperkalemia* is present in almost all cases of ARF in oliguric phase on account of excessive protein catabolism, breakdown of necrotic tissues, metabolic acidosis, and red cell hemolysis. Iatrogenic factors may also play a part when citrus and other fruit juices are allowed. Frequent *serum $K^+$* monitoring is therefore essential. Whenever values are higher than 6 mEq/L, or ECG changes suggestive of hyperkalemia are observed, emergent measures should be taken to control hyperkalemia (see section on "Clinical Electrolyte and Acid- Base Abnormalities").
- **Calcium, Phosphorus, and Magnesium:** These electrolytes are either well preserved or show only mild alterations that require no specific treatment. Significant hypocalcemia and hyperphosphatemia, if observed, may be treated with diet and phosphate-binding agents such as aluminum hydroxide 500 mg orally 3-4 times a day after meals. Additionally, oral calcium carbonate or citrate may be given. Restriction of dietary protein and fruits also help in reducing phosphate level. Hypermagnesemia results

from impaired excretion, and improves as diuresis sets in. Magnesium-containing antacids and cathartics should be avoided.
- ❖ **Acid-base homeostasis:** Metabolic acidosis is a common feature of ARF. It results from inability of the patient to excrete daily generated load of [H$^+$] ions (about 1 mEq/kg/day), as well as from inability to regenerate [HCO$_3$]. Additionally, sulfates, phosphates, and other organic anions accumulate. However, replacement therapy with NaHCO$_3$ should be employed cautiously, and preferably restricted to patients with pH <7.20. Severe acidosis warrants dialysis (*see* also section on "Clinical Electrolyte and Acid-Base Abnormalities").

*Nutrition*

Adequate nutritional support is essential, but since symptoms of uremia are related to level of BUN, protein intake is usually restricted. For the first few days of oliguria when rapid increase in BUN occurs due to tissue catabolism especially in the presence of sepsis, the diet should provide about 25–30 kcal/kg body weight with about 20 g high biologic-value proteins (**Table 5.13**). However, very low-protein diets (<20 g/day), which may temporarily decrease progression of uremia and delay/avoid dialysis are, in the long-term, counterproductive and possibly increase morbidity and mortality due to impaired nutrition. A fairly nutritious diet should therefore be given after the first few days of ARF as renal function improves or dialysis is started. At this stage both enteral and parenteral routes should be employed so as to provide a daily intake of 35–40 kcal/kg with 0.6–0.8 g/kg/day of protein.

*Dialysis*

This is the most rational method of treatment of ARF especially during the phase of oliguria/anuria. However, dialysis should be regarded as a supplement (and not a substitute) to efficient conservative management outlined above. Indications for dialysis are as follows:

**Table 5.13:** Liquid diet for enteral feeding in acute renal failure (Total calories: 1300).

| Foodstuff | Quantity | Carbohydrate (g) | Fat (g) | Protein (g) | Na$^+$ (mg) | K$^+$ (mg) |
|---|---|---|---|---|---|---|
| Milk (Cow's) | 400 mL | 20 | 36 | 12 | 76 | 360 |
| Egg (1) | 40 g | – | 5.3 | 5.3 | 15 | 27 |
| Rice water | 500 mL | 50 | – | 2.0 | – | – |
| Sugar | 70 g | 70 | – | – | – | – |
| Sago | 50 g | 44 | – | – | – | – |
| Butter (unsalted) | 25 g | - | 20.2 | – | – | – |
| | Total | 184 | 61.5 | 19.3 | 91 | 387 |

This diet can be given by nasogastric tube.

**Absolute indications**
- Appearance of uremic symptoms such as severe anorexia, vomiting, mental cloudiness, twitching, and convulsions
- Neurologic deficits with sensory or motor neuropathy
- Uremic pericarditis.

**Relative indications**
- Conservative treatment is unlikely to be successful
- Massive volume overload
- Hyperkalemia, especially if accompanied by ECG changes
- BUN value >100 mg/dL or creatinine value >10 mg/dL
- Severe metabolic acidosis (pH <7.2).

The current trend is towards early and aggressive dialysis. This is especially true for patients with sepsis, trauma, burns, diabetes, and postsurgical cases. Hemodialysis is generally preferred as it allows removal of large quantities of potassium and urea-nitrogen over a short time.

*Symptomatic measures*

- **Infection:** Every effort should be made to avoid introducing infection into the urinary tract. Catheterization should be done in only urgent situations, and indwelling catheters avoided as far as possible. Source of infection, if present, should be identified, bacteria isolated, and appropriate antibiotics instituted on the basis of sensitivity pattern. The dosage of antibiotic used, should be suitably adjusted keeping in view the creatinine clearance and the normal pharmacokinetic of the drug. For emergency use or when bacteriologic facilities are not available, third generation cephalosporin or quinolones may be used. For a given degree of azotemia, the dosage schedule for various antibiotics should be modified as given at **Table 5.14**.
- **Hypertension:** Hypertension is not uncommon in patients with ARF, and is due in large part to sodium retention and fluid overload. Initially therefore, salt restriction (<2 g/day) and loop diuretics should be used. Calcium channel-blockers and beta-blockers are the drugs of choice.

**Table 5.14:** Guidelines for antimicrobial therapy in renal failure.

| Dosage schedule | Drugs |
| --- | --- |
| No change | Azithromycin, carbenicillin, cephalexin, cefaclor, cefoperazone, ceftriaxone, clindamycin, doxycycline, erythromycin |
| Moderate reduction | Amoxicillin, ampicillin, clarithromycin, crystalline penicillin (G), quinolones |
| Marked reduction | Aminoglycosides, all cephalosporins except those in group 1, monobactams, piperacillin, ticarcillin, septran, vancomycin |
| Contraindicated | Nitrofurantoin, tetracycline |

ACE inhibitors and angiotensin II receptor blockers should be avoided especially if serum creatinine is >3 mg/dL.
- **General measures:** Drug history should be scrupulously reviewed in all cases of ARF, and any (possible) incriminating drug should be discontinued. Drugs, which are (largely or entirely) excreted through the kidney, should be avoided, or their dosage reduced appropriately. Troublesome nausea and vomiting may be relieved with prochlorperazine *(Stemetil)* or ondansetron *(Emeset),* but usually require dialysis. Anemia is a problem only if renal failure gets protracted. Administration of erythropoietin and packed red cells transfusion should be considered, if hemoglobin is <8 g%.

## Prognosis

Acute renal failure is a serious disorder with a high mortality especially in surgical setting (up to 70%). Advanced age and severe comorbid/multiorgan disease are associated with poor prognosis. It is to be realized that despite wide availability of dialysis, mortality rates remain high. This is a sobering fact and should *reemphasize the importance of prevention of ARF* (vide infra).

## Prevention

It is often possible to anticipate the occurrence of ARF in both medical and surgical settings if careful attention is paid to urine output. In all threatened cases urine output should be recorded every 3-4 hours, and maintained at a rate >30 mL/hour. Urine excretion less than 20 mL/hour is ominous, and should warrant detection and prompt correction of hypovolemia, treatment of associated infection, if any, and careful maintenance of blood pressure. It is important to remember that susceptibility to ATN is increased in pregnancy, obstructive jaundice, and hepatic failure. Risk of ARF can be decreased in such cases by prophylactic use of furosemide (and mannitol) as described earlier.

## Summary

- ARF can be of three types: prerenal, intrarenal, and postrenal
- Management of ARF is a complex problem. Postrenal ARF should be identified straight-away and managed appropriately, jointly with urologist.
- ARF is associated with a significant mortality (despite dialysis support) especially if it occurs in critically ill patients. Prevention is critical since no specific treatment (except dialysis and renal transplantation) is available once renal failure is established.
- Any patient at risk of prerenal or renal ARF should be identified early. Protracted hypoperfusion and nephrotoxic drugs account for majority of cases of intrinsic renal failure.
- In all patients of intrinsic renal failure, an attempt should be made to convert oliguric renal failure into nonoliguric type.

- ❖ **Carefully control:**
  - Fluid-volume homeostasis
  - Electrolyte and acid-base balance
  - Further renal insults of any type
  - Optimal nutrition and protein intake.
- ❖ Adopt judicious measures for any associated infection, hypertension, and anemia.
- ❖ Consider early dialysis in cases not responding adequately to conservative measures.
- ❖ **Avoid:**
  - All nephrotoxic drugs
  - All foods rich in potassium and phosphates, e.g., fruit juices, potato, meat, banana, and dry fruits
  - Diuretics until intravascular volume is corrected
  - Prolonged use of IV lines and indwelling catheter.

# 6 CHAPTER

# Hematological Emergencies

## INTRODUCTION

Compared to the frequency with which urgent problems arise in system-disorders described so far, hematological emergencies are rather uncommon. Their scope of presentation is also often limited to virtually two types: **(1) severe anemia and (1) bleeding disorders.** Either of these can, however, result from a variety of disorders, and obviously, appropriate treatment demands a precise diagnosis. While a careful history and physical examination are as important here as in any other acute medical disorder, certain basic investigations are invariably required to provide a clue to the nature of disease. These include *complete blood count, a hemogram, and a thorough study of peripheral blood film* (for reticulocytes, form and shape of red cells, platelet defects, and any abnormal cells). Bleeding and coagulation profile and a marrow smear are some other investigations often required to elucidate hematological problems.

## CLASSIFICATION

A proper understanding of the pathophysiology and type of anemia is essential for rational approach to its treatment. These are listed at **Tables 6.1 and 6.2** respectively.

## SEVERE ANEMIA

Severe anemia can be of two types:
1. **Severe anemia of acute onset:** This is due either to acute blood loss or acute red cell hemolysis.

| Table 6.1: Classification of anemia by pathophysiology. | |
|---|---|
| *Defects in synthesis* | *Increased blood loss* |
| *Hemoglobin synthesis / Intake/absorption of iron, folic acid, $B_{12}$ thalassemia* | Trauma, surgery, gastrointestinal, piles, menstrual, hematuria |
| • *Bone marrow disorders* Aplastic anemia, bone marrow infiltration (carcinoma, lymphoma)<br>• *Myeloproliferative disorders* | **Hemolysis**<br>Intrinsic/extrinsic<br>(for details, see **Table 6.3**) |

| Table 6.2: Classification of anemia by red blood cell (RBC) size (MCV).* ||
|---|---|
| **Microcytic** <br> • Iron deficiency <br> • Anemia of chronic disease <br> • Thalassemia | **Macrocytic** <br> • *Megaloblastic* <br> ➢ Folic acid deficiency <br> ➢ Vitamin $B_{12}$ deficiency |
| **Normocytic** <br> • Blood loss <br> • Pregnancy/lactation <br> • Hemoglobinuria | • *Nonmegaloblastic* <br> ➢ Liver disease <br> ➢ Myelodysplasia <br> ➢ Hypothyroidism |

*Normal mean corpuscular volume (MCV): 87 ± 7 cubic micron ($\mu m^3$)

2. **Insidious and progressive severe anemia:** Only acutely developing anemia is considered in this section, though some degree of overlap between the two types is not uncommon.

## Severe Anemia of Acute Onset

### Acute Blood Loss

*Pathophysiology*

Rapidly developing severe anemia is usually due to acute and massive blood loss as in trauma, gastrointestinal bleeding, postpartum hemorrhage, severe epistaxis, and following surgery. The consequences depend on the age of the subject, amount of blood lost, and more importantly on the *rate of blood loss. Symptoms usually arise when over 1 L of blood is lost in a short time.* These include marked fatigue, weakness, giddiness, blurred vision, and syncope. Tachycardia and hypotension occur in proportion to the degree of blood loss, and even shock and peripheral circulatory failure may supervene. Clinical features are likely to be more severe in the elderly because of compromised circulation in vital organs. An acute loss of over 2 L often proves fatal.

*Diagnosis*

This is usually obvious from the history and circumstantial/clinical evidence of acute blood loss. The amount of blood lost may, however, be more difficult to determine. *Hemoglobin estimation and hematocrit can be misleading in the immediate post-hemorrhagic phase* since the red cell mass and plasma volume are contracted in parallel. Certain postural signs may be useful. An increase in pulse rate by 25% or more, or a drop in systolic pressure by 20 mm Hg or more upon a change of posture from supine to sitting position, implies significant hypovolemia, and a loss of over 1 L of blood.

  **Laboratory data** usually reveal a normocytic anemia of varying severity. Other findings include some degree of leukocytosis with a "shift to the left", mild to moderate thrombocytosis, and an increase in reticulocytes with appearance of nucleated red cells.

## Treatment

The primary aim should be:
- ❖ *To control the source of bleeding as quickly as possible, and*
- ❖ *To restore the blood volume at the earliest*
  - **Immediate measures:** Foot end of the patient's bed should be raised by 9–12" to assist cerebral circulation. Mild tranquilizers may be used to allay patient's anxiety.
  - **Hemostasis:** Specific treatment of massive hemoptysis and hematemesis is described in Chapters 2 and 3, respectively. Suitable mechanical measures to control bleeding should be instituted when applicable (e.g., nasal pack in case of epistaxis).
  - **Restoration of blood volume:** While blood transfusions are being arranged, D5W or normal saline (preferably supplemented with dextran) may be given to correct hypovolemia. As soon as possible, blood should be transfused so as to restore blood pressure. Estimation of hemoglobin or hematocrit may be misleading in early stages (vide supra).
  - **General measures:** Oral fluid therapy should be permitted and in fact, encouraged during the acute phase. Suitable hematinic supplements should be given on a long-term basis to correct anemia and to replenish iron stores. A high protein diet is also advisable.

## Complications

- ❖ Acute renal failure
- ❖ Peripheral circulatory failure
- ❖ Congestive heart failure

### Acute Hemolytic Anemia

*Etiology*

Hemolysis of red blood cells (RBCs) in various disease states may be due to *intracorpuscular or extracorpuscular defects* **(Table 6.3)**. Intracorpuscular

**Table 6.3:** Important causes of hemolytic anemia.

| Intracorpuscular (intrinsic) | Etracorpuscular (extrinsic) |
|---|---|
| • *Membrane defects*<br>➤ Hereditary spherocytosis<br>➤ Hereditary elliptocytosis<br>➤ Paroxysmal nocturnal hemoglobinuria | • *Immunohemolytic*<br>➤ Autoimmune drug toxicity<br>➤ Lymphoproliferative disorders |
| • *Others*<br>➤ Hemoglobinopathies<br>➤ Enzyme defects: G6PD deficiency<br>➤ Pyurate kinase deficiency | • *Others*<br>➤ Microangiopathic DIC, HUS, TTP, CVH<br>➤ Hypersplenism<br>➤ Infections |

(CVH: cardiac valve hemolysis; DIC: disseminated intravascular coagulation; HUS: hemolytic uremic syndrome; TTP: thrombotic thrombocytopenic purpura)

| Table 6.4: Drugs causing hemolysis in G6PD-deficient subjects. | |
|---|---|
| Antimalarials | Primaquine, chloroquine, quinine |
| Sulfonamides | All sulfonamides |
| Analgesics | Phenacitin, paracetamol, aspirin |
| Miscellaneous | Probenecid, nitrofurantoin, nalidixic acid, quinidine, dapsone, chloramphenicol, L-dopa |

or intrinsic defects may involve any component of the RBC including the membrane, enzyme systems, and hemoglobin. Most of these defects are hereditary. Generally, the hemolysis is mild and chronic, but acute massive hemolysis **(acute hemolytic crisis)** may occur at any time and result in acute anemia. Such acute episodes are more common with autoimmune hemolytic anemia. Common examples are black water fever and mismatched transfusions. Occasionally, hemolysis following administration of certain drugs in G6PD deficiency subjects may also be severe **(Table 6.4)**. It is to be remembered that G6PD deficiency is an X-linked trait and predominantly affects men.

*Clinical features*

Acute hemolysis is characterized clinically by fever, headache, body pains, and a varying degree of circulatory collapse. Jaundice is invariably present with increase in indirect bilirubin, though its intensity may not reflect the severity of hemolytic process. Very severe cases may develop hemoglobinuria which may result in oliguria and acute renal failure.

*Diagnosis*

The diagnosis is often suspected from the clinical background of the case. Laboratory tests indicative of hemolysis include anemia of variable severity, increased reticulocyte count with associated neutrophilia and sometimes thrombocytosis, and decreased or absent haptoglobins (this is a normal plasma protein that binds and clears hemoglobin released in the plasma). Some degree of jaundice is common (indirect hyperbilirubinemia) but the total serum bilirubin does not ordinarily exceed 4 mg/dL. Higher levels should suggest some degree of hepatic dysfunction. Changes in red cell morphology **(Table 6.5)** may provide valuable clues as to the cause of hemolysis, but description of specific tests to elucidate the precise etiology of hemolytic anemia is beyond the scope of this text.

*Treatment*

General measures ordinarily employed in anemia of acute onset should be instituted. Any incriminating drug or toxic substance should be sought for and eliminated. Blood transfusions need to be given with extreme caution, especially in immune-hemolytic anemia (IHA). **Corticosteroids** should be considered in all such cases (of IHA). **Splenectomy** is the treatment of choice

## Chapter 6: Hematological Emergencies

**Table 6.5:** Red cell morphology in hemolytic anemia.

| Cell type | Possible diagnosis |
|---|---|
| Sickle cells (SC) | Sickling disorders |
| Elliptocytes | Hereditary elliptocytosis |
| Parasites | Malaria |
| Spherocytes | Hereditary spherocytosis, autoimmune hemolytic anemia |
| Target cells | Hemoglobin SC disease, liver disease |
| Bitten out cells | G-6PD deficiency |
| RBC fragments | Microangiopathic hemolytic anemia |

in patients with hereditary spherocytosis (these cases should also receive uninterrupted therapy with folic acid). It may also be considered in patients of IHA refractory to corticosteroids, or who relapse on tapering the dose.

In selected cases with severe acute hemolysis, high-dose **IV immune globulin** (1 g daily for 1 or 2 days) is sometimes highly effective, but the benefit is short-lived, and the treatment is expensive.

### *Aplastic (refractory) Anemia*

All hematopoietic cells, erythroid, myeloid, megakaryocytes/platelets, are derived from a pluripotent stem cell in the bone marrow. The clinical expression of marrow aplasia will depend upon the nature and severity of injury to this hematopoietic stem cell. Ordinarily, hypoplasia of bone marrow results in pancytopenia, but clinical features may be determined by the type of hematopoietic cell(s) chiefly affected. Conditions which result predominantly in aplastic anemia are listed in **Table 6.6**. Most of the cases are related to certain drugs. This association (between aplastic anemia and the incriminating drug) may be dose-related or idiosyncratic in nature. Chloramphenicol can result in both types of bone marrow depression. The former (dose-related effect) is more common and is reversible after discontinuation of the drug, while the latter (idiosyncratic) is extremely serious type of bone marrow failure, is usually irreversible, and ends fatally.

**Table 6.6:** Important causes of aplastic anemia.

| Drugs | Others |
|---|---|
| • Chloramphenicol | • Chemotherapy, radiotherapy |
| • Sulfonamides | • Toxins (insecticides, benzene, toluene) |
| • Phenylbutazone | • Systemic lupus erythematosus |
| • Phenytoin | • Viral hepatitis |
| • Carbamazepine | • Paroxysmal nocturnal hemoglobinuria |
| • Gold salts<br>• Tolbutamide | • Idiopathic (autoimmune) |

## Clinical features

The onset is usually insidious. Early symptoms are generally nonspecific (fatigue, malaise, weakness, shortness of breath), and increase progressively as hematological status worsens. Sometime during the course, purpura, epistaxis, petechiae, and bleeding from gums may occur. A few cases, especially those with acute onset, develop necrotic ulcers in the mouth, and irregular fever is not uncommon. At any stage cerebral hemorrhage may occur resulting in convulsions, coma and death. In cases who recover, a mild thrombocytopenia may persist for many years. *Lymphadenopathy and hepatosplenomegaly are notably absent.*

## Diagnosis

The *hallmark of aplastic anemia is pancytopenia,* though some cases may have depression of only two cell lines initially **(Table 6.7)**. There is no poikilocytosis or anisocytosis, and premature cells are absent. The most severe cases have granulocytes <500/mm$^3$, platelets fewer than 20,000/mm$^3$, and severe anemia with (corrected) reticulocyte index 0-1%. The bone marrow aspirate as well as marrow biopsy appear hypocellular with only few progenitors of normal hematopoietic cells. There are no abnormal cells.

## Treatment

There is no specific treatment for aplastic anemia. The causative factor (often a drug or a chemical agent) should be diligently sought and, if identified, removed. It is a safe policy to withhold all unnecessary drugs from the patient. Mild cases may be treated with supportive measures, but periodic RBC (and sometimes also platelet) transfusions are usually required.

The prognosis is poor in patients in the "severe category", the median survival in majority of untreated cases being no more than 3 months. The treatment of choice in young adults is bone marrow transplantation. In elderly patients immunosuppression with antithymocyte globulin (ATG) and cyclosporine has shown promising results. Androgens (oxymetholone 2-3 mg/kg orally in adults) have been occasionally successful as a maintenance therapy.

**Supportive measures:** These should aim at prevention of bleeding as far as possible, and include measures such as careful oral hygiene, use of laxatives

**Table 6.7:** Criteria for assessment of severity of aplastic anemia.

| Criterion | Severe | Moderate |
| --- | --- | --- |
| Reticulocytes | <20,000/mm$^3$ | <60,000/mm$^3$ |
| Granulocytes | <500/mm$^3$ | <1,000/mm$^3$ |
| Platelets | <20,000/mm$^3$ | <50,000/mm$^3$ |

**For diagnosis:** Two of the above values + a hypocellular or acellular marrow on bone marrow biopsy is required.

and, in thrombocytopenic patients, avoiding blades and razors (electric shaver may be safer). Menstruating females should be placed on suppressive doses of birth control pills.

*Infection is a common problem* in these patients especially if there is severe neutropenia. It may occur at unusual sites, may involve organisms of low pathogenicity, and be unaccompanied by fever and local inflammatory changes. Infection by *gram negative organisms* can result in fulminant sepsis with early cardiovascular collapse. Prompt and aggressive treatment with quinolones and broad spectrum antibiotics should be instituted and continued until granulocyte count increases by at least 200/mm³ even if the clinical signs of infection subside. Resistant cases may require **granulocyte colony-stimulating factor.** Once or twice weekly treatment is usually sufficient for a safe neutrophil count. More detailed treatment falls in the domain of the specialist.

ote

- Aspirin and all NSAIDs should be avoided since these may induce qualitative platelet defects (inhibit cyclooxygenase activity).
- *IM injections should be forbidden as these may cause deep tissue bleeding.*

## HEMOSTATIC DISORDERS

Hemostasis is maintained by a balance between *coagulation* (and clot formation) and *thrombolysis*. Defects in any of the two systems (coagulation or thrombolysis) can lead to either bleeding disorders or hypercoagulability. In this section, the focus is on the bleeding disorders.

### Etiology

Hemostasis is maintained by two key components, viz. *platelets and clotting proteins*. Integrity of the vascular endothelium is another factor required for hemostasis, but since it may be violated in a subtle manner in many conditions (surgery, trauma, sepsis) and is difficult to evaluate, only platelet defects and defective (fibrin) clot formation are considered here.

### Evaluation

Hemostatic disorders can be *usually picked up in clinical practice by three simple laboratory tests:* **platelet count, prothrombin time (PT), and partial thromboplastin time (PTT).** Other tests sometime required estimation of bleeding and clotting time, fibrinogen level and fibrin degradation products **(Table 6.8)**. PT and PTT respectively evaluate extrinsic and intrinsic pathways of coagulation cascade. Common clinical states in which PT and PTT may be prolonged are given at **Table 6.9**.

**Table 6.8:** Conventional tests for hemostasis.

| Test | Normal range | Remarks |
|---|---|---|
| Platelets | 150,000–400,000 | Spontaneous bleeding unlikely unless platelet count <20,000/mm$^3$ |
| Bleeding time (BT) | 2.5–10 min | Indicates interaction between platelets and subendothelium |
| Clotting time (CT) | 10–12 sec | Tests conversion of fibrinogen to fibrin |
| Prothrombin time (INR) | 12–14 sec (INR 1.0) | Tests extrinsic and common pathways |
| Activated partial thromboplastin time | 22–35 sec | Tests intrinsic and common pathways thromboplastin time |
| Fibrinogen level | 150–450 mg/dL | Fibrinogen is converted by thrombin (Ha) into soluble fibrin which is then converted into fibrin clot |
| Fibrin degradation products | <2.5 (depends on methodology) | Breakdown products of fibrinogen and fibrin |

(INR: international normalized ratio)

**Table 6.9:** Common causes of prolonged prothrombin time (PT) and prolonged partial thromboplastin time (PTT).

| Prolonged PT | Prolonged PTT |
|---|---|
| • Hepatic disorders<br>• Warfarin therapy<br>• DIC<br>• Vitamin K deficiency<br>• Salicylate poisoning<br>• Dilutional coagulopathy | • Laboratory errors<br>• Contact factors deficiency<br>• Factors XII and XI, factor IX (hemophilia B), factor VIII (hemophilia A, von Willebrand's disease)<br>• Circulating anticoagulants (anti-VIII, heparin, lupus) |

(DIC: disseminated intravascular coagulation)

## PLATELET DISORDERS

Platelet abnormalities may be quantitative (thrombocytopenia) or functional in nature (defective platelet functions). A very large number of drugs can result in such platelet disorders **(Table 6.10)**.

### Symptoms

Excessive bleeding is the common symptom in platelet disorders, especially in thrombocytopenia (platelet count <40,000, and especially if <20,000/mm$^3$). Typically, platelet disorders result in mucocutaneous bleeding, including purpura/petechiae, epistaxis, gum bleeding, menorrhagia, or gastrointestinal and genitourinary bleed. Coagulation factor deficiencies, on the other hand, usually result in deep muscle hematomas, and joint and retroperitoneal bleeding, though skin bleeding may also occur. A schematic approach to

**Table 6.10:** Medications which may alter platelet production or function.

| Decreased platelet production (thrombocytopenia) | Defective platelet function (prolonged bleeding time) |
|---|---|
| **Aspirin** | Aspirin and NSAIDs |
| Diuretics (thiazides, furosemide) | Antihistamines |
| Digoxin | Clopidogrel |
| **Ethanol** | Calcium channel blockers |
| **Gold salts** | Penicillins and cephalosporins |
| **Heparin** | Phenothiazines |
| H$_2$ blockers (cimetidine/ranitidine) | Propranolol |
| **Indomethacin** | Tricyclic antidepressants |
| **Quinine and quinidine** | |
| **Sulfa-containing drugs** | |
| Valproic acid | |

**Note:** Medicines in bold letters are relatively more important.

evaluation of purpura is given in **Flowchart 6.1,** and some common conditions associated with excessive bleeding are described in detail here under.

## Immune Thrombocytopenia

Immune (antibody mediated) destruction of platelets is commonly of two types: *(1) idiopathic thrombocytopenic and (2) drug-induced immune thrombocytopenia.*

### Idiopathic Thrombocytopenic Purpura

*Etiology*

Idiopathic thrombocytopenic purpura (ITP) is an **acquired immune disorder** characterized by formation of *IgG autoantibody that binds to platelets.* The antibody is mostly produced in the spleen, which also accounts for destruction of such antibody-coated platelets. The high rate of success of splenectomy in the treatment of ITP is a further proof of the important role played by spleen in the pathogenesis of ITP.

*Clinical features*

Idiopathic thrombocytopenic purpura occurs in all age groups and may have an acute or chronic onset. The course of the disease is different in children and adults. In **children (classical form),** ITP has an acute onset, and affects the two sexes equally. The disease is usually self-limiting and typically, recovery occurs spontaneously in half of the children in 6 weeks, and in over 80% within 6 months. Serious or fatal hemorrhage is rare. A few children are left with persistent disease but often with platelet counts 30,000/mm$^3$ or more, and with normal bleeding time. Such children may have few clinical symptoms,

# Chapter 6: Hematological Emergencies

**Flowchart 6.1:** Evaluation of purpura.

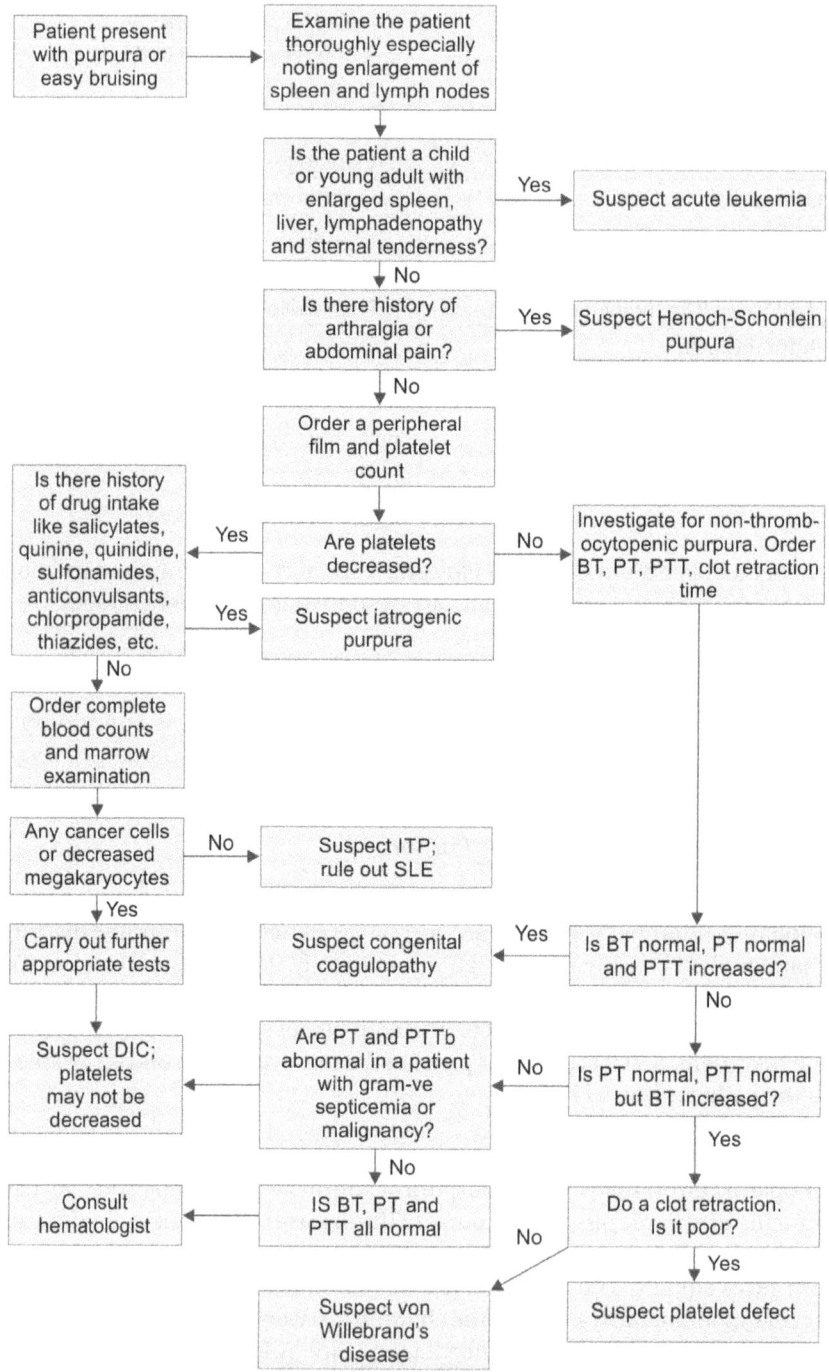

(BT: bleeding time; DIC: disseminated intravascular coagulation; ITP: idiopathic thrombocytopenic purpura; PT: prothrombin time; SLE: systemic lupus erythematosus; PTT: partial thromboplastin time)

are able to pursue their studies normally, and participate in nonviolent games. Most of these chronic cases improve gradually, and splenectomy is rarely required.

Classical ITP is uncommon in adults in whom it accounts for only about 10% of the cases. The **"adult" form** usually manifests between 20 and 50 years of age, is more common in women than in men in the ratio of 3:1, and is chronic in nature **(chronic ITP)** with frequent remissions. The onset of bleeding may be acute (as in children), or there may be a long preceding history of easy bruising or menorrhagia. Usually, multiple sites are involved but sometimes recurrent bleeding occurs from one site only. Sudden death due to internal bleeding, especially cerebral hemorrhage, may occur at any stage of the disease, the risk being greatest at the onset.

*On examination* patient appears well, there is no adenopathy, and *spleen is not palpable*. The only discernible finding may be bleeding from one or more sites in the form of purpura, ecchymosis, epistaxis, and bleeding gums.

*Diagnosis*

The platelet count is decreased and is usually below $20,000/mm^3$ (often <10,000). Spontaneous bleeding is rare with a count $>20,000/mm^3$ platelets, but at this level bleeding may occur with minor trauma. *A platelet count of $>50,000/mm^3$ in the face of extensive bruising and petechiae should suggest a diagnosis other than ITP.*

Hematological investigations reveal decrease in hemoglobin (proportionate with the degree of bleeding), prolonged bleeding time, poor clot retraction, normal clotting time, and a positive tourniquet test during the acute phase/relapse of the disease. Bone marrow has a normal morphology with normal or increased number of megakaryocytes.

Idiopathic thrombocytopenic purpura can be secondary to a number of drugs and diseases **(Table 6.11)**. These disease states should be carefully excluded before ITP is considered as primary disorder. A scrupulous drug history is mandatory.

*Management*

**Specific measures:** Most of the children with ITP respond satisfactorily to corticosteroids, and do not need splenectomy. In adults too, the initial response to corticosteroids is satisfactory, but relapses are common and finally, majority of such cases require splenectomy.

❖ **Corticosteroids:** Patients who are asymptomatic and have platelet counts $>50,000/mm^3$ do not require any treatment. Corticosteroids should be administered whenever the patient has more than minimal bleeding, and a platelet count $<30,000/mm^3$. *Treatment with prednisolone must be started if the platelet count is $<20,000/mm^3$ even if there is no bleeding.* Treatment is started with oral prednisolone 1–2 mg/kg, with a maximum of 100 mg/day in adults. A good clinical response appears within 1–2 days even before platelet count begins to rise (ascribed to enhanced vascular stability). Improvement in platelet count occurs a little later, and is usually

| Table 6.11: Diseases associated with thrombocytopenia.* ||
|---|---|
| **Defective production** | **Abnormal consumption** |
| **Bone marrow disorders** | **Immune-mediated** |
| • Aplastic anemia<br>• Hematologic malignancies<br>• $B_{12}$/folate deficiency<br>• Myelodysplasia<br>• Chronic alcoholism<br>• Radiation | • ITP drugs**<br>• SLE, CLL<br>• Lymphomas |
| **Non-marrow disorders** | **Nonimmune-mediated** |
| • Viral infections (including AIDS and dengue fever)<br>• Hemangiomas | • Microangiopathic<br>• Dilutional coagulopathy<br>• Prosthetic cardiac valves<br>• Hypersplenism<br>• Sepsis |

(CLL: chronic lymphocytic leukemia; SLE: systemic lupus erythematosus)
*Severe thrombocytopenia (<10,000/mm³) is most likely in ITP, acute leukemia, dengue fever, and aplastic crisis.
**Commonly incriminated drugs are heparin, sulfas, quinidine, digoxin, and methyldopa.

seen within 1–3 weeks of treatment, the response being quicker in younger patients and in those with a shorter duration of symptoms. The action of prednisolone is two-fold: (1) reduces the binding of the antibody to the platelet surface, and (2) decreases affinity of splenic macrophages for antibody-coated platelets.

Nearly all children and about 80% of the adults show satisfactory response to prednisolone, and platelet counts return to normal in 4–8 weeks. Thereafter prednisolone should be tapered gradually over 1–2 weeks. Younger patients usually recover completely but most adults with ITP relapse when prednisolone is withdrawn, and will require a maintenance dose of prednisolone.

Oral prednisolone is likely to prove inadequate in patients with *life-threatening bleeding. Such cases should be treated by IV methylprednisolone 1–2 g/day for 2–3 days.* After the first dose of methylprednisolone, platelets should be transfused as required. *It is worth noting that platelet count need not be increased to near normal level;* the risk of bleeding is generally small if platelet count can be maintained >50,000/mm³.

- ❖ **Splenectomy:** This should be seriously considered in adult patients with ITP, since this is the definitive treatment, and a majority of adult cases seem to need it eventually. This is the only treatment available whenever the patient fails to respond satisfactorily to prednisolone, or requires unacceptably high doses of steroids to maintain adequate platelet count. The procedure should not be unduly delayed since it provides complete or near complete remission in most of the adult patients of ITP. Presence of accessory spleen(s) should however, be excluded by radioimaging prior to surgery.

❖ **Other measures:** Intravenous immunoglobulin in high doses (1 g/kg) for 1 or 2 days has been used to tide over emergencies, and is successful in raising platelet count in most of the patients. The treatment is, however expensive, beneficial effect lasts for only 1–2 weeks, and therefore immunoglobulin therapy is advised only in emergency situations. It may be combined with IV methylprednisolone. Conjugated estrogen, 25 mg intravenously one time, can be administered to patients with severe uterine bleeding.

*Prognosis*

This is generally excellent in children with classical ITP, but in adults it is very poor if they fail to respond to corticosteroids and splenectomy. Danazol and immunosuppression are some other measures for such cases but these are best used only by onco-hematologists.

*General measures*

These are similar to those described in the section on "aplastic anemia". Any antiplatelet medication [e.g., aspirin, nonsteroidal anti-inflammatory drugs (NSAIDs)] should be stopped, "fall" risks taken care of, optional surgical procedures avoided, and only electric shavers used for shaving. *Platelet infusions are not of much use in ITP since transfused platelets will survive no better than the patients' own platelets.* These can at best serve as a temporary measure for life-threatening situations, and should be given after the first dose of methylprednisolone or immunoglobulin. *Packed RBC transfusions* are indicated in patients who develop significant anemia.

*Summary*

❖ ITP is characterized by isolated thrombocytopenia, the other hematopoietic cell lines being normal. It can affect both children/adolescents, and adults. Such patients have no systemic illness, spleen is not palpable, and bone marrow is normal.
❖ The overall prognosis in ITP is good, especially in younger patients. In most of the cases bleeding can be controlled with prednisolone. Splenectomy offers a definitive treatment, and is generally required in adult patients of ITP in whom it is usually successful in inducing complete or significant remission.
❖ The main risk during acute phase of the disease is bleeding into a vital organ, especially cerebral hemorrhage, if platelet count falls below 10,000/mm$^3$.

## *Drug-induced Immune Thrombocytopenic Purpura*

Several drugs can cause thrombocytopenia but **heparin** (unfractionated or low-molecular weight) is most commonly associated with this condition. Platelet counts typically start falling from the 5th day of therapy, usually to below 100,000/ mm$^3$, but in some cases may reach as low as 20,000/mm$^3$.

The symptom-complex in these cases is very different from ITP. Instead of bleeding, such patients develop thromboembolic complications such as deep venous thrombosis, pulmonary embolism, and stroke (the very diseases in which heparin is used as a therapeutic measure).

**Treatment** lies in stopping heparin whenever platelets drop below 100,000/ mm³, or >50% from baseline. Platelet transfusions may also be considered.

Many other drugs can, on rare occasions, result in immune thrombocytopenic purpura. Important ones are platelet glycoprotein IIb/IIIa receptor antagonists, sulfonamides, penicillins, and cephalosporins. In such cases platelets start falling after about 1 week of therapy, may drop to <30,000/ mm³ and result in petechiae, mucosal bleeding, or even significant bleeding following minor surgery.

# HENOCH–SCHONLEIN PURPURA (ANAPHYLACTOID PURPURA)

This is primarily a disease of the blood vessels, a **hypersensitivity vasculitis,** in which plasma and RBCs pass across vessels into various tissues, notably the skin, joints, and gastrointestinal and urinary tracts.

## Clinical Features

Henoch–Schonlein purpura usually occurs in children, though no age is exempt. The disease generally has a subacute onset and is characterized by palpable purpura (especially on buttocks and around ankles), joint pains, gastrointestinal features, and glomerulonephritis. Hematuria is often present and may be accompanied by mild and transient azotemia and hypertension. Remissions and relapses are common, but most patients recover spontaneously and completely. Occasionally, the disease presents as a medical emergency (mimicking acute abdomen) with colicky abdominal pain, vomiting, diarrhea or constipation, and passage of blood per rectum.

## Diagnosis

The diagnosis clinical, and can be confirmed with biopsy. Platelet count, Hess capillary test, bleeding and coagulation time are all normal. Once the typical rash appears, the nature of the disease becomes obvious; in its absence a confident diagnosis is difficult. When taking a biopsy of the skin lesions, it is important that the periphery of the lesion be sampled and specifically stained for IgA deposits. Kidney biopsy may also be useful in making the diagnosis.

## Treatment

Besides usual symptomatic measures, prednisone should be tried in a daily dose of 1 mg/kg. Antihistamines are of no proven value. In patients presenting with acute abdomen, if a correct diagnosis has been made, surgery should be avoided unless obvious obstruction is present.

## Complication
Renal failure

# HEMOPHILIA

Hemophilia is a disorder of coagulation affecting the **intrinsic pathway** of the coagulation cascade **(Flowchart 6.2)**. It results from deficiency or defect in one of the two plasma proteins; *(1) clotting factor VIII [the classical disorder—hemophilia (A)], or (2) factor IX (Hemophilia B/Christmas disease)*.

**Flowchart 6.2:** Schematic diagram of the procoagulant phase of coagulation, depicting the cascade sequence in three steps designated as extrinsic coagulation pathway, intrinsic coagulation pathway, and common pathway of coagulation. Tissue damage activates the extrinsic pathway; the intrinsic pathway is stimulated by the presence of collagen on walls of damaged vessels. The extrinsic and intrinsic pathways converge with the formation of activated factor X. This formation initiates a series of cascade steps in the common pathway, culminating in the formation of a fibrin clot.

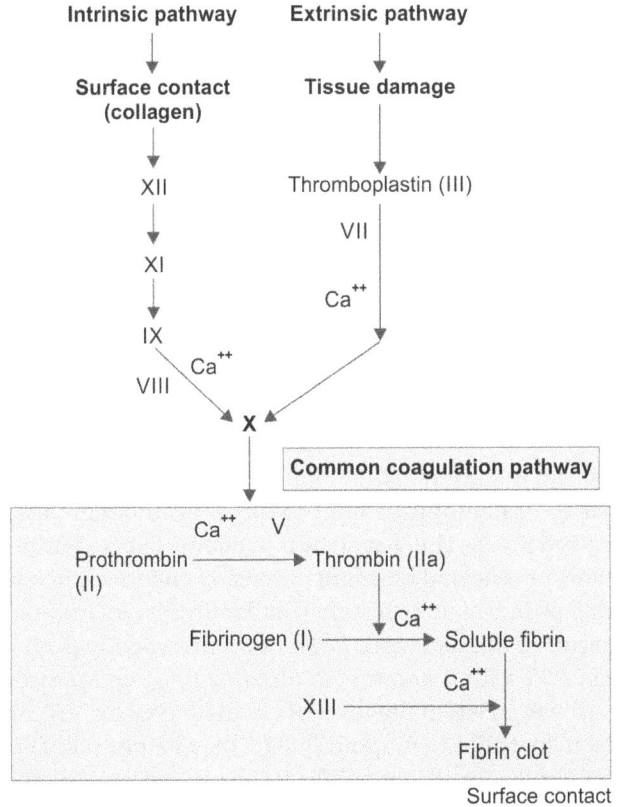

(XII: Hageman factor; XI: plasma thromboplastin; XIII: fibrin stabilizing factor; $Ca^{++}$: calcium)

The former is much more common and accounts for about 85% of cases of hemophilia. Both are X-linked recessive disorders, affecting as a rule only males but transmitted by females. Recognition of female carriers is important. Most of such carriers are heterozygotes, and produce sufficient quantity of clotting factors. Occasionally, however hemophilia carriers have factor VIII levels much less than 50%, and such asymptomatic carriers may bleed with major surgery or during menstruation.

## Clinical Features

The disease usually manifests in childhood or adolescence, though in some patients with mild deficiency in clotting factors, the disease may remain undetected until a severe hemostatic challenge occurs. Clinical severity of the disease closely parallels degree of deficiency of factor VIII or IX. The disease is regarded as *severe (spontaneous bleeding)* if the clotting factor is below 1% of normal, *moderate (bleeding occurs only on trauma or surgery)* if the level is between 1 and 5%, and *mild (few bleeding problems)* when the level is 5–50% of normal. The pattern of deficiency usually breeds true in hemophilic families. Many hemophiliacs also suffer from chronic hepatitis (type B and/or C), and some are infected with HIV as a result of repeated exposure to blood and blood products.

The *bleeding characteristically occurs in the deep tissues (muscles and joints), and hemarthrosis* is a very common manifestation of hemophilia (usually weight bearing joints). However, any part of the body, external (skin and mucus membrane of mouth, nose, etc.) or internal (gastrointestinal and urinary tracts, central nervous system, etc.) may be involved. Emergency situations may arise rapidly in several ways: (i) loss of large amount of blood within a short time, (ii) intra-abdominal emergency, and (iii) hemorrhage in a vital organ like brain which may end fatally; such instances are however, rare.

## Diagnosis

Unlike purpuric disorders which manifest clinically as mucocutaneous bleeding, cases of hemophilia tend to bleed from larger vessels into the deep tissues and joints. The diagnosis is usually suspected from a history of prolonged and/or repeated bleeding from early childhood in a male patient usually with a positive family history (but family history may be negative in about a quarter of the patients). *Laboratory investigations typically reveal an abnormal PTT with a normal PT, bleeding time, and platelet and white cell counts.* However, when the level of circulating factor VIII or IX is >30% of normal activity (mild hemophilia), PTT may be normal. Differentiation between hemophilia A and hemophilia B can be made only by specific assays of factors VIII and IX. A precise diagnosis should always be made in order to decide the specific replacement therapy.

## Management

Every hemophilic patient should be instructed to carry a proper card for identification in the event of an emergency. He should also be instructed to report to the hospital at the earliest sign of a bleeding.

### Replacement Therapy

Whenever there is more than minimal hemorrhage, measures will be required to combat the bleeding tendency by providing the missing coagulation factor, in one form or another. Two types of factor replacements are available: (1) plasma derived and (2) recombinant **(Table 6.12)**.

Specific factor replacement is currently the standard treatment for hemophilia. Compared to plasma-derived factors, recombinant factors are more pure and safer (virtually eliminate the risk of viral transmission), but are more expensive. Another problem with plasma-derived factors is that some of the preparations may contain other coagulation factors. Prolonged use of less pure concentrates may therefore increase the risk of disseminated intravascular coagulation (DIC), and may even cause paradoxical clotting.

*Whole blood,* once a major standby for bleeding, should now be used only when acute bleeding continues and circulatory support is required. Even in such a situation it should be used in conjunction with specific factor concentrates. Likewise, *fresh frozen plasma (FFP)* and *cryoprecipitate* should be reserved only for very urgent situations when specific replacement factors are not readily available.

The **dosing of replacement factors is standardized.** The desired level depends both upon the severity and the site of bleeding. One unit of factor represents the amount present in 1 mL of plasma. Rise in level of clotting factor is about twice in hemophilia A compared to hemophilia B, e.g., 1 unit/kg of the *specific clotting factor* increases the plasma level by 0.02 U/mL (2%) in hemophilia A, and by 0.01 U/mL (1%) in hemophilia B.

❖ Mild bleeding usually requires raising the missing factor 25% in hemophilia A and 40–50% in hemophilia B.

| Table 6.12: Replacement factors available for hemophilia treatment. | | |
|---|---|---|
| *Hemophilia type* | *Replacement factor* | *Remarks* |
| Hemophilia A | Human-plasma derived factor VIII **(Humate-P)** | Low risk of hepatitis and HIV transmission |
| | **Recombinant factor VIII (Recombinate)** | Low risk of hepatitis or HIV |
| Hemophilia B | Factor IX complex products | HIV seroconversion is possible |
| | Activated factor IX products | Low risk of viral transmissions |
| | Purified factor IX products | Low risk of hepatitis and HIV |
| | Recombinant factor IX | No known risk of viral transmission |

- Moderate bleeding such as in deep tissues requires factor VIII level to be raised initially to 50%, and maintained at >25% for 2-3 days, by repeated transfusions, and
- Patients with gastrointestinal bleeding, major trauma (such as head injury, with or without neurological features), or those requiring surgery should have factor VIII levels increased to 100%, and then maintained at >50% for 10-14 days. The amount of clotting factor required in such situations for control of bleeding in hemophilia B will be 50-100% more than in cases of hemophilia A.
- Local measures should be supplemented in cases with superficial cutaneous or mucosal injuries.

## Other Measures

- **Desmopressin** (DDAVP: desamino-d-arginine vasopressin) has been used in some mild cases of hemophilia who have minor bleeding or require minor surgical procedures. In a dose of 0.3 g/kg (maximum, 20 **g**) over 30 minutes every 24 hours, it can raise factor VIII levels 2-3 times for several hours by release of the coagulant factor VIII from endothelial storage sites. The advantages of DDAVP are its ease of administration (can be given subcutaneously or by intranasal spray in home setting), and negligible risk of viral transmission since it is not a blood product.
- **Antifibrinolytic agents E-aminocaproic acid** (EACA) in a dose of 75-100 mg/kg in children (6 g in adults) has been found useful in cases of bleeding from the mouth when given along with factor replacement. In fact, EACA *alone* may be able to control bleeding from superficial mucosa injuries in mild cases of hemophilia.
- **General measures:** Topical hemostatic agents should be used to control oral or nasal bleeding. These include absorbable gelatin sponges, thrombin, and microfibrillar collagen hemostats. Infections should be treated with appropriate antibiotics but **IM injections should be avoided** because of risk of deep seated hematomas. Pain may be a common accompaniment and should be treated with paracetamol or propoxyphene; *aspirin and NSAIDs must be avoided.* Long-term measures will include administration of oral hematinic, and avoidance of cuts and injuries as far as possible.

## Summary

- Both hemophilia A and B are inherited X-linked recessive disorders affecting males only.
- The basic defect is deficiency of factor VIII coagulant in hemophilia A, and factor IX in hemophilia B.
- The two types of hemophilia can be recognized only by specific factor testing; clinical differentiation is not possible.
- The disease is characterized by spontaneous bleeding especially in deep tissues such as joints and muscles.

❖ Availability of specific coagulant factors has vastly improved the prognosis. The risk of viral infections is negligible with recombinant factor products.

# DISSEMINATED INTRAVASCULAR COAGULATION

## Etiology

Disseminated intravascular coagulation is a syndrome in which there is widespread activation of both coagulation system (fibrin formation), and fibrinolytic system (breaking down of fibrin clots). Though thrombosis and hemorrhage can occur simultaneously, in an individual patient, one manifestation usually predominates, and the more common one is bleeding. DIC is associated with a number of serious illnesses **(Table 6.13)**, the most frequent being sepsis.

Activation of the coagulation cascade leads to deposition of fibrin (small thrombi) throughout the microvasculature. Fibrin deposition in excess of normal stimulates plasmin-mediated fibrinolysis in an attempt to maintain vascular patency. *This continued process of fibrin formation (clotting) and fibrinolysis leads to consumption (depletion) of platelets, fibrin, and factors V and VII to such a degree that it outstrips their production, resulting in loss of hemostasis with consequent diffuse bleeding.*

## Clinical Features

Disseminated intravascular coagulation can occur on the background of any of the disorders mentioned in **Table 6.13,** and can result in both bleeding and thrombosis. The process usually starts acutely, and spontaneous bleeding may occur at one site, or at multiple sites such as needle puncture or catheter sites, surgical wounds, gastrointestinal tract (hematemesis/melena), or from other mucosal surfaces. Thrombosis usually manifests as digital ischemia or gangrene, but may involve internal organs resulting in catastrophic events such as renal cortical necrosis (leading to acute renal failure), and hemorrhagic adrenal infarction (leading to peripheral circulatory failure).

Occasionally, the process of DIC occurs in a subacute manner as in patients with malignancies. Such cases usually present with recurrent superficial

| Table 6.13: Important causes of disseminated intravascular coagulation. ||
|---|---|
| **Infections/sepsis** | Bacterial (especially gram negative), viral, fungal, parasitic (malarial) |
| **Obstetric** | Amniotic fluid embolism, septic abortion, retained dead fetus, eclampsia |
| **Severe tissue injury** | Burns, head injury, frostbite |
| **Malignancy** | Mucinous adenocarcinomas, acute leukemia |
| **Miscellaneous** | Hemolytic blood transfusion reactions, black water fever, envenomation, fat embolism |

and deep vein thromboses, but may also have mild mucosal bleeding and bruising.

## Diagnosis

Disseminated intravascular coagulation should be suspected strongly in the event of diffuse bleeding or clotting developing in a patient suffering from any serious medical illness. The clinical features are related to a complex coagulopathy. However, the laboratory diagnosis can be made precisely by a characteristic constellation of *thrombocytopenia, hypofibrinogenemia, increase in fibrin degradation products (FDP), and a prolonged PT.* Partial thromboplastin time may or may not be prolonged. The platelet count is usually <150,000/mm$^3$, and fibrinogen level <150 mg/dL. *The most characteristic finding of DIC is increase in the level of FDPs, of which D-dimer is the most sensitive.* Some cases develop microangiopathic hemolytic anemia, and will show fragmented red cells, especially if DIC involves renal microvasculature.

The laboratory picture of *subacute DIC* is quite different. Fibrinogen level and PTT are normal, and the only abnormality in such cases is thrombocytopenia and elevated D-dimer. The results of other organ-specific laboratory work-up will depend upon the basic disease responsible for DIC.

## Management

The chief aim of management should be to diagnose and *treat the underlying disorder* responsible for DIC. In cases with obvious clinical manifestations of DIC, hypoxia, hypotension and oliguria are invariably present and will need active and knowledgeable management, preferably in an intensive care unit. The main constituents of treatment are: (i) maintenance of vital functions, (ii) treatment of basic initiating factor, (iii) replacement therapy, and (iv) control of thrombotic process, if obvious.

The underlying disorder (usually an infection) should be searched diligently and treated aggressively, as far as possible. Once it is controlled/corrected, the bleeding problem will subside as the body's continuing manufacture of clotting factors will restore normal levels, usually within 2-3 days. In the interim period, specific deficiencies should be replaced. This will comprise **platelet infusions** to maintain a platelet count >30,000/mm$^3$, and infusion of **FFP** to replace coagulation factors. Fibrinogen deficiency, if marked will require cryoprecipitate, the aim being to raise its level to 150 mg/dL (1 unit of cryoprecipitate increases fibrinogen level by 6-8 mg/dL). Such measures will be especially required when the initiating factor is either not identified or is not rapidly reversible.

**Heparin therapy** in DIC is controversial. It should be considered in patients with documented DIC in whom thromboembolic complications dominate the clinical picture. However, it must be used in combination with

**replacement therapies** since heparin alone will result in increased bleeding. Smaller doses are usually sufficient (500–750 units/hour), and successful therapy is indicated by a rising fibrinogen level (results of PTT may be variable). Obviously, heparin should be used selectively, and only in clinical units with facilities for detailed hematological monitoring and specialized expertise.

## NEUTROPENIA

This is a serious illness characterized by a marked decrease in neutrophils as measured by absolute neutrophil count (ANC) which is normally >1500 cells/mm$^3$. Severe neutropenia is diagnosed when ANC is <500 cells/mm$^3$. The disorder can result from a number of drugs/chemicals, and bone marrow or other disorders **(Table 6.14)**, but the most common agents are drugs used to treat malignancies.

### Clinical Features

Aside from congenital neutropenia which is usually benign, the onset of (acquired) neutropenia is usually sudden with fever, chills, extreme weakness and aching pains. There may be necrotic ulcers and brownish-gray exudate in the throat resulting in dysphagia. In fact, patient may present simply as a case of sore throat. Ulceration may also occur in respiratory tract, vagina and rectum. Sometimes severe neutropenia is a part and parcel of pancytopenia, and such cases may additionally have features of severe anemia coupled with tendency for easy bruising and bleeding.

*The course of the disease* is variable, from acute and fulminant cases which are rapidly fatal, to chronic and recurrent mild neutropenia. The latter type of cases may be asymptomatic except for some debility and an increased tendency to infections.

| Table 6.14: Important causes of neutropenia. | |
|---|---|
| **Bone marrow disorders** | Aplastic anemia, pure white cell aplasia, lymphoma, tumors, fibrosis |
| **Drugs** | Amidopyrine, chloramphenicol, sulfas, semisynthetic penicillins, cephalosporins, phenytoin, methimazole, chlorpropamide, oxyphenbutazone, penicillamine, gold salts, cimetidine, procainamide, antiretrovirals* |
| **Antibody related** | Autoimmune neutropenia |
| **Hereditary** | Cyclical neutropenia, dysgammaglobulinemia |
| **Others** | Felty's syndrome, hypersplenism, sepsis, HIV infection certain bacterial infections (e.g., typhoid, brucellosis, pertussis, protozoal infection, megaloblastic anemia) |

*This is not an all-inclusive list.

## Diagnosis

Neutropenia is diagnosed when absolute neutrophil count (ANC) is <800/mm$^3$, and it is graded "severe" when ANC is <500/mm$^3$. Red cells and platelets are not affected. Bone marrow is hypoplastic and only a few early myeloid cells are seen; red cell series and megakaryocytes are normal.

## Treatment

- **Various drugs, chemicals or toxins** to which the patient may have been exposed should be meticulously reviewed, and any suspected agent discontinued at once.
- As far as possible the patient should be isolated and **"barrier nursing"** employed.
- **Supportive measures** include good oral hygiene, adequate fluid intake, and use of mild laxatives and avoidance of cuts and abrasions.
- **Infections** are common, and often serious especially when due to enteric gram negative bacteria. Blood and urine culture as well as culture from any obvious infection site should be obtained and IV antibiotics used according to sensitivity reports. While waiting for culture reports or in case the cultures are negative, empiric antibiotic therapy should be started using multiple antibiotic regimens. Generally, any of the newer cephalosporin is used in combination with a fluoroquinolone (levofloxacin), or a carbapenem with vancomycin. A rise in neutrophil count by even 200/mm$^3$ during antibiotic therapy implies an improved response.
- **Granulocyte transfusions** have been used in severely neutropenic patients especially when infection is the overwhelming problem. However, because of the difficulties involved in arranging such transfusions, their temporary benefit, and the cost involved, granulocyte transfusions are seldom advised except perhaps as a supportive therapy in patients in whom neutropenia can be reversed and who have a reasonable chance of recovery.
- **Myeloid growth factors** often prove useful especially in cases of idiopathic or autoimmune neutropenia. Parenteral administration once or twice a week often increases the neutrophil count to safe levels.

# Endocrinal and Metabolic Emergencies

## THYROID GLAND

Acute medical conditions which may occur in thyroid disorders are given in **Table 7.1**.

## THYROID CRISIS ("STORM")

Thyroid crisis is an extreme form of thyrotoxicosis that can occur in untreated or partially treated patients of long duration (rather than in newly diagnosed cases). It is rarely seen in current clinical practice.

### Precipitating Factors

Thyroid crisis occurs when an already thyrotoxic patient (commonly due to Graves' disease, multinodular goiter, and toxic adenoma) develops any type of acute serious concurrent illness, or trauma. Common precipitating factors include surgery, sepsis, stroke, myocardial infarction, amiodarone therapy, emotional upsets, pregnancy/pre-eclampsia, or the patient discontinues antithyroid medication. The exact mechanism of thyroid crisis is not known. It is not just an acute increase in the severity of thyrotoxicosis; rather it results from a sudden *shift from protein-bound to free hormone, brought* by any systemic illness/stress. Occasionally, it may be precipitated as a delayed reaction, in predisposed subjects, after iodine administration as in radioactive iodine therapy, cardiac catheterization, and intravenous pyelogram (IVP). This is probably because iodine initially increases $T_4$ production and then temporarily suppresses its release. However, as serum iodine level falls in 10-14 days, large amount of newly formed $T_4$ is discharged into the circulation.

| Table 7.1: Common thyroid emergencies. | |
|---|---|
| *Hyperthyroid states* | *Hypothyroid state* |
| • Thyroid crisis<br>• Malignant exophthalmos<br>• Thyrotoxic hypokalemic periodic paralysis<br>• Cardiac arrhythmias and heart failure | Myxedema coma |

## Clinical Features

Clinical features which may appear in thyrotoxic crisis are as follows:
- **Fever:** This is invariably present and may be in the range of hyperpyrexia (>40°C).
- **Cardiovascular:** Marked tachycardia, tachyarrhythmias, *atrial fibrillation*, and (high output) congestive heart failure. Blood pressure is often elevated with a wide pulse pressure, but may be low in very advanced stage of thyroid crisis.
- **Central nervous system:** Usual manifestations include restlessness, agitation, confusion and even frank psychosis. Rarely, however, there may be apathy and prostration ending in coma.
- **Gastrointestinal:** Severe vomiting, diarrhea and dehydration are frequent. Occasionally, abdominal pain occurs mimicking acute surgical abdomen.

Other physical examination features may include thyromegaly (caution with exam due as aggressive palpation of the thyroid can lead to *more* release of thyroid hormone), exophthalmos, tremor, and warm/moist skin.

## Diagnosis

A search should be made for features suggestive of previous thyroid disease such as enlarged thyroid with or without a bruit, fine tremor, stare, etc. Free triiodothyronine ($T_3$), thyroxin ($T_4$) and thyroid-stimulating hormone (TSH) should be evaluated, and also serum cortisol levels. Thorough investigations are required and include complete blood count, renal and hepatic functions, serum electrolytes, glucose, and (whenever possible) arterial blood gas analysis. A chest X-ray (CXR) and urine and blood cultures are also indicated to look for precipitating cause.

Thyroid-stimulating hormone will be markedly low and free $T_4$ elevated in most of the cases. Since result of thyroid tests will not be available immediately, and also because these may not correlate with the severity of thyrotoxicosis, the diagnosis of thyroid storm has to be clinical. An electrocardiogram (ECG) is usually abnormal, common findings including sinus tachycardia, atrial fibrillation or flutter, and less frequently conduction defects. Presence of fresh myocardial damage may also be discovered.

## Management

### *Emergency Measures*

Immediate measures should be instituted to stabilize vital signs. Hypotension is usually due to volume depletion from fever. Intravenous (IV) fluids should therefore be administered (normal saline or lactated Ringer's solution), rapidly in first 1-2 hours (1-2 liters) to combat volume depletion. Fluid therapy should thereafter be adjusted according to central venous pressure (CVP) which should be maintained between 12 and 14 cm $H_2O$. Fluid overload should be prevented since many of these patients have high output cardiac failure.

## Chapter 7: Endocrinal and Metabolic Emergencies

Vasopressors may be required if hypotension persists despite adequate volume replacement. Aggressive fluid resuscitation should be balanced with the risk of volume overload from high-output congestive heart failure.

Fever should be managed promptly and adequately (*see* section on "hyperpyrexia"). Certain drugs should be avoided in these patients such as iodinated contrast agents, amiodarone, nonsteroidal anti-inflammatory drugs (NSAIDs), and pseudoephedrine.

Beta-blockers should be given immediately to control the adrenergic symptoms.

### Antithyroid Drugs

- **Hormone synthesis blockers:** In those with frank thyroid storm, a thionamide should be used to block new hormone synthesis, and an iodine solution should be used to block release of the thyroid hormone. The iodine solution should be given 1 hour *after* thionamide so that the iodine is not taken up by the thyroid gland and used to make more thyroid hormone. The two most commonly used thionamides are propylthiouracil **(PTU)** and methimazole. Both *block thyroid hormone synthesis*. The usual dosage is 150-200 mg of PTU or 15-20 mg Néomercazole (NMZ) orally every 6 hours. PTU is preferred in thyroid storm as it also blocks peripheral conversion of $T_4$ to its biologically active form $(T_3)$, and it can be given in IV form for critically ill patients. Consider transitioning patient to methimazole once stable due to the longer half-life of this drug. However, the use of PTU is limited by its multiple side effects, some of which may be serious [e.g., aplastic anemia, agranulocytosis, systemic lupus erythematosus (SLE), acute arthritis, and acute hepatitis]. Both *these drugs may however, take about a week to lower serum $T_3$ level significantly.*
- **Hormone release blockers:** *Iodine* is the main drug in this subgroup, and should be given in large doses IV or orally beginning 1 hour after the initial dose of NMZ/PTU to avoid further hormone production. Its action starts within a few hours of administration. Iodine is given as Lugol's solution (saturated solution of potassium iodide) 10 drops three times a day for 24 hours, and then 3 drops a day for 7-10 days. In emergent situations, iodine can be given IV as sodium iodide 1.0 g in 1 L of normal saline over 3-4 hours. An alternative approach is to administer iodinated X-ray contrast agent, sodium ipodate 500 mg per day orally 1-2 hours after PTU or NMZ. It has the additional advantage of inhibiting peripheral conversion of $T_4$ to $T_3$. Although rare, iodine can cause gastric and duodenal mucosal irritation and should be given with food or diluted.
- **Hormone action blockers:** Beta-blockers block the peripheral effects of excess of thyroid hormone with dramatic results. Metoprolol is usually used, and in urgent situations should be given IV 0.5-1 mg slowly (under ECG control) every 15-20 minutes until heart rate is adequately controlled. Thereafter it should be repeated IV after 4-6 hours, or may be given orally 50 mg every 6-8 hours. All through this period patient should be closely

observed for signs of pulmonary edema, worsening heart failure, or bronchospasm. When doubt exists with regard to the safety of the drug, therapy may be started with an ultra-short beta-blocker *(esmolol)* orally in a dose of 50 mg every 12 hours.

### Corticosteroids

Since biological half-life of cortisol is shortened and adrenocortical reserve is reduced in thyroid crisis, hydrocortisone should be given IV 100 mg initially followed by 50 mg every 6 hours with rapid reduction as clinical condition improves. Corticosteroids block hormone release from thyroid gland, impair peripheral conversion of $T_4$ to $T_3$, and provide adrenal support.

### Other Measures

Bile acid sequestrants such as cholestyramine may be used to decrease hepatic recirculation of thyroid hormones.

Atrial fibrillation is common in thyrotoxic crisis, and should be managed with antithyroid measures, digoxin, and beta-blockers. Electrical cardioversion is unlikely to be successful while the patient is severely thyrotoxic. Restlessness and anxiety should be controlled with diazepam/alprazolam. Oxygen administration at fast rates is also beneficial. Any precipitating factor(s) should be identified and treated appropriately. Infection in one form or another is a common precipitating cause, and hence broad spectrum antibiotics are routinely administered in such case.

## Prevention

Thyroid crisis is to a large extent preventable if: (i) reasonable care is taken to keep the disease under control in thyrotoxic patients, (ii) precipitating factors are quickly identified and treated, and (iii) surgery (thyroid or any other) is avoided until the patient becomes euthyroid. If emergency surgery is required, the same may be undertaken under effective beta-blockade and iodine therapy, as described earlier.

## Complications

- ❖ Hyperpyrexia
- ❖ Shock
- ❖ Tachyarrhythmias and congestive cardiac failure

## THYROID-ASSOCIATED OPHTHALMOPATHY

Certain ophthalmic changes, particularly lid retraction are common features of thyrotoxicosis. However, some cases especially those with Graves' disease may develop specific eye signs which have been described as Graves' ophthalmopathy or thyroid-associated ophthalmopathy (earlier called malignant exophthalmos). Though not a medical emergency in the strict sense, it is sometimes sufficiently severe and rapidly progressive to constitute a threat to vision. It is important to realize that the *severity of ophthalmopathy does not correlate closely with the severity of thyrotoxicosis,* and that some patients with Graves' ophthalmopathy may even be clinically euthyroid.

The patient may already have mild ocular features such as lid lag and a varying degree of proptosis. What marks the beginning of Graves' ophthalmopathy is rapid progression of proptosis along with chemosis, conjunctivitis, and periorbital swelling. With increasing severity, serious complications may supervene such as corneal ulceration, papilledema, optic neuritis, and optic atrophy with threatened loss of vision. Eye changes may sometimes be asymmetrical or even unilateral.

## Management

Mild or moderate cases of ophthalmopathy require no specific treatment since most of them recover spontaneously. More severe cases may be managed along following lines.

- ❖ **Local and general measures:** Primary disease should receive appropriate treatment so that level of thyroid hormones is optimally controlled. Smoking (active or passive), should be prohibited, and dark glasses advised. Dryness and gritty feeling in eyes can be ameliorated by protection from dust and wind, and by local instillation of 1% methylcellulose eye drops, and gels. Elevation of the head of the bed by about 6 inches may be required in more severe cases. Use of diamox 200 mg three times a day is advised when intraocular pressure is raised.
- ❖ **Corticosteroids:** High dose prednisolone (60-80 mg daily) is generally effective, and should be administered for 2 weeks. Thereafter the dose should be gradually reduced to the lowest level that maintains improvement. Severe cases should receive *pulse therapy with IV methylprednisolone* (1 g dissolved in 250 mL of normal saline and infused over 2 hours) daily for 1 week followed by oral prednisolone. Corticosteroids relieve ophthalmopathy primarily by decreasing edema and infiltrative component. Care must be taken to *avoid topical use of corticosteroids particularly in instances of corneal involvement.*
- ❖ **Other measures:** Intravenous immune globulin is of great benefit in severe cases of thyrotoxic ophthalmopathy. The usual dose is 1 g/kg IV for two consecutive days followed by a similar dose every three weeks for 2-4 months. Progressive and refractory cases may require orbital radiation and even orbital decompression.

## THYROTOXIC HYPOKALEMIC PERIODIC PARALYSIS

Acute symmetrical flaccid paralysis of sudden onset occasionally develops in thyrotoxic patients even though signs of thyrotoxicosis are minimal. The condition is usually associated with hypokalemia and hypophosphatemia.

It often presents abruptly, and may be precipitated by vigorous exercise, administration of IV dextrose, or high carbohydrate diet. Recurrent attacks are possible, each attack lasting for about 12-72 hours.

### Treatment

It starts with oral **propranolol** in an initial dose of 2-3 mg/kg. It normalizes serum potassium and phosphate levels and results in a quick reversal of paralysis (often within 4-6 hours). Intravenous potassium and/or phosphate are ordinarily not required, and *IV dextrose or oral carbohydrates are contraindicated.* For long-term management propranolol 40-80 mg every 8 hours should be continued for a few weeks, and then tapered off. Simultaneously, thyrotoxicosis should be treated with NMZ.

## MYXEDEMA COMA

Myxedema coma is a rare complication of severe hypothyroidism (most often Hashimoto's thyroiditis) with certain characteristic features such as *hypothermia, central neurological dysfunction,* and hypotension, not ordinarily seen in simple hypothyroidism. It is encountered mostly in the elderly (>60), and such as hypothyroidism, occurs much more often in women than in men (4:1). The underlying cause of hypothyroidism may be idiopathic, autoimmune thyroiditis, radioiodine therapy, or thyroidectomy. It is a medical emergency with a high mortality rate.

### Precipitating Factors

Prolonged *exposure to severe cold* is the most important precipitating factors. In predisposed patients (severe hypothyroidism), it may also be precipitated by several other conditions such acute infection (especially pulmonary), trauma, injudicious use of iodides, sedatives and antidepressants, gastrointestinal bleeding, cardiovascular events, cerebrovascular accident, and discontinuation of therapy.

### Clinical Features

The usual features of hypothyroidism such as pallor, puffy face, periorbital swelling, dry skin, coarse hair, and non-pitting edema are present in variable degree. In such patients, onset of myxedema coma is marked by a variety of symptoms such as increasing lethargy, hypothermia, hypoglycemia, altered consciousness, hypoventilation, bradycardia, hypotension, and severe ileus presenting as bowel obstruction. More severe cases may manifest frank psychosis with hallucinations and delusions accompanied by phases of excitement, so called *myxedema madness.* Seizures have also been reported. It carries a high mortality, but if recognized and treated appropriately, 3 out of 4 cases can be saved.

## Diagnosis

Fluid and electrolyte disturbances are common, the most important being *severe hyponatremia*. Thyroid function tests (TFT) will typically show low $T_3$ and $T_4$, values of TSH can vary. It is usually high in primary hypothyroidism, but can be low in secondary hypothyroidism. However, TFT alone may not distinguish between hypothyroidism and myxedema coma. Moreover results of TFT are rarely available in emergency situation.

Other laboratory abnormalities can include low blood sugar, anemia, hyperlipidemia, respiratory (or mixed) acidosis, and hypoxemia (with hypercapnia) on arterial blood gas study.

## Management

### Specific Measures

- **Thyroid hormone, levothyroxine ($T_4$)**, which is partially converted in the body to $T_3$, the more active thyroid hormone, is the treatment of choice as replacement therapy. It is given IV 300–500 µg as a loading dose over the first hour, followed by 50–100 µg IV daily for a few days. IV route is indicated whenever any of the serious complications of hypothyroidism is present. Clinical improvement is usually evident within 48 hours. Lower dosing is recommended to avoid cardiac complications. Anyway, IV thyroid hormones should always be given under continuous ECG control.
  **Liothyronine ($T_3$)** when available is better and is preferred in young, healthy patients. It is given in a loading dose of 5–25 µg IV or orally, and then 5–10 µg every 8 hours till sufficient improvement occurs.
- **Corticosteroids:** Adrenal corticoids have been found to be deficient in myxedema coma and, therefore, should be replenished especially if hypotension is a problem. Hydrocortisone 100 mg is given IV initially, followed by 50 mg 3-4 times daily until the patient's condition is stabilized. It should be administered before or concomitantly with levothyroxine.
- **Rewarming:** Hypothermia should be corrected gradually by means of blankets, hot water bottles, and by increasing room temperature. A rise in temperature by about 0.50°C every 1–2 hours is optimal. Acute elevation in core temperature should be avoided as it can precipitate vascular collapse.

### General Measures

Care of the comatose patient (*see* section on "The Unconscious Patient", Chapter 4), and fluid and electrolyte balance under CVP monitoring are basic measures. **Hyponatremia** should be treated with fluid restriction, and **hypoglycemia** with infusion of 10% dextrose. Respiratory depression can be severe and may require intubation and mechanical ventilation. A watch should also be kept on the bowels and bladder as ileus and bladder atony may develop. Furthermore, the precipitating cause should be identified and treated appropriately.

> ote
>
> (i) In all patients with hypothyroidism, other causes of coma (e.g., cerebral stroke) must be excluded before diagnosing myxedema coma. (ii) Phenothiazines and antidepressants should be avoided in severely hypothyroid patients.

## ACUTE ADRENOCORTICAL INSUFFICIENCY

Adrenal cortex synthesizes three principal types of hormones: *(1) glucocorticoids* (e.g., cortisol), *(2) mineralocorticoids* (e.g., aldosterone), and *(3) Androgens* [e.g., dehydroepiandrosterone (DHEA)]

### Etiology

❖ **Primary adrenocortical insufficiency (Addison's disease):** It arises from inhibition or destruction of adrenal glands most commonly autoimmune in nature, or due to some chronic infection such as tuberculosis (most common type in India and some other developing nations), and AIDS. Infrequent causes include metastatic carcinoma, trauma, hemorrhage, and medications. Occasionally, acute adrenal insufficiency is the result of hemorrhagic destruction of both adrenal glands due to some fulminating infection or meningococcal septicemia (Waterhouse–Friderichsen syndrome). Rarely, adrenal hemorrhage may be anticoagulant-induced or due to coagulopathy.

❖ **Secondary adrenocortical insufficiency:** It is due to some pathology of the hypothalamus and pituitary. This is most commonly seen after prolonged use of steroids which impairs corticotropin-releasing hormone and adrenocorticotropic hormone (ACTH) release. Consequently, there is dysfunction of the hypothalamus-pituitary-adrenal axis.

In both these subgroups, features of adrenocortical insufficiency may suddenly worsen and develop into a medical emergency (**Addisonian crisis**) whenever: (i) steroids are withdrawn rapidly, or (ii) there is some concurrent event requiring larger output from adrenal glands as in acute infections, surgery, or trauma.

### Clinical Features

In untreated patients, the onset of acute adrenal crisis is suggested by intensification of pre-existing symptoms such as weakness, anorexia, nausea, and vomiting. Abdominal pain may develop and may be puzzling. As the situation worsens, blood pressure begins to fall progressively, sometimes to unrecordable levels. *Unexplainable hypotension* developing in any of the situations outlined above is a warning sign of impending **acute adrenal crisis.** The *temperature is variable.* It is often normal but may be low when peripheral circulatory failure sets in. Not infrequently, however, patient has moderate to high fever which, in the presence of shock, is highly suggestive of associated acute infection. *Progressive adrenal failure results in tachycardia, altered sensorium, oliguria, and hypovolemic vascular collapse.*

## Investigations

Mild hypoglycemia, elevated blood urea nitrogen and serum potassium, and low serum sodium are common findings. Electrolyte changes are mostly restricted to cases of primary adrenal insufficiency in which aldosterone secretion is impaired. Some degree of volume depletion and normocytic normochromic anemia can be seen in both types of adrenal insufficiency. Additional laboratory abnormalities may be present according to the nature of the precipitating cause.

**Adrenal function tests:** Serum cortisol level will be low in both types of adrenal insufficiency. Morning serum cortisol level <3 µg/dL is confirmatory of adrenal insufficiency, while a level >20 µg/dL (in a random blood sample) makes the diagnosis unlikely. Primary and secondary adrenocortical insufficiency can be differentiated by ACTH stimulation test. Failure to observe a brisk rise in cortisol level (increment >9 µg/dL) will suggest primary type of adrenal failure.

## Management

Any patient suspected of acute adrenocortical insufficiency should be hospitalized in an ICU. The key elements in the treatment of acute adrenal insufficiency are replenishment of intravascular volume and administration of corticosteroids.

- ❖ **Volume replacement:** Volume depletion, hyponatremia, and hypoglycemia invariably exist together in acute adrenal insufficiency. The fluid deficit often exceeds 6% of the body weight. 5% dextrose in normal saline is the fluid of choice and should be infused initially at a rate of 500–1,000 mL/h, the therapy being guided by an hourly record of pulse, blood pressure, and central venous pressure. Hyperkalemia usually responds to administration of glucose, corticosteroids, and fluids.
- ❖ **Corticosteroids:** Hydrocortisone provides the best steroid replacement as it has both glucocorticoid and mineralocorticoid activity. An initial bolus of 200 mg IV should be followed by 100 mg (1.5 mg/kg) every 6–8 hours. Hydrocortisone has an immediate onset of action, but has a relatively short half-life (1–2 hours). It should be continued for 24 hours after recovery from adrenal crisis which usually takes 24–48 hours. Thereafter, oral prednisolone should be substituted in a daily dose of 20–40 mg, and later tapered to maintenance dose. Treatment with hydrocortisone provides both gluco- and mineralocorticoid effect, and therefore mineralocorticoid supplementation is not always required. If mineralocorticoid deficiencies are still present despite hydrocortisone treatment, maintenance fludrocortisone should be added.

## Prevention

All patients on long-term steroid therapy or those with adrenal insufficiency, primary or secondary, should be advised to increase their maintenance dose of steroids by 25% during minor infections and by 50% during any acute illness necessitating hospitalization. If any surgery is required, the maintenance dose should be supplemented by 100 mg hydrocortisone two or three times a day, the first dose being given preoperatively.

ote

> Dexamethasone and prednisolone lack effective mineralocorticoid activity, and should not be used in the initial management of adrenal crisis.

## ▉ DIABETIC COMA

Acute impairment of cerebral functions leading to drowsiness and coma may occur in a diabetic patient due to: (i) **ketoacidosis,** (ii) **hypoglycemia,** (iii) **hyperosmolality,** and (iv) **lactic acidosis.** The first two types are relatively common, and it is vital to differential them since the treatment is diametrically opposite **(Table 7.2).** Coma may also occur in a diabetic patient from causes unrelated to the basic metabolic disorder, e.g., cerebral infarction, head injury, cerebral malaria, encephalitis, uremia, etc. Such conditions can usually be differentiated by a careful assessment of the overall clinical picture and relevant laboratory data.

**Table 7.2:** Differential diagnosis between ketoacidotic and hypoglycemic coma.

| | *Ketoacidotic coma* | *Hypoglycemic coma* |
|---|---|---|
| • History | Inadequate insulin; some precipitating factor often present | Excessive insulin; little or no food with usual dose of antidiabetic drug |
| • Onset | Relatively gradual | Quick |
| • Symptoms | Abdominal pain, epigastric discomfort, vomiting, anorexia | Sinking sensation |
| • Signs | Dry skin and tongue, fever, feeble pulse, low BP, deep labored breathing (acidotic), diminished deep reflexes | Moist skin and tongue, full and bounding pulse, normal BP, normal breathing, brisk tendon reflexes |
| • Laboratory tests | | |
| ➢ Urine: | Glycosuria and ketonuria | No ketones; usually no sugar |
| ➢ Blood sugar: | Usually >350 mg/dL | Usually <50 mg/dL |

(T1 DM: type 1 diabetes mellitus)

**Note:** If some doubt still persists, 50 mL of 50% glucose should be administered IV after colecting a blood sample for sugar estimation. In case the coma is hypoglycemic, patient will rapidly recover consciousness; if ketoacidotic, no serious harm would have been done.

## Diabetic Ketoacidosis

Diabetic ketoacidosis (DKA) is one of the most serious medical emergencies. It is more common in type I diabetes but may also occur in type 2. In both the types, DKA is associated with absolute (type I) or relative insulin deficiency. Lately, with the advent of the sodium-glucose cotransporter 2 drugs for treatment of diabetes and heart failure, there has been a rise in the number of cases of *euglycemic* DKA.

### *Pathogenesis*

Diabetic ketoacidosis is a complex syndrome resulting from interplay of two factors: *(1) severe insulin deficiency,* which may be endogenous (as in type 1 patients) or exogenous [inadequate administration of insulin/oral hypoglycemic agents (OHA) in a known diabetic], and *(2) relative excess of counter-regulatory hormones* (growth hormone, cortisol, glucagon, catecholamines).

With decrease or failure of insulin production in the pancreas, glucose utilization is decreased creating a situation like relative starvation. Counter-regulatory hormones are thereby stimulated which promote glycogenolysis and gluconeogenesis. Since cellular uptake of glucose cannot occur in the absence of insulin, these mechanisms continue to increase glucose levels. Marked hyperglycemia results and induces osmotic diuresis leading to loss of significant quantities of water and electrolytes chiefly $Na^+$, $K^+$, and $Mg^{++}$. Volume depletion impairs glomeruli filtration of glucose, further creating a cycle of progressive hyperglycemia.

Along with increasing blood sugar, these (counter-regulatory) hormones also *increase lipolysis,* which converts adipose to free fatty acids (FFA). Instead of being metabolized to carbon dioxide (or stored), the incoming FFA are converted by the liver into ketone bodies (acetone, acetoacetic acid and beta-hydroxybutyric acid) which react with the buffer system of the body resulting in **metabolic acidosis** (with increased anion-gap).

All these metabolic and hemodynamic changes, if left untreated, collectively result in varying degree of impairment of cerebral functions, prerenal azotemia, cardiovascular collapse, and finally death.

### *Precipitating Factors*

Besides sudden stoppage or reduction in the dose of insulin or OHA, many other situations can precipitate DKA. These include any infection (most important), pancreatitis, surgery, digestive disturbance, medications (corticosteroids, thiazides, or sympathomimetics), ethanol or drug abuse, acute vascular catastrophe (coronary or cerebral), or acute emotional disturbance. In many cases, however, no precipitating factor may be obvious.

### *Clinical Features*

Diabetic ketoacidosis usually has a ***subacute onset*** developing over 24 hours. *Anorexia, nausea and vomiting* are important early symptoms and their presence in a case of diabetes should immediately suggest the possibility of DKA. A prominent feature occasionally is *abdominal pain* which may be due to gastric distension, stretching of the liver capsule, or underlying medical or surgical condition. Hyperglycemia leads to osmotic diuresis and secondary loss of electrolytes. In due course volume depletion results in *hypotension and tachycardia*.

*Kussmaul respiration* (attributed to respiratory compensation for metabolic acidosis) may be observed, and breath acquires a *"fruity odor"* due to presence of acetone. At this stage the patient may be conscious or may have already slipped into *stupor and coma*. The level of consciousness varies widely in such cases, and correlates best with the severity of *hyperosmolality*. Some degree of pyrexia is not uncommon and suggests infection; however, its absence does not exclude this possibility.

### Diagnosis and Investigations

Diabetic ketoacidosis comprises **a triad of hyperglycemia, ketosis, and metabolic acidosis** *(increased anion gap)*. Blood glucose is invariably more than 250 mg/dL (often in the range of 400–600 mg/dL) though the degree of hyperglycemia may not correlate with severity of acidosis. Acidosis is reflected by pH <7.3, and bicarbonate level 15 mEq/L or less. Serum $K^+$ is often elevated (secondary to acidosis which drives potassium out of cells) despite total body $K^+$ depletion due to polyuria and protracted vomiting. Serum ketones are present in a dilution greater than 1:2, and ketonuria is marked. The latter is detected semiquantitatively by nitroprusside solution, or reagent strips.

It is important to remember that *nitroprusside test reflects the concentration of only acetone and acetoacetate, and does not measure the level of beta-hydroxybutyric acid*. Normally the ratio of beta-hydroxybutyric acid to acetoacetate (acetone is generally much less significant) is 3:1, but under certain circumstances (in DKA) the ratio may be greatly elevated so that a patient with even significant ketosis may show only a weak positive nitroprusside test for ketones. Furthermore, *nitroprusside test is also a poor indicator of the patients' response to therapy*. It may continue to be strongly positive long after apparent biochemical recovery from DKA sets in because beta-hydroxybutyric acid is slowly converted to acetoacetate, and also because the acetone that might have accumulated in the DKA patient is excreted rather slowly.

**Other investigations** recommended in DKA include white cell count, estimation of blood urea, serum creatinine, electrolytes, chest X-ray, and ECG. *White cell count even up to 25,000/$mm^3$ with a shift to the left is not uncommon in DKA per se*. Serum creatinine and BUN are elevated commonly because of dehydration-induced decrease in glomerular filtration rate. *Serum amylase is often raised* and may result in an inaccurate diagnosis of pancreatitis. Increased amylase is usually of salivary origin. *Serum lipase* may be more useful if a diagnosis of pancreatitis is a genuine possibility.

Other causes of ketosis include starvation ketosis and alcoholic ketoacidosis (bicarbonate >15 mEq/L). However, in both these conditions plasma glucose is not elevated. On the other hand, coma associated with marked hyperglycemia may be of the hyperosmolar (but non-ketotic) type, absence of ketosis being ascribed to presence of circulating insulin enough to suppress ketosis but not enough to control blood glucose level.

## Management

As soon as DKA is suspected the patient should be hospitalized, preferably in ICU. The degree of dehydration, state of consciousness, acidosis, and any other associated illness should be assessed quickly. Blood sugar should be determined rapidly by dextrostix, and a blood sample sent for laboratory confirmation. A sample of urine should also be collected and examined for ketones, sugar, albumin, and microscopically for pyuria. As far as possible these investigations should be carried out urgently, and then repeated at regular intervals.

It is useful to maintain a therapeutic flow chart listing vital signs, and time sequence of diagnostic laboratory values in relation to therapeutic measures instituted. All patients of DKA in coma require central venous pressure recording, an indwelling catheter (to maintain proper fluid balance), and gastric intubation (to relieve any gastric retention that may lead to vomiting/aspiration). The broad principles of management are:

- Aggressive replacement of fluids
- Correction of electrolyte imbalance
- Appropriate insulin therapy
- Treatment of precipitating cause(s)

## Specific Measures

### Fluid therapy

Volume depletion is an important feature of DKA, usual *fluid deficit* being 5–8 liters (80–100 mL/kg body weight) with sodium deficit about 300–500 mEq. Intravenous fluid therapy should therefore be started at the earliest. Initially, 2 liters of fluid should be given in the first hour, followed by 250–500 mL/h until the blood pressure is stabilized and adequate urine flow is established. Ordinarily 3–4 liter fluid is required in 8 hours with the aim to restore 50–75% of the deficit within 24 hours. Excessive fluid replacement (>5 liters in 8 hours) should be avoided since it may result in respiratory distress syndrome or cerebral edema. Persistence of oliguria despite adequate fluid therapy is ominous and may indicate acute tubular necrosis. Hypotension unresponsive to volume and pH correction should warrant a search for complications such as gastrointestinal or retroperitoneal bleeding, septic shock, adrenal insufficiency, myocardial infarction, or pancreatitis.

**Type of fluid:** Normal saline solution is the fluid of choice in the initial stages as it quickly restores intravascular volume and avoids a rapid fall in extracellular osmolality. If serum sodium is high, 0.45% saline is recommended after initial 2-3 liters of normal saline infusions to avoid severe hypernatremia. If serum sodium is low or normal, 0.9% saline should be continued.

As the blood sugar falls below 250 mg/dL, infusion of 5% dextrose in 0.45% saline is the fluid of choice at a rate of 200-300 mL/h. If the serum sodium remains low, D5N should be infused. This will prevent hypoglycemia and reduce the risk of cerebral edema which can result from too rapid a decline in blood glucose. If hypotension persists despite adequate fluid replacement dopamine infusion may be required.

*Insulin therapy*

*Regular insulin* is required to: (i) *control hyperglycemia* by restoring carbohydrate utilization in muscles and adipose tissues, (ii) *block lipolysis,* and (iii) *correct electrolyte imbalance.* The guiding principle should be to supply insulin at a regular rate and in doses which *avoid acute lowering of blood sugar.* Large bolus doses of insulin must be avoided, and patients treated with *small dose regimen which is now the standard therapy in DKA.* Such a regimen results in circulating insulin levels approximately 100 µU/mL which is the optimal physiologic concentration of insulin for treatment of DKA.

**Advantages of small-dose insulin therapy** are: (i) the timing of insulin injections is straightforward, and the rate of fall in plasma glucose in any one patient is even and predictable; (ii) the residual IM pool of insulin when plasma glucose approaches normal level is small and predictable so that there is little risk of late hypoglycemia; (iii) pronounced changes in plasma potassium are less of a problem; and (iv) a lower incidence of cerebral edema. Two routes are available for small-dose insulin therapy.

- **Intravenous (small-dose) regimen:** This is the regimen recommended as initial therapy. After an initial bolus of 0.2-0.5 units/kg of *regular* insulin, continuous infusion should be set up delivering insulin at a rate of 0.1 unit/kg/hour through infusion pump. If infusion pump is not available comparable results may be obtained by giving insulin infusion through microdrip adjusting the rate of flow so as to deliver 5-10 units of insulin per hour.

  With such a regimen blood sugar may be anticipated to fall by 50-100 mg/dL/h. If the response is inadequate, rate of insulin infusion should be doubled. If the decline in blood glucose is >100 mg/dL/h, rate of insulin infusion should be decreased by 25-50%. Once blood sugar reaches 250-300 mg/dL, saline infusion should be replaced by D5W and rate of insulin infusion gradually decreased to 1-2 units/hour until ketosis is resolved. *Since plasma insulin has a half-life of only 4-5 minutes IV insulin should not be given as frequent bolus injections.* Such injections result in wide fluctuations in insulin levels with greater chance of a rapid increase in anti-insulin hormones.

- **Intramuscular (small-dose) regimen:** This is the method of choice for insulin therapy in DKA whenever continuous insulin infusion is not

possible. Regular insulin 20 units should be administered IM initially followed by hourly injections of 8–10 units. *Insulin has a half-life of about 2 hours in muscle,* and with this regimen optimal insulin concentration is reached in <3 hours. Intramuscular regimen is thus not unduly slow, and since the method is quite simple and convenient it works out quite well in general practice. As the blood glucose level falls to 250 mg/dL or less, dosage of IM insulin should be decreased by half, and fluids administered as infusion D5W instead of normal saline. When the patient is able to take food orally, blood glucose is below 250 mg/dL, and ketone bodies are negative, small dose insulin therapy (IV or IM) should be discontinued and regular **insulin given by subcutaneous route every 6–8 hours in appropriate dosage until patient's original diabetic regimen is established.**
- ❖ **Subcutaneous insulin:** In rare cases of very mild DKA in which the patient is hemodynamically stable, awake, alert, and oriented, and the anion gap is small, it might be safe to consider subcutaneous long-acting insulin with mealtime short-acting insulin to manage the DKA.

## *Practical Approach*

**As soon as DKA is diagnosed 20–40 units of soluble insulin should be given, half IV and half IM, depending upon the severity and duration of ketosis, and the degree of impairment of consciousness. The patient should then be transferred to a hospital** *with a note stating clearly the amount and route of administered insulin.*

On arrival at the hospital, a blood sample should be taken for estimation of glucose and electrolytes. If the patient has not received any insulin so far, 20 units of soluble insulin should be given, half IV and half IM. Thereafter, small-dose insulin therapy should be started by IV or IM route as feasible (preferably by IV route since it assures rapid dose adjustment according to blood glucose level which should be monitored every 1 hour).

*Following points are worth noting:*
- ❖ There is neither a hard and fast rule nor any simple formula that can help to determine the exact amount of insulin required in a given case.
- ❖ Regular insulin 15–20 $\mu U/mL$ shifts $K^+$ to intracellular compartment, up to 30 $\mu U/mL$ prevents lipolysis, up to 100 $\mu U/mL$ increases amino acid synthesis, and 100–200 $\mu U/mL$ effects glucose transport.
- ❖ Blood sugar should be lowered gradually especially when it is around 250 mg/dL.
- ❖ Ketones may persist in plasma and urine in sufficient concentration to be detectable long after blood glucose level begins to fall. Therefore, insulin should not be discontinued as blood sugar concentration approaches normal, rather glucose should be infused and insulin continued until ketosis clears.

ote

*(i) Only soluble (regular) insulin should be used **in patients with DKA and given IV/IM** (not SC). (ii) **IM insulin should be given in deltoid muscle** (not in gluteal region)*

*Control of electrolytes*

- **Potassium:** Considerable amount of potassium is lost during the course of therapy in DKA as renal perfusion improves and urine output increases. Hypokalemia in such cases is also accounted for by migration of potassium along with glucose into the cells under the influence of insulin. Potassium should, therefore, be introduced into the regimen as soon as insulin is being dosed. 10–20 mL of 15% potassium chloride (20–40 mEq) should be given with each liter of normal or 1/2 normal saline slowly (in not <4–6 hours). The precise dosage should be guided by repeated serum potassium estimation.
- **Sodium:** Large amount of sodium is also lost in DKA but this is usually adequately replaced along with fluids in the form of normal or 1/2 normal saline.
- **Bicarbonates:** Acidosis results mainly from ketone body production, but poor tissue perfusion is also an important factor. In most of the patients, however, this is easily corrected with insulin and fluid replacement, and bicarbonate therapy is seldom required.
- Electrolytes and beta-hydroxybutyrate levels should be checked every 4–6 hours. Once the anion gap has closed, IV insulin can be transitioned to subcutaneous insulin.

*Control of precipitating factor(s)*

The most common precipitating factor being some type of infection, it is advisable to give broad spectrum antibiotics in every case of DKA, even though evidence of overt infection may be lacking. A search should simultaneously be made for source and type of infection, or other precipitating factor(s) which, if discovered, should receive appropriate treatment.

### Subsequent Measures

As soon as ketosis is controlled and patient has recovered sufficiently to take fluids by mouth, oral feeding of carbohydrates and liquids should be started while continuing part of the fluid therapy by IV route. The latter should be gradually reduced and finally stopped in about 48 hours as oral feeds are better tolerated. When the acidosis has resolved, deliver 0.1 mg/kg of subcutaneous long-acting insulin glargine, then after 1 hour shut off the continuous insulin infusion. Glucose should be checked every hour for the next 6 hours, and metabolic profile and beta-hydroxybutyrate should be check at 4–6 hours after transitioning to subcutaneous insulin dosing. If the anion gap reopens (acidosis returns), IV insulin should be restarted.

As already stated, oral potassium should be continued during this phase. Regular insulin is continued and is given, for first few days, three times a day, the exact dose of insulin being guided by frequent urine/blood sugar estimation. After 48–72 hours of recovery it should be possible to put the patient on appropriate diet and original antidiabetic regimen.

## Complications
- Irreversible shock
- Acute tubular necrosis
- Acute myocardial infarction and/or cerebral thrombosis
- Aspiration pneumonia
- Septicemia and/or disseminated intravascular coagulation
- Lactic acidosis
- Coma
- Death

## Summary
The syndrome of diabetic ketoacidosis is characterized by a triad of hyperglycemia (blood sugar >250 mg/dL), acidosis (blood pH <7.3) and ketonuria. The onset is usually subacute, and patients generally present with abdominal pain, vomiting, fruity odor in breath, and varying degree of hypotension. The principles of treatment may be summarized as follows:
- Hospitalize the patient at the earliest.
- Replace fluids effectively and rather rapidly during the first 3 hours.
- Initiate small-dose (regular) insulin regimen by IV infusion through an infusion pump (IM if infusion-facility is not available).
- Monitor potassium levels and administer potassium as required after diuresis begins and blood glucose level begins to fall.
- Introduce 5% glucose as replacement fluid once blood glucose falls to 250 mg/dL.
- Assess acidosis after correction of dehydration, but avoid excessive bicarbonate administration.
- Search for precipitating factor(s), but broad-spectrum antibiotics should be administered routinely.

# ■ HYPEROSMOLAR HYPERGLYCEMIC NONKETOTIC COMA

## Etiology
Hyperosmolar hyperglycemic nonketotic coma (HHNC) is usually a complication of noninsulin dependent diabetes mellitus and is generally encountered in elderly people with mild and often previously unknown diabetes. It is much less common than DKA but carries a higher mortality probably because of delay in diagnosis. A large number of conditions may

**Table 7.3:** Clinical states and drugs implicated in hyperosmolar hyperglycemic nonketotic coma (HHNC).

| Clinical states | Drugs |
|---|---|
| Chronic renal insufficiency | Diuretics |
| Pneumonia | Corticosteroids |
| Myocardial infarction | Anticonvulsants |
| Gastrointestinal bleeding | Propranolol |
| Gram negative sepsis | Diazoxide |
| Pulmonary emboli | Cimetidine |
| Cerebrovascular accidents | Chlorpromazine |
| Severe burns | Immunosuppressants |
| Heat stroke | |
| Pancreatitis | |
| Recent surgery | |
| Hemodialysis | |

complicate or be associated with HHNC. Several drugs have also been implicated in its pathogenesis **(Table 7.3)**.

### Pathophysiology

Three major components of the syndrome are pronounced *hyperglycemia (usually >600 mg/dL), hyperosmolality (>310 mOsm/L), and absence of ketosis.* Hyperglycemia is due both to a relative lack of insulin and a relative excess of anti-insulin factors. In addition, elderly patients often have some degree of *renal insufficiency* which accounts for relatively lesser excretion of glucose in urine. Severe hyperglycemia induces osmotic diuresis with consequent dehydration which further worsens hyperglycemia. A vicious circle is thus established that leads to HHNC. Patients with hyperosmolar coma have higher blood glucose (>600 mg/dL vs. >250 mg/dL) and more pronounced volume depletion (8-9 L vs. 3-5 L) than patients with DKA because of more incipient onset and longer duration of symptoms before therapy is instituted.

The absence of ketosis is generally attributed to **less severe insulin deficiency** in HHNC so that while hyperglycemia is uncontrolled, lipolysis remains inhibited (lipolysis is prevented with as little insulin as 30 µU/mL whereas up to 200 µU/mL is required for glucose transport). Another possible factor is comparatively lower level of growth hormone and cortisol (which are lipolytic hormones) in HHNC compared to patients with DKA.

**Precipitating factors** include any superadded metabolic stress (myocardial infarction, burns, surgery, etc.) which may stimulate catecholamine release and glucagon secretion with consequent increase in hepatic glucose output. Hyperglycemia is likely to be worsened by diuretic therapy (excessive fluid loss), **and any acute or chronic illness (inadequate fluid intake), besides renal insufficiency as stated above.**

## Clinical Features

Hyperosmolar hyperglycemic nonketotic coma usually occurs in type II elderly diabetics (generally >65) with some degree of renal insufficiency. The onset is usually insidious stretching over a few days or even weeks with nonspecific early symptoms such as weakness, polyuria, and reduced fluid intake. Because of severe fluid deficit, tachycardia and orthostatic hypotension are common. With increasing fluid loss, lethargy and altered mental status develop which may progress into coma. Other neurological abnormalities which may be encountered are convulsions (sometimes Jacksonian) and Babinski sign mimicking cerebrovascular accident. In addition, there may be features of associated/complicating disease (vide supra). However, signs of ketosis such as fruity odor and Kussmaul respiration are not seen. It is important to remember that *HHNC may occur in patients who are not overtly diabetic, especially in elderly subjects.*

## Diagnosis

Hyperosmolar hyperglycemic nonketotic coma should be suspected in any elderly patient who develops altered sensorium. Laboratory confirmation is achieved by finding very high blood glucose values (over 600 mg/dL, may be as high as 1,000 mg/dL) though glycosuria may be only modest. Except in the very initial stages, serum sodium is normal or even increased (because of dehydration), potassium level is normal unless renal failure is present, serum osmolality* is increased (usually >330 mOsml/L), blood urea is moderately increased (usually prerenal), and acetonuria is absent or minimal (when detected, it is usually secondary to starvation). Metabolic acidosis is absent or mild (serum $HCO_3$ >15 mEq/L).

*Osmolality is measured either by an osmometer or calculated by the formula:
$$mOsm/L = 2(Na^+ + K^+) + \frac{Glucose\ (mg\%)}{18} + \frac{BUN\ (mg\%)}{2.8}$$
(Normal value: 280–300 mOsm/L)

## Management

**This comprises: (i)** *aggressive fluid replacement,* **(ii)** *control of hyperglycemia,* **and (iii)** *diagnosis and treatment of precipitating event(s).* **It may be noted that *HHNC carries a high initial mortality (more than 10 times that of DKA)* chiefly because it occurs in elderly patients who may have significant comorbidities and who usually have severe dehydration because of delays in diagnosis and treatment. Careful treatment in ICU with continuous**

monitoring of vital signs and mental status is therefore required for first 48 hours.
- **Fluid and electrolyte therapy:** Usual fluid loss in HHNC is 100–150 mL/kg (average 9 L). Therefore, large amount of fluids (4–6 liters) may be required in the first 12 hours, of which half should be given in first 3–4 hours. Fluid therapy should be initiated with normal saline, and 1–2 L administered as bolus in cases with circulatory collapse, aim being to restore systolic pressure to at least 90 mm Hg. Thereafter, attempt should be made to reverse the water deficit by employing ½ normal saline as the body fluids in such patients are markedly hyperosmolar. As blood glucose falls to about 250 mg/dL, fluid replacement should include D5W.
- Insulin therapy as in DKA, small-dose insulin therapy is employed. In fact because of absence of (significant) ketosis, smaller doses of insulin are required in these cases. Some cases may not even require insulin, and may resolve with fluid replacement only. However, if blood sugar is high, a standard practice is to give at the start 10 units of soluble insulin IV along with 5 units IM and then 5 units IM every hour (or IV insulin 3–6 units/hour) until blood sugar reaches approximately 250 mg/dL. Subsequently, insulin requirement should be assessed on individual basis.
- **Other measures:** Potassium depletion is usually much less in HHNC than in DKA, and therefore less potassium replacement is needed. A search should be made for any associated illness/precipitating factor. This is most likely to be an infection which should be identified and appropriately treated.

## Summary

- HHNC is characterized by severe hyperglycemia, profound dehydration (increased serum osmolality), and altered mental status that may progress to coma. Absence of acidosis (pH >7.3), normal anion gap, and serum bicarbonate usually >15 mEq/L are other features of the syndrome. It carries a much higher mortality than DKA.
- HHNC occurs most commonly in elderly subjects with mild type II diabetes who have some renal impairment. It is usually precipitated by an acute illness.
- Management comprises aggressive fluid replacement, low-dose insulin therapy, and treatment of the precipitating illness.

## LACTIC ACIDOSIS

### Etiology

Lactic acidosis can occur in any serious illness associated with tissue hypoxemia and decreased lactic acid clearance. Common causes include sepsis, shock, respiratory, renal, hepatic and cardiac failure. Other causes are multiple injuries and (rarely) certain drugs such as metformin, isoniazid, cocaine, and HIV medications.

## Pathogenesis

Principal sources of lactic acid are erythrocytes (which lack enzymes for aerobic oxidation), skeletal muscle, skin, and brain. Lactic acidosis is not a specific disease but a pathological state that can occur *whenever cellular oxidation of glucose is impaired.* Under such conditions pyruvate derived from glucose in muscles and other tissues is preferentially converted to lactate, and released into the blood stream. Lactic acid is removed from circulation chiefly by conversion to glucose (and its oxidation) principally in the liver, but also by the kidneys. Accumulation of lactic acid may therefore occur with its overproduction (tissue hypoxia) or deficient removal (hepatic failure), or both as in circulatory collapse.

## Clinical Features

Symptoms of lactic acidosis *per se* may be minimal in the initial stages. The single most important feature of lactic acidosis is *hyperventilation.* Lactic acidosis should be suspected in any seriously ill and susceptible patient who develops hyperventilation, lethargy, and abdominal pain. Sometimes, varying degree of *impaired consciousness* may supervene. Features of precipitating or contributing illness invariably coexist.

## Investigations

Classical findings *include metabolic acidosis (blood pH <7.30) with decreased plasma bicarbonate (<15 mEq/L) and high anion-gap* [normally, serum sodium - (serum chloride + bicarbonate anions) should not be >15]. Differentiation will be required from other conditions which may result in high anion-gap acidosis such as diabetic ketoacidosis, uremia, or certain drug intoxication (salicylates, methyl alcohol, and ethylene glycol). In lactic acidosis ketones are absent in urine and plasma. Confirmation of diagnosis requires *estimation of plasma lactic acid level* (normally <2 mMol/L). While collecting blood sample it is important that the sample is chilled immediately and centrifuged quickly to prevent continued lactic acid production by red and white blood cells.

## Treatment

Management of the *underlying cause* is the most appropriate treatment of lactic acidosis. This will vary according to the basic pathology in lactic acidosis, and can range from intensive antibiotic therapy for sepsis to specific procedures for possible etiologic factor(s) such as cardiogenic shock, etc.

Specific treatment for acidosis comprises *IV administration of bicarbonates,* but the entire concept of bicarbonate therapy is controversial. It can be considered when pH is <6.9 and the patient has some complication of acidosis. It is administered as sodium bicarbonate 2-3 ampoules (4 mEq/ampoule), the target being pH >7.20. Significant risks of bicarbonate therapy include hypernatremia, hyperosmolality, volume overload, and cerebral edema.

Restoring *intravascular volume* to improve *tissue perfusion* by rapid infusion of 1 L normal saline, and oxygen therapy at high flow rates are equally important. In some cases hemodialysis may be required. Vasopressors such as dopamine may also be required to achieve adequate systolic pressure to help overall perfusion, but their vasoconstrictive properties (which may worsen tissue hypoxemia) should be kept in mind.

## HYPOGLYCEMIA

Hypoglycemia, when abrupt can rapidly impair cerebral functions since, unlike other organs, brain relies mainly on glucose for its energy requirements. Consequently, brain metabolism suffers and patient quickly develops various symptoms.

### Etiology

Hypoglycemia is commonly defined as serum glucose <50 mg/dL. It is severe when <30 mg/dL, and invariably presents as an emergency. A large number of conditions can result in hypoglycemia **(Box 7.1)** which is of two main types: (1) *fasting* (2) *postprandial (reactive)*.

### Clinical Features

**Two clinical patterns are recognized:**
1. ***Features of adrenergic discharge*** such as anxiety, pallor, sweating, hunger, tachycardia, palpitation, and decreased concentration. Such symptoms are most prominent when blood glucose falls rapidly as in *reactive (postprandial)* hypoglycemia, and are due to rapid gastric emptying of large amounts of concentrated calories resulting in rapid increase in serum glucose and thereby, excess insulin. This type of hypoglycemia is usually seen in patients with gastrointestinal surgery, especially after gastrectomy *(dumping syndrome)*. Occasionally, it may be encountered as a *psychosomatic problem* in patients with hyperactive parasympathetics and vagal overactivity.
2. **Neuroglycopenic symptoms:** These comprise mental confusion, delirium, unsteady gait, memory defects, abnormal behavior, involuntary movements (sometimes resembling epilepsy), focal neurological deficits (e.g., hemiplegia) suggestive of acute stroke, and loss of consciousness. Such symptoms reflect brain dysfunction due to inadequate energy supply and are *usually seen when hypoglycemia is of gradual onset* (e.g., after administration of insulin or oral hypoglycemic agents). Not infrequently, the two groups of symptoms coexist but only neuroglycopenic features manifest, the other (sympathetic) symptoms being masked by either coexisting diabetic neuropathy or simultaneous use of beta-blockers.

# Chapter 7: Endocrinal and Metabolic Emergencies

**Box 7.1: Principle causes of hypoglycemia.**

**Fasting hypoglycemia**
- **Primary overutilization of glucose**
  - *Hyperinsulinism*
    - Pancreatic beta cell tumor
    - Exogenous insulin
    - Oral hypoglycemic agents
  - *Normal insulin levels*
    - Extrapancreatic tumors secreting insulin-like substances
    - Acute starvation
- **Primary underproduction of glucose**
  - *Hormone deficiency*
    - Adrenal insufficiency
    - Hypopituitarism
    - Hypothyroidism
    - Glucagon deficiency
  - *Liver disease*
    - Severe hepatitis
    - Cirrhosis
  - *Drug induced*
    - Alcohol
    - Salicylates
    - Quinine in falciparum malaria
  - *Renal failure*

**Postprandial (reactive/alimentary) hypoglycemia**
- Postgastrectomy
- Functional (increased vagal tone)
- Early diabetes (delayed insulin release)
- Hepatic enzyme deficiency (fructose intolerance)
- Idiopathic

## Diagnosis

Classically, a diagnosis of insulinoma is based on *Whipple's triad* which consists of: (i) a history of hypoglycemic symptoms, (ii) documented laboratory evidence of blood glucose 40 mg/dL or less, and (iii) immediate recovery upon administration of glucose. Difficulties may arise, however, since neuroglycopenic symptoms may be rather late in onset, and sympathetic symptoms of hypoglycemia are nonspecific. In any doubtful situation therefore, blood glucose level should be rapidly assessed by glucometer and action taken accordingly. The firm diagnosis is made by performing an observed fasting or postprandial challenge (depending in which state the patient observes symptoms). A 72 hour fast (while time and resource intensive), can be essential to diagnosing the cause of hypoglycemia. To complete this test, blood glucose, insulin, c-peptide, proinsulin, and beta-hydroxybutyrate should be collected every 6 hours during a 72 hour fast. The patient may have noncaffeinated and zero-calorie drinks during the fast. The fast ends when plasma glucose reaches 45 mg/dL or the patient becomes symptomatic. In an insulinoma, the plasma c-peptide proinsulin, and insulin levels should be elevated when the plasma glucose levels are low, indicating excessive pancreatic production of insulin. Note that sulfonylurea drugs can also produce the same laboratory results, so serum screening for sulfonylurea should be done to rule-in or rule-out medication toxicity as the cause of hypoglycemia. If the c-peptide is not elevated, exogenous insulin administration should be considered as the cause of hypoglycemia.

## Management

The aim of treatment is to restore blood glucose to normal levels as rapidly as possible. A practical approach is outlined here.

### Immediate Management

- Patients who exhibit only sympathetic symptoms but are fully conscious (mild hypoglycemia) can be managed with oral glucose solution. As the symptoms begin to resolve, more complex carbohydrate foods should be supplemented.
- Patients who present with neuroglycopenic symptoms, especially when in stupor or coma, should be given 25 g glucose IV (50 mL of 50% glucose solution or 100 mL 25% glucose). Thereafter mental status and blood sugar should be estimated (by glucometer) and if required a second bolus injection of hypertonic glucose given. This should be followed by continuous infusion of 10% glucose especially if there is risk of recurrent hypoglycemia as is often seen after overdoses of insulin or oral hypoglycemic agents. *A guiding principle in such cases is to provide approximately 20 g of glucose per hour.*
All through this period of hypertonic glucose administration a careful watch should be kept on fluid (avoiding volume overload) and electrolyte balance (avoiding hypokalemia). Oral feeding should be resumed as soon as patient's condition permits. *Remember to administer 100 mg of thiamine IV or IM in alcoholic patients to prevent Wernicke's encephalopathy.*
- In cases with *refractory hypoglycemia,* **glucagon** can be used in a dose of 1 mg IM. The response should be obvious within 20–30 minutes. Intravenous administration is not recommended because blood glucose may fall rapidly, after an initial rise, due to a brisk increase in serum insulin level. Since hypoglycemia may be refractory in some cases, due to *adrenal insufficiency,* it is a good practice to administer hydrocortisone 100–200 mg IV.

### Subsequent Management

Most of the cases of hypoglycemia are due to overdose of insulin or oral hypoglycemic drugs, and therefore proper adjustment of antidiabetic medications and regular meal times will avoid further episodes of hypoglycemia. In fact many diabetic patients become familiar with early features of hypoglycemia and can prevent serious symptoms by ingesting concentrated sugar in some form. In nondiabetic patients the etiology of hypoglycemia should be investigated and appropriately treated. When a precise cause is not discovered or is not amenable to specific therapy, symptomatic improvement is possible by long-term treatment with diazoxide 5-20 mg/kg body weight daily by mouth especially if combined with small doses of chlorothiazide.

# ACUTE GOUTY ARTHRITIS

## Pathogenesis

Gout is a chronic disorder of uric acid metabolism associated with hyperuricemia. The elevated level of urates may persist in an asymptomatic form for many years without progression. However, hyperuricemia is often associated/punctuated by attacks of acute gout. *Development of acute gouty arthritis usually evolves through two stages:*

1. **Deposition of urates into joint tissues:** Saturation point of urates in biological fluids is approximately 6.8 mg/dL, and elevated serum urate level is the basic underlying cause of gout. Prolonged hyperuricemia results in deposition of *monosodium urate crystals into the joints.* The higher the serum urate level, greater are the chances of crystal deposition. It should be noted, however, that hyperuricemia, even for extended periods, may not by itself result in arthritis. Certain *local factors aid in crystal deposition.* These include: (a) mechanical stress (e.g., first metatarsophalangeal joint), or irritation (as in olecranon bursa from leaning on the elbow), (b) areas of lower temperature as in helix of the ear, and (c) previously diseased joints such as osteoarthritis in the fingers (Heberden node).
2. **Release of deposited urates into joint space:** Onset of acute arthritis follows sudden release of urates into joint space either by some metabolic change, such as increase or decrease in serum urate levels, by mechanical trauma, or by some unknown factor. In the joint space, urate crystals are phagocytized by synovial lining cells and initiate a complex inflammatory process ending in acute attack of gout.

## Clinical Features

Hyperuricemia may remain asymptomatic throughout life but is usually punctuated by acute attacks of gout. Such acute episodes are generally self-limited and resolve either spontaneously (especially early in the course of the disease) or with medication. Acute arthritis is *sudden in onset* and is characterized by warmth, swelling, redness of the joint, and often severe pain. Occasionally, symptoms such as lethargy and a sensation of burning, tingling or numbness in the affected joint may herald the acute episode. The patient may in fact be familiar with such prodromal features, their importance lying in that it may be possible to ward off an acute attack if treatment is initiated at this stage.

## Diagnosis

A presumptive diagnosis of gout can usually be made on the basis of typical clinical features and the presence of hyperuricemia. Occasionally, serum urate level may not be high when measured during an acute attack of arthritis. In such cases a repeat estimation at 2 weeks will often reveal hyperuricemia if the patient does indeed has gout. Synovial fluid aspiration and analysis remains, however the gold standard for diagnosis of gout but is seldom necessary or practical in clinical practice.

## Management

Comprehensive treatment of acute gouty arthritis should have three goals: (1) terminate the acute attack and relieve pain, (2) prevent further acute recurrences, and (3) treat associated conditions.

- ❖ **Treatment of acute attack:** Several drugs are available to control acute gouty arthritis. These include NSAIDs, colchicine, and corticosteroids. All these drugs, singly or combination, can **effectively control pain and terminate the acute attack.** *What is critical however, is how rapidly the acute episode is brought under control.* **The choice of a particular anti-inflammatory agent should be guided by the patient's concurrent medications and comorbidities such as renal disease.**
  - **Nonsteroidal anti-inflammatory drugs:** These are the first-line drugs in the management of acute gouty arthritis and have largely replaced colchicine because of their better tolerance and increased duration of action. When used in full anti-inflammatory dose, all NSAIDs appear to be equally effective, and are the drugs of choice if the patient has no significant gastrointestinal, renal or cardiovascular disease. The usual initial dosage of some commonly prescribed NSAIDs is as follows: (i) *indomethacin* 150–200 mg daily in 3 or 4 divided doses, (ii) *diclofenac sodium* 50 daily three times a day, and (iii) *naproxen* 500 mg twice daily. Any of these drugs should be administered in full dosage until the symptoms resolve completely and then tapered gradually over the next 7-10 days. Simultaneous use of a proton pump inhibitor can improve gastrointestinal tolerance of NSAIDs.
  - **Colchicine:** Once in the fore-front for treatment of acute gout, use of colchicine is now restricted to patients who, having experienced past attack(s) of gout, can start the drug at the first hint of an acute attack. The standard dosage schedule is 0.6 mg every 1 hour (up to a maximum of 10 doses) till the pain subsides or side effects (such as nausea, vomiting, abdominal discomfort, diarrhea) appear. Since the drug has a low therapeutic index, and very few patients may be able to follow

this schedule, a regimen of colchicine 0.6 mg administered three times daily often proves effective while obviating GI side effects. The drug is ineffective if started more than 24 hours after the onset of acute attack.
- **Corticosteroids:** In patients with polyarticular gout corticosteroids are often used especially when contraindications exist to administration of NSAIDs or colchicine, i.e., renal failure or history of GI bleed. The optimal dose is prednisone 40 mg per day until the flare resolution begins then a slow taper over the course of a week. If symptoms begin to flare again, consider elongating the taper to 2–3 weeks. Corticosteroids may also be injected intra-articularly when only one or two joints are involved. This route may be especially useful in patients who have some contraindication to use of systemic corticosteroids.
- **Urate lowering therapies:** It is recommended to continue urate-lowering therapies through a flare if a patient had previously been taking them regularly.

❖ **Prevention of recurrences:** 2–3 weeks after all the symptoms of acute attack settle, serum urate level should be estimated. If high levels persist, specific urate-lowering drugs should be started to decrease levels below 5 mg/dL (preferably <4 mg). When these low levels are maintained for 1–2 years, urate crystals get depleted from inside the joint(s) and recurrences are prevented. Urate-lowering therapy, however, is generally a life-long commitment. Three drugs are available to decrease urate levels: (i) Allopurinol which is a xanthine oxidase inhibitor and blocks synthesis of uric acid; (ii) Probenecid which works by increasing urinary excretion of urates; (iii) Febuxostat which is also a xanthine oxidase inhibitor but much more costly.

If starting allopurinol de novo, it is recommended to start low at 100 mg per day and titrate up every 2–4 weeks to an optimal dose of around 300 mg daily. During the initial titration, colchicine or NSAID prophylaxis should be considered to prevent an acute gout flare.

Once an optimal level is established, serum urates should be checked once or twice a year to ensure a satisfactory level. Since rapid alterations in serum urate concentration (even a decrease) may precipitate acute attacks, anti-inflammatory prophylaxis should be employed whenever urate-lowering therapy is initiated. In this setting any NSAID or colchicine may be prescribed at lower than full anti-inflammatory dose.

❖ **General measures:** Alcohol consumption, intake of meat and dairy products should be curtailed as all of them are known to increase serum urate levels. Commonly associated conditions such as hypertriglyceridemia, obesity, and hypertension should also be prevented or reversed.

# CHAPTER 8

# Emergencies in Infectious and Tropical Diseases

## DENGUE FEVER

Dengue fever (DF), also called break-bone fever, is an acute febrile illness prevalent in many parts of the world especially in tropical countries. A major outbreak of serious form of the disease occurred in 1996 in the Northern parts of India especially affecting Delhi and its adjoining areas.

### Etiology

The disease is caused by dengue virus *(arbovirus)* transmitted to man through Aedes mosquito, the most common species being *Aedes aegypti*. The female species bites man during the day mostly a couple of hours after the daybreak and before sundown. After feeding on infected person the mosquito transmits the disease either immediately by changing the host or after a week or so during while the virus multiplies in its salivary glands. Four serotypes of dengue virus have been identified, which are not quite identical antigenically, and therefore immunity after infection by one serotype does not provide full immunity against the other three serotypes.

### Pathogenesis

Dengue fever principally involves blood vessels, bone marrow, lymphoid tissue, and cells in the liver, spleen, kidneys, thymus, and lungs. The infected monocytes release *vasoactive mediators which increase vascular permeability* resulting in loss of plasma with consequent hemoconcentration. In severe cases plasma volume is reduced by 20% or even more leading to hypotension and shock **[Dengue Shock Syndrome (DSS)]**. However, this is only a transitory functional disturbance in capillary permeability, and no inflammatory or destructive vascular lesions have been observed.

Bone marrow suppression occurs early resulting in neutropenia and thrombocytopenia. Hemostasis is also disturbed, and levels of fibrinogen, prothrombin, and various clotting factors are decreased with possibility of multiple and extensive hemorrhages in skin and mucosal surfaces **[Dengue Hemorrhagic Fever (DHF)]**. However, classical markers of disseminated intravascular coagulation are usually absent.

## Clinical Features

Dengue fever affects mostly children and young adults though no age is immune. Incubation period averages 5 days with a range of 3–10 days. Initial symptoms are usually nonspecific such as fever, malaise, and headache *(viral syndrome)*. More severe cases develop a triphasic fever with arthralgia and leukopenia with or without petechiae. The severest forms of disease are characterized by shock (DSS) or multiple hemorrhages (DHF).

*Classical illness* is marked by an abrupt rise in temperature often preceded by prodromes like conjunctivitis, upper respiratory catarrh, retro-ocular pain, severe muscle, and joint pains, and ocular soreness (pain on moving the eyes). Between third to fifth days a *characteristic rash* usually appears initially over the trunk, and spreads peripherally. It may be pruritic and ends generally in 3–5 days with desquamation. *Tourniquet test is often positive.*

In more *severe cases,* petechiae become extensive, and epistaxis, bleeding gums, easy bruising, and bleeding at venipuncture sites occur. Hematuria and gastrointestinal hemorrhage are possible. Other features may include epigastric discomfort, tender hepatomegaly, abdominal pain, lymphadenopathy, serous effusions, and even encephalitis.

The fever and associated symptoms usually last for 5–6 days and then subside rapidly. In many cases a short-lived (about 2 days) remission occurs on the third or fourth day, to be followed by recurrence of fever *(saddle back fever)* and other symptoms which are, however, not as severe as in the early part of illness. There are generally no residual signs and symptoms except for some fatigue and debility, which may persist for a few weeks.

### Dengue Shock Syndrome

Besides usual features of "classic" dengue fever, DSS is characterized by a varying degree of shock, which may be heralded by fall in temperature usually between the third to fifth days of disease. More severe cases rapidly develop features of profound shock with imperceptible pulse, severe hypotension, and may die within 12–24 hours. Such cases usually also exhibit hemorrhagic features of the disease, and may terminally develop metabolic acidosis and disseminated intravascular coagulation (DIC).

The pathogenesis of "shock syndrome" is multifactorial, predominant factor being increased vascular permeability with contraction of plasma volume *(hypovolemic shock)*. A contributory factor is blood loss due to bleeding from various sites. In patients who survive the shock stage, complete recovery occurs within a few days.

## Diagnosis

In milder cases the disease can be suspected only during an epidemic of DF. In more severe cases, the diagnosis should rest upon: (1) high continuous fever of acute onset and, (2) hemorrhagic manifestations. Serous effusions and

hypoalbuminemia provide additional evidence of disease. *The identification of DHF requires four criteria:*
1. Fever, occasionally biphasic
2. Hemorrhagic tendencies
3. Thrombocytopenia (<100,000/mm$^3$), and
4. Evidence of plasma leakage in the form of hypoalbuminemia, or serous effusions.

Once diagnosed, the severity of DHF can be graded as follows:
**Grade 1:** High fever associated with muscle and bone pains, other nonspecific constitutional features, and a positive tourniquet test/thrombocytopenia.
**Grade II:** Manifestations of grade 1 + spontaneous bleeding like purpura, epistaxis, and gastrointestinal/vaginal hemorrhaged.
**Grade III and IV:** Features of grade II DHF + hypotension and cold extremities (grade III) or vascular collapse (grade IV).

## Investigations

Moderate to severe thrombocytopenia is the classical laboratory finding. Platelet count is invariably <100,000/mm$^3$ and often less than 50,000/mm$^3$. Significant bleeding however occurs only when platelet count drops to 20,000/mm$^3$ or less. **Serological confirmation** is by enzyme immunoassay technique, which qualitatively detects IgM and IgG antibodies to dengue virus in serum or plasma. *The test can also differentiate between primary and secondary infection.* The **primary dengue infection** is characterized by rise in IgM antibodies by 5th day of the onset of symptoms, and may persist as long as 3 months. IgG antibodies in such cases appear after 2 weeks of infection and may persist for many years. In **secondary infection,** on the other hand, it is the IgG antibodies that rise within 1–2 days after the onset of symptoms, whereas IgM antibodies are induced after 20 days.

## Treatment

This is entirely symptomatic. In milder and even in "classic" cases the predominant symptom is fever and myalgias both of which can be relieved by paracetamol. *Salicylates and nonsteroidal anti-inflammatory drugs should not be used* since these can alter hemostasis and cause bleeding.

Ordinarily, cases of DF can be treated at home provided close clinical observation and serial study of platelet count and hematocrit is possible. *Hospitalization will become necessary,* if patient develops any of the following features: (1) hemorrhages, (2) restlessness/lethargy, (3) fall in BP and/or a narrow pulse pressure (20 mm Hg or less), (4) rapid feeble pulse, (5) fall in platelet count to <100,000/mm$^3$, and (6) sudden increase in hematocrit. In serious cases typified by DHF and DSS, management is guided by main pathophysiological abnormalities. Plasma volume and platelet counts should therefore be maintained within safe limits by IV fluids and platelet transfusions, respectively.

## Fluid Therapy

Careful clinical monitoring and serial study of hematocrit and platelet count is mandatory in all cases of DF. *The critical period is during the transition from the pyrexia to the apyrexial phase, which usually occurs after the third day.* Adequate fluids should be administered orally and/or intravenously (normal saline or D5W) keeping a watch on urine output and, simultaneously avoiding pulmonary overloading. In cases of continuing or profound shock, plasma transfusion (20-30 mL/kg body weight) or plasma expander (dextran 40) may be useful. Usually, parenteral fluid therapy is not required beyond 48 hours of termination of shock.

## Platelet Infusions

Platelet concentrates are prepared either by centrifugation of platelet-rich plasma from single units of blood (yield $6 \times 10^{10}$ platelets) or by plateletpheresis, which yields six such platelet units from one donor. If properly handled, one unit of platelet infusion should increase platelet count in an adult by 5,000 cell/mm$^3$. *Platelet transfusions should be monitored by platelet counts carried out 1 hour and 24 hours after infusion.*

Platelet transfusions are indicated in all cases of DF with spontaneous bleeding. Most of such cases will have platelet counts less than 20,000 (often <10,000). In patients without obvious bleeding, prophylactic platelet infusions are generally recommended to maintain platelet counts above 20,000/mm$^3$. However, it may be safer to maintain platelet count above 40,000 since defects in hemostasis in these cases may be at multiple levels (capillary leakage, thrombocytopenia and coagulopathy).

## Complications

- Encephalitis
- Acute liver failure
- Renal failure
- Dual infections with other endemic diseases, such as falciparum malaria, leptospirosis, or viral hepatitis.

# CHIKUNGUNYA FEVER

## Epidemiology

Chikungunya fever has been reported sporadically from various parts of India since 1963 but has assumed clinical importance after an epidemic break in 2005-06. Worldwide, epidemics of chikungunya fever have occurred repeatedly during past 50-60 years in several countries, mostly in Africa and Asia.

## Transmission

Chikungunya fever is caused by "Chikungunya virus", which is transmitted through the *bite of an infected Aedes mosquito* (which also transmits dengue fever and yellow fever). The virus is transmitted from human to human via *Aedes aegypti* mosquito (cycle of the disease is human-mosquito-human). Explosive urban epidemics occur during rainy season (same as for dengue fever). Direct human to human transmission is not known but maternal-fetal transmission has been documented.

## Clinical Features

"Chikungunya" is a word in the spoken language of ethnic residents of Tanzania and Mozambique, and translates to "dry up or become contorted". This refers to the principal manifestation of the disease in which the patient "bends up" and develops a stooped posture due to rheumatologic manifestations of the disease.

Chikungunya fever affects all age groups and involves both sexes equally. After a short incubation period of 2-4 days (from 3 to 12 days), the disease starts abruptly with *high grade fever with chills* associated with myalgias, arthralgia, headache, photophobia, flushed face and pain in throat. **Arthralgias** are polyarticular, migratory and mostly involve small joints, though larger joints such as knee and shoulder may also be affected. The joints are swollen, extremely tender, and greatly restrict mobility. Papular or maculopapular *skin rashes* typically appear on the trunk and limbs, often during the 2nd to 5th day of the illness. The rash may be even petechial but the hemorrhagic manifestations of dengue fever are either absent or minimal. Mild conjunctivitis and generalized lymphadenopathy (especially cervical) may also be seen. Rare manifestations include meningoencephalitis and fulminant hepatitis. Twin outbreaks of dengue fever and chikungunya fever have been reported.

## Course of Disease

Chikungunya fever is by and large a self-limiting disease. In most of the patients fever settles in a few days and joint pains subside in 1-3 weeks. Occasionally however, pyrexia assumes a biphasic pattern lasting 2-3 weeks with a short-afebrile phase in between. Likewise, in some patients arthralgia may persist for several months or even up to 1-2 years.

## Diagnosis

Chikungunya fever usually occurs during the fall and rainy season, which is also the period for outbreaks of dengue fever, leptospirosis, and malaria. Clinical differentiation between these diseases may be virtually impossible in the first few days. Compared with serious cases of dengue hemorrhagic fever, patients with chikungunya fever usually present with polyarthralgia. In fact history of fever may have been forgotten, and presentation may resemble more like rheumatoid arthritis. Such cases will require laboratory testing to distinguish chikungunya fever from other conditions.

Confirmation of chikungunya fever requires isolation of the chikungunya virus by culture techniques. A more rapid method of definitive diagnosis is the reverse transcription-polymerase chain reaction (RT-PCR). Besides isolation of the virus, serodiagnostic methods are also available by detecting IgM and IgG antibodies against chikungunya virus.

## Treatment

In the absence of any specific drug the treatment of chikungunya fever is totally symptomatic and supportive. Analgesics are often required to treat arthralgia, but aspirin and NSAIDs should be avoided because of their side effects on platelets. Paracetamol and dextropropoxyphene can be safely used. Hydroxychloroquine has been found useful in the treatment of arthropathy, if prolonged. Supportive measures in the febrile phase include adequate fluid intake and electrolyte regulation. Complete recovery ensues eventually. Corticosteroids are of no use.

# EBOLA VIRUS DISEASE

**Ebola virus disease (EVD),** or simply **Ebola,** is a disease of human and other primates caused by (four of the five viruses of the) genus *ebola virus*. The disease was first identified in 1976 in two simultaneous outbreaks in Sub-Saharan Africa, one in Nazara, and the other in Yambuku, a village near the Ebola River from which the disease takes its name. Outbreaks of the disease occur intermittently in tropical regions of Sub-Saharan Africa. The largest outbreak is the recent one (2014-15), which has involved many countries around the world affecting more than 25,000 cases with mortality rate of about 40%.

## Clinical Features

The incubation period varies from 2 to 21 days, usually 4–10 days. Symptoms typically start suddenly with flu-like features characterized by fever, sore throat, muscular and joint pains, and headaches. This is soon followed by high fever, abdominal symptoms, and shortness of breath, chest pain, and confusion. Liver and kidney functions are deranged along with some decreased blood clotting resulting in both external and internal bleeding, usually 5-7 days after the first symptoms. Bleeding in the skin causes petechiae, ecchymosis or hematomas, especially around needle injection sites. Mucosal bleedings can result in hemoptysis, hematemesis, or blood in stool. Heavy bleeding is uncommon.

Death, if it occurs, follows 6–16 days after the first symptoms and is usually due to hypotension from fluid loss. In general, bleeding indicates a worse prognosis. Patients are often in coma near the end of life. Those who survive the illness start recovering between 7 and 14 days after first symptoms, and are often left with muscular and joint pains, some hearing loss, and constitutional symptoms, such as decreased appetite, weakness, and fatigue.

## Transmission

The disease *spreads from person-to-person mostly by direct contact* with blood, vomit and feces. However, other body fluids such as saliva, mucus, vomitus, feces, sweat, breast milk, urine, and semen can also transmit the virus, and so also contact with an item recently contaminated with body fluids including syringes, needles. The *entry points* for the virus are generally nose, mouth, eyes, open wounds, cuts and abrasions. *Human-to-human transmission of Ebola virus through air has not been reported.* However, dead bodies remain infectious. Therefore, people around a person with the disease as also those handling human remains must have *appropriate protective clothing,* such as masks, gloves, gowns, and eye protection, and *wash hands* as often as required. Healthcare personnel treating Ebola patients are at greatest risk of infection.

## Treatment

No specific treatment or vaccine has been available so far, but very recently (2015) a *vaccine* has been developed that is reported to be 100% effective in disease prevention in trials in Africa.

In all cases supportive efforts are most important, and often improve outcomes. These include providing plenty of fluids as oral rehydration and IV fluids so as to avoid hypotension; blood transfusions may be required. Additionally, symptomatic measures should be adopted for relief. All health personnel in contact with the patient must also practice protective measures as outlined above.

## ■ INFLUENZA A: VIRUS INFECTION

**Influenza A virus** has two subtypes—**H1N1 and H1N2,** depending on the type of H or N antigens they express. Recently (2009) there has been a pandemic of a new strain of H1N1 virus also called **swine flu.** This strain affects a small percentage of all human flu-like infections, and is endemic in pigs (so the name "swine flu").

Swine influenza *(swine flu)* virus is common in pig population throughout the world. *Transmission* of the virus from pigs to humans is not common, but people at regular exposure to pigs are at increased risk of swine flu infection. The meat of an infected pig, when properly cooked, is not a risk of infection.

In 2009, an outbreak of influenza-like illness (H1N1) occurred in the United States and Mexico, and soon acquired pandemic proportions. In India swine flu was reported in late 2014 and early 2015. It affected more than 20,000 people and claimed over 1,000 lives. The risk of contacting infection is greatest in pregnant women.

Swine flu is **contagious,** and spreads in the same manner as the seasonal flu. The virus spreads through droplet infection, and also if a person touches a surface (such as door knob or sink) that an infected person has recently touched.

## Clinical Features

People who have swine flu can be contagious 1 day before they have any symptoms, and as much as 7 days after they get sick. Children can be contagious for a longer period, as long as 10 days.

As far as symptoms are concerned these are the same as in seasonal flu. These include cough, sore throat, fever, stuffy or running nose, body aches, fatigue, and chills. Serious complications such as pneumonia and respiratory failure can occur in some patients, especially pregnant women or patients with comorbid states such as diabetes or asthma.

## Diagnosis

It is hard clinically to differentiate between swine flu and seasonal flu, because of common clinical features. Patients with swine flu may be more likely to have *gastric symptoms* such as nausea and vomiting compared to those with ordinary flu. Presence of symptoms like *shortness of breath,* severe vomiting, abdominal pain, dizziness, or confusion is ominous.

A laboratory test is the only way to make a certain diagnosis. A rapid flu test done in doctor's office can be misleading.

## Treatment

*Symptomatic measures often provide great relief,* when severe disease is likely, **vaccination** is recommended. *Swine flu is one of the viruses included in the vaccine.* Vaccination is recommended for all pregnant women as *prophylaxis* against influenza virus, but should be avoided when pregnant women become infected with influenza. Patients with moderate to severe illness should wait until they recover before taking the vaccination.

Two **antiviral medicines** are available (on prescription)—*oseltamivir* **(tamiflu)** and *zanamivir* **(relenza)**. They work best when taken within two days of becoming sick. The latter is preferable since resistance to *tamiflu* is being increasingly reported.

## ▌LEPTOSPIROSIS

Leptospirosis is an acute systemic disease caused by *Leptospira* genus. Leptospires are obligate aerobes, thin, and motile (flagellate), and constitute the smallest and most tightly coiled of the pathogenic spirochetes. These characteristics enable the organism to burrow in deep organs. The pathogenic species is *L. interrogans,* which has more than 200 serotypes. The disease is being increasingly reported from large cities in this country, other tropical regions, and even in some developed nations.

## Epidemiology

Leptospirosis is a worldwide zoonotic infection (much more so in tropical regions), affecting more than 150 mammalian species. The most common host animals are cattle, rats, pigs, swine, sheep, dogs, cats, squirrels, raccoons, and mongooses. In animals, the disease is usually subclinical, even when excreting leptospires in urine. The organisms often develop a symbiotic relationship with the host and can persist in renal tubules for years.

*Human infection* may result from direct contact with urine, blood, or tissue from an infected animal or indirectly via contaminated water or soil usually through abraded skin, the conjunctivae, or oral mucus membranes. *Person-to-person transmission is very rare,* though breastfeeding has been associated with transmission of leptospirosis.

## Pathology

Leptospirosis is typically a **biphasic disease.** In the initial phase of the disease **leptospiremia** develops after organisms enter through the abraded skin or mucus membrane. Infection spreads to all organs and multiplication occurs in both blood and organ tissues including central nervous system (CNS). At this stage organisms can be recovered from blood and cerebrospinal fluid (CSF) (during the first 4–12 days of illness) though very few cases develop features of meningitis. The *second phase* (leptospiruric phase) follows a brief period of 2–4 days and is characterized by a **systemic immune reaction** (involving endotoxin, hemolysin, and lipase). This is the febrile phase in which IgM antibodies appear in the circulation. The consequent *immunological injury accounts for most of the clinical manifestations of the disease.* This second phase may persist from a few days to several weeks.

Pathologically, two types of lesions have been described: (1) *capillary vasculitis* and (2) *adherence to cell surfaces and cellular toxicity.* As a result of these lesions the tissue damage can be extensive and any organ may be involved, the maximum impact being on the liver and kidneys. *Hyperbilirubinemia* is common but not entirely due to hepatic lesions; contributory factors include muscle damage (releasing myoglobin), intra-and- extravascular hemolysis, and hemorrhages. Some degree of centrilobular necrosis may occur but histological changes are generally not striking.

The most common *renal lesions* are interstitial nephritis and tubular necrosis. *Pulmonary changes* are largely due to alveolar capillary damage and resultant edema and bleeding. In severe cases acute respiratory distress syndrome (ARDS) is a possibility. *Skeletal muscles,* especially calf muscle, are also a common site of inflammation, which accounts for calf muscle pain and local tenderness in some patients. With the formation of antibodies, leptospirae are eliminated from all tissues except the eye (chronic or recurrent uveitis) and renal tubules where they may persist for months or years.

## Clinical Features

The incubation period is usually 7-12 days but may range from 2 to 20 days. In most of the patients (about 90%) the disease presents as an acute self-limited, anicteric disease with features simulating influenza. Fever may be the only symptom or there may be accompanying chills, myalgias, headache, and vomiting. This leptospiremic phase usually lasts for about a week, and in some patients may be troublesome with intense headache (especially retro-orbital) and severe myalgias chiefly affecting the calves, back, and abdomen. Development of cough and chest pain sometimes associated with hemoptysis will reflect pulmonary involvement. Some cases may also develop mental confusion.

Physical examination may reveal (besides fever) relative bradycardia, conjunctival suffusion (without purulent discharge), and muscle tenderness. Some type of rash is not uncommon and may take maculopapular, urticarial, petechial, or hemorrhagic form. Lymphadenopathy, splenomegaly and hepatomegaly are uncommon.

Most patients become symptom-free and recover in about a week (with disappearance of leptospirae from blood and CSF). However, after 1-3 days the *immune or leptospiriuric phase* begins when antibodies appear and leptospira can be recovered only from urine. Fever, headache, and myalgias return but are milder than the first phase. However some cases at this stage develop *uveitis and aseptic meningitis*. Occasionally, leptospirosis acquires a serious form and present as certain special syndromes.

- ❖ **Weil's syndrome** *(leptospira icterohemorrhagica):* This is the most severe form of the disease, which may develop in 5-10% of cases with a mortality of 5-15%. The initial symptoms are uncharacteristic and resemble the milder form of the disease. However, after 4-10 days (during the second phase) symptoms reappear with higher fever, and features of *hepatic, renal, and cerebral dysfunction*. The liver and spleen, especially the former, are enlarged; *marked direct hyperbilirubinemia* develops (multifactorial, as explained above) with only mild or modest increase in liver enzymes (AST and ALT). *Multiple small hemorrhages due to diffuse small vessel vasculitis* are common. *Renal damage* is common and reaches its peak early in the second phase of illness. It is manifested by proteinuria, hematuria, and azotemia. Most severe cases develop oliguric acute tubular necrosis and renal failure due to vasculitis and also possibly hypovolemia. Most serious cases develop *hepatorenal syndrome* which invariably proves fatal.

  Other less common manifestations include hemolysis, epistaxis, purpura, hemoptysis, gastrointestinal bleeding, rhabdomyolysis, myocarditis, heart failure, pancreatitis, and ARDS.

- ❖ **Aseptic meningitis:** This may be seen in 5-15% of cases of leptospirosis. As already stated leptospira may be isolated from the CSF during the first (leptospiremic) phase, and there may be even some symptoms suggestive of meningeal involvement, but there is no pleocytosis, which distinguishes it from viral meningitis. Pleocytosis develops during the second phase, and the cell count may range from 20 to 1000/mm$^3$. CSF glucose is normal but protein level is usually increased, sometimes above 100 mg/dL (which is unusual in viral aseptic meningitis).

## Investigations

There are two ways to establish a *definitive diagnosis of leptospirosis:*
1. Isolation of the organisms by culture from blood or CSF during the initial phase (first 10 days of illness), and from urine during the second phase, and even for some months after recovery. Use of *polymerase chain reaction for Leptospires,* when possible, is very useful in early diagnosis of disease.
2. **Microscopic agglutination test (MAT):** In cases with strong clinical suspicion of infection a single serological antibody titer of 1:400 to 1:800 may be considered diagnostic, but preferably a fourfold or greater increase in antibody titer should be demonstrated between specimens collected in the acute and convalescent stages of the disease.

Routine laboratory investigations yield nonspecific results. In anicteric cases, white cell count may be reduced, normal or elevated, but there is usually a shift to the left. In Weil's disease however, there is marked leukocytosis. Platelets are often decreased but not critically except in very severe infection. Liver functions are invariably deranged as described already. Hyperbilirubinemia is mostly of conjugated type. Urine examination reveals a varying degree of proteinuria and hematuria, and renal functions are deranged in proportion to the severity of the disease.

## Differential Diagnosis

Milder anicteric cases of leptospirosis are difficult to diagnose and can be suspected only when there is history of exposure to infected material. The disease should be differentiated from any acute febrile illness associated with severe headache and myalgia such as influenza, malaria, dengue, enteric fever, and viral hepatitis. Presence of significant thrombocytopenia will exclude last two conditions. In viral hepatitis, unlike leptospirosis, serum bilirubin is usually equally divided between conjugated and unconjugated fractions, and aminotransferases are invariably >400 IU. Severe forms of the disease show multiorgan involvement.

## Prognosis

Most patients with leptospirosis recover, and hepatic and renal functions become normal. Mortality is unusual except in some patients who are elderly and in those with Weil's syndrome. In pregnant women there is a high risk of abortion and fetal death.

## Management

Mild anicteric cases of leptospirosis are generally difficult to diagnose, and anyway require no more than symptomatic treatment. With strong suspicion of the disease, treatment should be started preferably within 4 days of the onset of illness. The antibiotic of choice is not yet defined, but oral doxycycline or amoxicillin are usually prescribed. Severe cases should be treated with IV penicillin G (1.5 million units four times a day) or ampicillin/amoxicillin 1 g IV every 6 hours. The medication should be started carefully, preferably in an intensive care unit, since, here is a chance (though remote) of developing Jarisch-Herxheimer reaction. Patients with Weil's disease may require whole blood transfusions, platelet infusions, and sometimes hemodialysis when renal failure supervenes.

## ENTERIC (TYPHOID) FEVER

Enteric fever continues to be one of the most common infectious diseases prevalent in India and many other tropical countries. Once a grave disease, its course has been completely modified and prognosis vastly improved, first by the introduction of chloramphenicol more than half a century ago, and more recently by quinolones. Nevertheless, serious complications still occur. The disease is encountered most often during rainy season and in autumn months.

### Clinical Features

The presenting symptom is moderate to high remittent or continuous fever. However, since *paracetamol is commonly administered* nonspecifically in such cases, the fever acquires an intermittent character settling soon after the drug and then rising again after a few hours, often with chills. Associated features include congested conjunctivae, and coated tongue with clear reddish tip and margins.

Untreated cases develop marked toxemia *("typhoid state")* characterized by mental confusion, delirium, and abdominal distension. At this stage dehydration is common, pulse becomes soft and rapid, blood pressure is precarious, and circulatory collapse may occur. However, these extreme features are very uncommon in contemporary medicine (except in completely neglected cases) because of the common use of quinolones in almost all cases of pyrexia of uncertain origin.

### Diagnosis

Any pyrexia of more than a week's duration associated with above mentioned features and without evidence of any other infection should suggest a diagnosis of enteric fever. A mild neutropenia is highly suggestive, and hepatic enzymes may be slightly elevated. However, frank icterus is not seen.

The standard test for confirmation of diagnosis is blood culture. However, cultures become positive only during or after 2nd week of illness. A rapid diagnosis is now possible with *Typhi-DOT* tor, which estimates IgM and IgG antibodies against *S. typhi*. Even after repeated emphasis to generations of students, *Widal test continues to be ordered widely, and generally misinterpreted. The test can be of value only if rising titers can be demonstrated, and anamnestic reactions are kept in mind.*

## Management

**Chemotherapeutic agents:** Fluoroquinolones are currently the preferred drugs, with some exceptions (vide infra). These compounds have excellent antibacterial activity against *S. typhi.*, are free from dreaded hematological side effects of chloramphenicol, and have the additional advantage of decreasing "relapse rate" and "carrier state" because of their excellent penetration into the gallbladder, bile, and gut.

The most commonly used drug is *ciprofloxacin* administered orally in a daily dose of 1,500 mg divided in 2 or 3 doses. In gravely ill patients, or when oral therapy is not possible, it is given by slow IV infusion—100 mL (containing 200 mg ciprofloxacin) over 30 minutes. Defervescence occurs usually within 2-3 days but may be delayed up to 7 days. Thereafter, the drug should be continued 500 mg twice daily for another 7-10 days.

**Ciprofloxacin resistant *S. typhi* (CRST)** have been noticed recently. In these patients fever takes longer to clear or does not respond to ciprofloxacin therapy. In such cases, and also in critically ill patients, ciprofloxacin should be combined with a third generation cephalosporin. Unfortunately, it is not possible to identify patients infected with CRST on the basis of clinical features.

*Fluoroquinolones are contraindicated* in children, pregnant/lactating mothers, and in patients with encephalopathy or past history of seizures. In such cases the drug of choice is a 3rd generation cephalosporin *(ceftriaxone or cefotaxime)*. Ceftriaxone is preferred and is administered IV 4 g daily in two divided doses for 2 days and then 2 g daily for 5 days (in children 80 mg/kg). If patient is allergic to ceftriaxone, ampicillin can be given IV 6-8 g daily in four divided doses (150-200 mg/kg in children).

### General Measures

The availability of quinolones has much simplified the treatment of typhoid fever. Frequent record of temperature, pulse and blood pressure should be maintained, and abdomen examined periodically to detect any serious complication. Delirium, if present, should be controlled with diazepam. Due care should be paid towards oral hygiene, nutrition and fluid and electrolyte control.

In an average uncomplicated case, liberal oral fluids and soft foods are allowed. However, in the presence of severe toxemia, most of the fluid and caloric requirement should be met through infusion of 10% glucose and normal saline for a few days. In such cases oral feeding should be restricted (for risk of producing gastric distension) to plain water, oral rehydrating solutions, diluted curd, and lemonated-sweet water till the patient's condition improves. Liberal amount of fluids should be provided to ensure adequate urine output.

## Complications

Most of the complications occur during 2nd or 3rd week of illness or thereafter. These are:
- Intestinal hemorrhage
- Intestinal perforation
- Encephalopathy
- Paralytic ileus
- Peripheral circulatory failure

## CHOLERA

Cholera is a grave infectious disease characterized by acute severe diarrhea, which can result in profound and progressive dehydration, hypovolemic shock, and death.

### Etiopathogenesis

Majority of the cases are due to *V. cholerae* type 01, which exists in two biotypes—**"classical" and "El Tor"**. The *non-01 types* comprise a large number of other members of species *V. cholerae*. These are much less pathogenic, and rarely produce acute severe diarrhea.

The infection is conveyed through feco-oral route. After ingestion, *cholera vibrio* multiplies rapidly in the lumen of the gut, but do not invade the blood stream or the gut wall. An *enterotoxin* is produced which stimulates adenylate cyclase in the intestinal epithelial cells leading to increased synthesis of intracellular cyclic "AMP". As a result sodium absorption is inhibited and chloride secretion activated resulting in accumulation of sodium chloride in the intestinal lumen. *Water moves passively to maintain osmolality, and thus isotonic fluid accumulates in the gut lumen. Intestinal fluid and electrolyte loss in cholera is thus the result more of a functional rather than anatomical alteration of the intestine.* The choleric stool is isotonic, with sodium and chloride concentration slightly less than plasma, bicarbonate concentration nearly twice, and potassium concentration nearly 3–5 times that of plasma.

### Clinical Features

Incubation period of the disease is usually 2 days but may vary from a few hours to 5 days. There are generally no prodromal symptoms. The clinical spectrum can range from asymptomatic carriers through cases with only mild diarrhea to fulminant disease causing vascular collapse and death within a few hours. On the whole, asymptomatic and minor infections are more often associated with the El Tor than with the classical biotype.

In majority of clinically overt cases, the onset is abrupt with profuse diarrhea, which is painless. Adults may lose as much as 1 L/hour, and children 10 mL/kg/hour in the first 24 hours. The stool may initially contain some fecal matter, but soon acquires a typical gray, slightly cloudy fluid with flecks of mucus, and non-offensive watery character *(rice-water stool)*. Vomiting generally follows but may occasionally precede the onset of diarrhea. This is effortless and not preceded by nausea. There is usually no fever but muscle cramps may occur due to potassium depletion.

Examination at this stage reveals features that parallel volume depletion. Thirst is observed at 3–5% fluid loss, postural hypotension, tachycardia, weakness, and decreased skin turgor at 5–8%, and oliguria, weak to absent pulses, sunken eyes, wrinkled skin, and drowsiness progressing to coma with a fluid loss in excess of 10% of normal body weight. If treatment is delayed or is inadequate, death occurs rapidly from vascular collapse, acute tubular necrosis and renal failure.

## Diagnosis

Cholera should be suspected in any patient who has an abrupt onset of profuse painless watery diarrhea associated with varying degree of shock. A naked eye examination of the stool is often helpful. Dark field or phase microscopy of fresh stool reveals typical motile "comma"-shaped bacilli.

Routine laboratory data may be normal or reveal mild neutrophil leukocytosis, and some elevation of blood urea and serum creatinine *(prerenal azotemia)*. Serum electrolytes are normal but bicarbonate is markedly reduced, and anion gap is increased due to increase in serum lactates and phosphates. Arterial pH is usually low (about 7.2). However, the treatment should not be held up for laboratory results, and all suspected cases must be treated as cholera.

## Management

It may be emphasized that the *clinical manifestations of cholera are solely the consequence of massive gastrointestinal loss of fluid and electrolytes.* Treatment comprises: (1) rapid rehydration, and (2) administration of adequate potassium and bicarbonate to prevent hypokalemic acidosis. With early and efficient treatment the mortality rate should be less than 1%.

- ❖ **Fluid replacement:** The rate and amount of fluid replacement will depend upon the amount of fluid loss. **In mild and moderate cases,** *oral rehydration therapy* (ORT) is most appropriate and usually adequate since intestinal absorptive capacity is preserved in cholera. Approximately ½ to 1 L of such fluid should be given orally per hour for the first few hours. ORT is quite safe since the precise requirement is physiologically regulated by thirst and urine output. If prepacked oral rehydration compound is not available, a simple homemade alternative is to combine 5 g sodium chloride (about one level teaspoon) and 40 g sucrose (or 50 g precooked rice cereal) in 1 L of drinking water. In this situation potassium has to be supplied separately either in the form of orange juice or *"coconut water".* **Severe cases** may lose as much as 1 L of isotonic fluid per hour during the first 24 hours. *Large amount of fluids* should be given in such cases, initially at a rate of 25–50 mL/min, until a good volume pulse is restored, systolic pressure rises to about 90 mm Hg and urine flow is established. This ordinarily requires 5–6 L of fluid during the first 3–4 hours. Once the hypovolemic shock has been corrected, subsequent fluid replacement may be continued by either IV route or ORT, so as to balance further gastrointestinal losses.

The **type of fluid** used for infusion is based on the knowledge of the nature of gastrointestinal losses. Since the choleric stools contain bicarbonates roughly twice that in plasma, the resulting metabolic acidosis is best treated by infusion of normal saline and Ringer lactate in a 2:1 ratio. If the latter is not available, fluid losses should be replenished by N saline alone. In either case potassium supplements (preferably orally) are required to replace K$^+$ loss from stool.

❖ **Antimicrobial therapy:** Antibiotics help in hastening the clearance of organisms from the stool, and also reduce the duration as well as volume of diarrhea, thus decreasing by nearly one-half the amount of replacement fluids. Several antibiotics are effective against *V. cholerae* including tetracycline, doxycycline, cotrimoxazole, and fluoroquinolones.

With the above mentioned measures, diarrhea usually ceases within 24 hours and a quick recovery ensues. Thereafter, a period of convalescence must be allowed to avoid recurrence of shock.

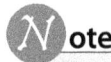ote

The shock and vascular collapse in cholera are entirely due to hypovolemia, and fully respond to adequate fluid and electrolyte replacement. Corticosteroids and vasopressors are not required, and may actually be harmful.

## Complications

❖ Acute renal failure
❖ Acute coronary or cerebral vascular episode

## MUMPS

### Etiopathogenesis

Mumps is an infection of worldwide distribution, and is caused by a virus, which especially affects glandular and nervous tissues. The virus is transmitted through infected salivary secretions, and less commonly through urine. The period of greatest infectivity extends from 1-2 days before the onset of parotitis to 5-7 days afterward. The virus enters through respiratory route and has an incubation period of 12-24 days. Virus is disseminated through blood stream initially to parotid glands and meninges, and later to other organs such as gonads, liver, pancreas, kidneys, thyroid, breasts, and heart. Life-long immunity is usually conferred by an attack of mumps irrespective of whether it is marked by unilateral or bilateral parotitis.

## Clinical Features

Mumps usually affects children and young adults, and is rare before 2 years of age. The disease itself is usually benign comprising a short febrile illness followed within 2-3 days by unilateral or bilateral painful parotid swelling with or without involvement of other salivary glands. Serious manifestations of disease include orchitis, meningitis, pancreatitis, hepatitis, oophoritis, thyroiditis, neuritis, arthralgias, myocarditis, and thrombocytopenic purpura. The entire course of the disease seldom exceeds 2 weeks, and fatalities are rare. The first two of these complications (orchitis and meningitis) are described hereunder in some detail.

### *Epididymo-orchitis*

This occurs in about a quarter of cases of mumps, mostly in postpubertal males. Testicular inflammation and swelling usually appear 1-2 weeks after the parotid swelling but may precede or appear simultaneously with parotitis. Occasionally, orchitis is the sole manifestation of the disease. It is usually unilateral (bilateral in about 25%), and is often associated with epididymitis.

The onset of orchitis is marked by high fever and chills. The affected testicle is acutely painful, hot, tender and swollen, and the epididymis is often palpable as a swollen tender cord. The symptoms resolve in about a week, but the main risk is of subsequent sterility due to testicular atrophy, especially if bilateral.

## Treatment

Scrotum should be supported by a suspensor bandage or toweling "bridge", and analgesics administered as required. IV hydrocortisone for 2-3 days has been used to reduce the inflammation but is without proven benefit. Other measures including incision of tunica, estrogen therapy, or broad-spectrum antibiotics have not been found to be consistently useful.

### *Meningoencephalitis*

While some increase in cells, mostly lymphocytes in CSF is common, clinical evidence of CNS involvement is unusual. Neurological features may develop prior to parotid swelling or 2-3 weeks later, or even in the absence of parotitis.

Clinically, neurological involvement manifests as meningitis, starting with acute headache, vomiting, high fever, and neck stiffness. The course is usually benign. Less commonly, the clinical picture comprises varying combination of acute encephalitis, myelitis and polyneuritis, sometimes ascending in character *(Landry Guillain-Barré syndrome)*.

## Treatment

There is no specific treatment, and corticosteroids have no proven role. Symptomatic measures should be adopted as indicated.

## TETANUS

This is an acute and extremely serious disease with a worldwide distribution, but especially common in underprivileged countries. It is caused by infection with *Clostridium tetani* which is a *strict anaerobe*. The organisms usually gain entry into the body through minor injuries and wounds, IM injections with infected syringes, during childbirth under unsanitary conditions and, rarely, after surgery (from contaminated catgut and dressings). Not infrequently, it occurs in the new born (***T. neonatorum***) due to poor obstetric conditions. In 10-20% of cases there may be no history of injury.

### Pathophysiology

Tetanus toxin *(tetanospasmin)* is synthesized at the contaminated site, and reaches the spinal cord and brain by intra-axonal transport. Clinical features result from powerful exotoxin, which has a special affinity for nervous tissue. The earliest symptom is trismus *(lockjaw)* due to painless spasm of masseter muscles bilaterally. The disease may remain confined to this stage, but more often is followed after a variable period, by increasing spasm of facial muscles *(risus sardonicus),* muscles of the neck, abdominal wall, and back *(opisthotonus)*.

Gradually, the muscle spasms increase in extent, frequency and severity. In more severe cases powerful reflex spasms *(convulsions)* occur, either spontaneously or on being precipitated by some external stimuli such as noise, strong light, and moving or feeding the patient. These may last from a few seconds to even 2 or 3 minutes. Additionally, severe cases may show features of *sympathetic overactivity* characterized by hypertension, tachycardia, arrhythmias, hyperpyrexia, and profuse perspiration. Ominous features include hyperpyrexia, hypotension, and bradycardia. Death may occur due to any of these features, or aspiration pneumonia and asphyxia.

### Prognosis

It is always useful to assess the *severity of illness,* which is graded as *mild* (muscle rigidity with few or no spasms), *moderate* (trismus, rigidity, dysphagia, and recurrent spasms), or *severe* (frequent explosive spasms). Though prognosis is generally better with lesser severity of illness, it is to some extent unpredictable once lockjaw has developed. It is relatively better if:

- The *incubation period* (interval between the date of injury and onset of first symptom) is over 2 weeks.
- Trismus is not severe and oral feeding is possible.
- Generalized spasms either do not occur or are only occasional and mild.
- *"Period of onset"* (interval between onset of lockjaw and appearance of convulsions) is 1 week or more (generally, spasms occur within 24-72 hours of the first symptom).
- Muscle spasm is confined to the site of injury *(local tetanus)*.
- Patient is under 50 years of age.

## Management

As soon as a diagnosis of tetanus is made, the patient should be transferred to a hospital, preferably with a separate tetanus ward, and facilities for intensive respiratory and cardiac resuscitation. Unfortunately, there are very few such units in India. The *principles of treatment* are:
- Neutralize circulating toxin and unbound toxin in the wound
- Eliminate source of toxin by antibiotic therapy
- Control and prevent muscle spasms
- Provide nutritional, antibiotic, and cardiorespiratory support till recovery occurs.

### Specific Measures

- **Immunotherapy:** This is aimed at neutralizing the circulating toxin and toxin in the wound; toxin already bound to the nervous system is unaffected. To be effective therefore, it should be undertaken as early as possible. Tetanus immune globulin (TIG) is preferred over equine antiserum which it has now replaced. Usual dose is 3,000-6,000 units deep IM in divided doses at different sites (because of large volume). Some authorities also recommend simultaneous administration of 500 units of TIG *intrathecally*. Hypersensitivity reactions do not occur with TIG and, therefore, pretreatment testing is not required. When treatment with TIG is not possible either because of nonavailability or high cost, heterologous (viz. equine) antitoxin serum (ATS) in a dose of 10,000 units should be given IM after the patient has been tested for sensitivity. Higher doses (up to 100,000 units) given earlier do not seem to have any additional advantage. Since anaphylaxis may occur despite negative sensitivity test, patient must be carefully observed for 12 hours after administration of ATS.
- **Antibiotics:** *Penicillin G* has been the standard antibiotic therapy in tetanus and is given in a dose of 10-12 million units daily for 10-12 days. However, recent studies show that it is not the drug of choice since penicillin is a known antagonist of GABA (like tetanus toxin). *Metronidazole* is reported to have equal or even better antimicrobial activity against *C. tetani*, and should be given 2.0 g IV daily divided in 2-4 doses for 10 days. Complicating infections, if present should be treated with specific antibiotics according to culture and sensitivity results.

- **Control of muscle spasms:** (a) *Sedation:* Diazepam is the mainstay for control of muscle spasms. It is GABA-agonist, and directly antagonizes the tetanus toxin. The dosage varies from 0.5 to 10.0 mg/kg/day depending upon the severity of the disease. It may be given IV in bolus doses of 5 mg every 10-15 minutes in a freely running drip or as a continuous IV infusion. Higher doses can result in lactic acidosis probably as a result of the solvent vehicle-propylene glycol.
  Alternative sedatives include lorazepam, which has a longer duration of action, and midazolam, with a short half-life. Throughout the therapy a close watch should be kept on the patient's respiration and circulation, and dosage decreased, if features of cardiorespiratory depression appear. Phenobarbitone and chlorpromazine are second-line drugs, and can be used IM in doses varying between 100-200 mg, and 50-75 mg, respectively, every 4-6 hours, **(b)** If severe spasms continue despite full medication, and especially if these threaten ventilation, *neuromuscular blocking agents along with mechanical ventilation* should be considered. This approach is highly effective but can be utilized only in intensive care units.
- **Respiratory care:** *Intubation or tracheotomy,* combined with *mechanical ventilation,* can be lifesaving in severe cases as it protects the patient from life-threatening laryngeal spasms. This will also decrease the risk of aspiration, and help in maintaining a clear airway. The procedure is usually required in all severe cases of tetanus, and should be performed electively and early rather than as a late emergency measure.
- **Care of the wound:** If the site of wound is obvious, a small amount of antiserum (250 units of TIG or 3,000-6,000 units of ATS) should be infiltrated proximal to and around the wound. The wound should be thoroughly cleansed (after antitoxin has been administered) and necrotic material or foreign bodies removed, but major surgery should be postponed till the patient's condition stabilizes. Any abscess if present, should be opened, irrigated and drained.

### General Measures

These are of utmost importance. The patient should be kept in a dark quiet room, and disturbed as little as possible. However, periodic changes in posture and suction of nasopharyngeal secretions must be done to avoid bed sores and aspiration pneumonia, respectively.

Some patients develop marked **sympathetic overactivity** in the form of perspiration and tachycardia. Beta-blockers are not safe, but **Clonidine** (a centrally acting anti-adrenergic drug), and **morphine sulfate** may be used. A proper fluid and electrolyte balance, and adequate caloric intake should be maintained. It may be emphasized that patients of tetanus are in severe **catabolic state,** and this may be associated with marked fluid loss. Initially, this can be corrected by administration of IV fluids. However, as the illness gets prolonged, Ryle's tube feeding or IV hyperalimentation may be required to meet the nutritional requirement of these patients which may be as high as 4,000-5,000 calories/day. Additionally, all vitamins should be supplied in appropriate dosage. Low dose heparin therapy has been recommended to prevent deep vein thrombosis and pulmonary embolism.

Pyrexia is generally not a problem but occasionally high fever and even hyperpyrexia may occur due to frequent generalized spasms and/or complicating infection. It should be controlled by conventional measures.

### Prevention

Despite all the advances in treatment, the disease still carries a high mortality. Furthermore, death may occur suddenly and unexpectedly in a patient who otherwise appears to be responding to treatment. Prevention of disease is, therefore, of utmost importance (for details, *see* section on "Emergency Personal Prophylaxis" in this Chapter). So far as the patient himself is concerned, surprisingly, *the disease does not confer immunity against subsequent infection.* Active immunization must, therefore, be started during the recovery stage of the disease itself by administering 1.0 mL of tetanus toxoid IM. The same dose should then be repeated at 6 weeks' and 6 months' intervals. In areas where tetanus is endemic (as in India) life-long immunity can be maintained by booster doses of such toxoid every 5-10 years.

## RABIES

Rabies is basically a type of **viral encephalitis** transmitted by infected saliva of certain animals. More than 99% cases of rabies in countries where dogs commonly have the disease are caused by dog bites. The disease can also be transmitted by bats and animals such as monkeys, raccoons, foxes, cattle, bears, wolves, and cats. The virus is introduced through the bite of an infected animal, or when saliva from an infected animal comes into contact with the open cuts or wounds in skin, and mucus membranes such as mouth, nose (also eyes). Simple contact (e.g., petting) with a rabid animal, and contact with the blood, urine or feces of a rabid animal does not by itself constitute an exposure, and is not an indication for prophylaxis. Human to human transmission is extremely rare. Small rodents such as squirrels, hamsters, guinea pigs, rats and mice, and also rabbits and hares are almost never found to be infected with rabies, and are not known to transmit rabies to humans.

The virus travels through the afferent nerves to brain where it multiplies, rapidly causes encephalitis, and then migrates along the efferent nerves to the salivary glands. Rabies may also inflame the spinal cord, producing transverse myelitis.

### Clinical Features

The *incubation period* (**IP**) between the infection and the first flu-like symptoms is typically 2-12 weeks in humans. Incubation periods as short as 4 days or more than 6 years have been reported, depending on the location and severity of the contaminated wound and the amount of virus introduced.

Pain or paresthesia occurring at the site of the bite is ominous and highly suggestive of impending disease. As symptoms progress (from initial flu-like features), the patient becomes anxious, confused, agitated, and develops abnormal behavior, paranoia, terror, and hallucinations, progressing to delirium (with periods of lucid intervals in which the patient is well-oriented but extremely anxious). Slight or partial paralysis occurs, and spasms of muscles of deglutition supervene.

The spasms involve pharynx, larynx, and to a lesser extent all the respiratory muscles, and may be precipitated initially by attempts at eating and drinking, and later by slightest stimulus such as sudden movement, any noise, a smell or even sight or thought of water **(hydrophobia).** This is commonly associated with *furious rabies* that affects 80% of the infected people. The remaining 20% may experience a *paralytic form of rabies* that is marked by muscle weakness, loss of sensation, and paralysis. Death almost always occurs 2-10 days after the first symptoms. Survival is rare once symptoms have presented, even after administration of proper and intensive care.

## Diagnosis

In a fully developed case, there is little difficulty in arriving at a correct diagnosis. In the initial stages however, when there is acute anxiety and apprehension, a diagnosis of hysteria may mistakenly be made. Symptoms such as lockjaw and "hydrophobia" should decide the issue. The disease is basically a type of encephalitis and in the paralytic stage all causes of meningoencephalitis should be considered. In fact, one wishfully hopes that the patient's illness may turn out to be some other type of viral encephalitis with a better prognosis.

The specific test recommended by WHO for diagnosis of rabies is the fluorescent antibody test (FAT). The diagnosis can be reliably made from brain samples taken after death. The diagnosis can also be made from saliva, urine, and CSF samples, but this is not as sensitive and reliable as brain samples. Cerebral inclusion bodies called *Negri bodies* are 100% diagnostic but are found in only about 80% cases.

### *Postexposure Prophylactic Treatment*

Once the symptoms of rabies have developed tragically, little can be done to control it, and *death occurs within 2-4 days.* Symptomatic measures consist of isolation of the patient, and controlling the spasms by diazepam, phenobarbitone, and midazolam. Prompt postexposure treatment can however prevent the disease if administered within 10 days of infection.

- ❖ **Cleaning of the wound:** The first and the most important step is *thorough flushing of the wound and scratches* as soon as possible with soap and water, approximately for 5 minutes. This is effective in reducing the entry of viral particles substantially. Thereafter, povidone iodine *(betadine)* or alcohol *(40-70%)* should be applied locally. This further reduces the number of viral particles. Primary suture or cauterization of the wound is not advocated because of the possibility of inoculating rabies virus deeper into the wound. If the wounds are extensive, appropriate antibiotics should be given additionally.

❖ **Passive immunization:** It varies according to the severity of animal bites and wounds, which are divided into three classes:

| Class I *(Minimal risk)*<br>Class II *(Moderate risk)** | Slight or negligible contact; licks on intact skin, (i) All bites except on neck, face, head, palm, and fingers, (ii) Licks on fresh cuts and scratches |
|---|---|
| Class III *(Grave risk)* | All bites on neck and above, palm and fingers, lacerated wounds anywhere on the body, multiple bites (5 or more wounds), and bites by wolf, jackal, or other wild animals |

***Note:** Any case in this category who has delayed treatment by 14 days or more should be considered as class III for purpose of management.

Human rabies immunoglobulin (HRIG) is the first line of defense. It should be administered immediately to provide protective antibodies. HRIG is given only once, 20 units/kg. If the patient is seen within 24 hours of the bite, half of this dose should be infiltrated around the wound and the other half given IM (at a site distant from the wound) into the gluteal region. If the patient reports after 24 hours local administration may be of no use, and full dose of HRIG should be given IM.

Serum therapy is of little use if the patient is seen more than 7 days after the bite. If HRIG is not available, equine antirabies serum should be given IM in a dose 40 units/kg after testing for sensitivity. It is to be noted that HRIG/equine serum and rabies vaccine should never be administered in the same syringe or into the same anatomic site. Passive immunization is not necessary in Class I and Class II bites (vide infra), if tissue culture vaccines are used.

❖ **Active (postexposure) immunization:** Tissue-culture vaccines are used except in very tight economic situation when Semple vaccine is employed. The best culture vaccine is inactivated Human Diploid Cell Vaccine (HDCV) [Verorab, (Cadilla) or Verovax-R (Aventis)]. Five injections of 1 mL each are given IM in the deltoid (not in gluteal region) on days 0, 3, 7, 14, and 28 (irrespective of the weight or age of the patient). The first dose should be given on the day of exposure or as soon after as possible. An additional 1 mL dose may be given on day 90 in cases with severe bites. Patients who have previously received pre-exposure vaccination do not require HRIG; they need only postexposure vaccinations on days 0 and 2.

ote

Patient should not be receiving chloroquine concomitantly with vaccination as it may interfere with antibody response to vaccine.

**Table 8.1:** Dosage schedule for Semple vaccine.

| Nature of bite | Dosage | | Duration of treatment | Booster |
| --- | --- | --- | --- | --- |
| | Adults | Children* | | |
| Class I | 2 mL | 2 mL | 7 days | Nil |
| Class II | 5 mL | 2 mL | 14 days† | One similar dose 3 weeks after the last injection |
| Class III | 5 mL | 2 mL | 14 days† | Two similar doses 7 and 21 days after last injection |

*Weight 30 kg or less
†Stop treatment, if animal remains healthy for 10 days.

### Semple Vaccine

This is a suspension of beta-propiolactone (BPL) or phenol inactivated virus in sheep or higher mammalian brain. It is given deep SC, and the conventional site is anterior abdominal wall since this area provides enough space for large quantities of the vaccine to be injected. The dosage schedule recommended by Central Research Institute, Kasauli, is given in **Table 8.1**.

This vaccine is much cheaper than tissue-culture vaccines but has two important shortcomings: (1) it is comparatively less potent, and (2) it carries a significant risk of neuroparalytic complication. Because of this, its use has been almost abandoned.

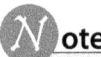ote

Neither pre-exposure nor postexposure prophylaxis is associated with fetal abnormalities, and therefore pregnancy *is not a contraindication to vaccination.*

### Booster Doses

Booster doses are required in cases exposed again to rabies even when they have received full immunization in the past. The regimen varies according to how far back the previous vaccination was received. Two vaccinations (days 0 and 3) are required, if the interval is <1 year, 3 (days 0, 3, and 7), if the time interval is between 1 and 5 years, and a full course of five injections, if the previous vaccination was more than 5 years ago. HRIG is not given in such cases. When further exposures are feared, booster vaccination should be administered regularly—one dose of HDCV 1.0 mL IM every 2–5 years.

### Care of the Dog

If the offending dog is living and can be traced, it should be isolated and watched for signs of disease. In the event of dog surviving for more than 10 days, it may be presumed that it was not rabid at the time of the bite, and in such a situation further inoculation should be stopped. However, *specific prophylactic vaccination should never be delayed while waiting for proof of the disease in the dog.*

### Complications of Antirabic Treatment

Besides local infection at the site of injection, mild fever and body pains, inoculations with sheep brain vaccine can result in serious neurological complications (*see* section on "Acute Viral Encephalitis", Chapter 4). These usually manifest after about a week of start of inoculation, and may take the form of polyneuritis (sometimes ascending type), radiculitis, myelitis, or encephalitis. If such complications appear, further injections should be immediately stopped, complete bed rest advised and a course of corticosteroids instituted. Antirabies treatment should thereafter, be completed with tissue culture vaccines, which are, by and large free from the risk of neuroparalytic complications.

## MALARIA

Malaria is widespread in India and other tropical and subtropical regions of the world. According to World Health Organization, there were 198 million cases worldwide in 2013 with an estimated mortality of 584,000–885,000. The disease is transmitted most commonly by the bite of an infected *female Anopheles mosquito*. Five species of *Plasmodium* can infect humans. Of these most deaths are caused by *P. falciparum* and *P. vivax*. The species *P. ovale* and *P. malariae* result in only a mild illness while *P. knowlesi* rarely causes disease in humans. The disease generally results in a mild-moderate illness, but occasionally serious complications result necessitating emergency treatment. Malaria parasites can also be transmitted by blood transfusion, although this is rare.

World Health Organization has **classified malaria into two types—"severe" and "uncomplicated".** It is deemed severe when **any** of the following complications is present: (i) impaired consciousness, (ii) breathing problem, (iii) low blood pressure (<70 mm in adults), (iv) circulatory shock, (v) kidney failure, (vi) hemoglobinuria, (vii) bleeding problems, (viii) severe anemia, (ix) breathing problem, and (x) blood glucose <40 mg/dL.

### Special Features of *P. falciparum* Infection

❖ Infection by *P. falciparum* is associated with a *very high parasitemia* because of its ability to invade erythrocytes of all ages, unlike other forms of malarial parasite, which show a marked predilection for either old red cells or reticulocytes.
❖ Unlike *P. vivax*, *P. falciparum* does not have any *dormant forms in liver* and therefore once the infection is cured, there is no relapse.
❖ In contrast to *P. vivax* infection in which all stages of development from ring forms to schizonts and gametocytes take place in peripheral blood,

in falciparum malaria only the ring and early trophozoite stages develop in peripheral blood. For development of schizont and gametocyte *P. falciparum* must invade deeper circulation. This leads to *sequestration of millions of parasitized red blood cells in deep internal organs* especially in brain, but also in liver, lungs, kidneys, etc.

- ❖ Because of such sequestration *only the younger ring forms of P. falciparum are seen in the peripheral blood.* This explains a rather low peripheral parasitemia compared to severity of infection, and also for a negative blood film so often encountered in falciparum infection.
- ❖ During asexual cycle, mature forms of the parasite in host cells in deep organs send out adhesive proteins to the surface of red blood cells forming "knobs" which mediate attachment of such erythrocytes to vascular endothelium. This is the process of *"cytoadherence",* which is specific to *P. falciparum* infection, and *has important pathologic implications:*
    - It results in *microcirculatory obstruction* with resulting hypoxia especially in deep internal organs where red blood cells are lying sequestrated in millions. Even uninfected erythrocytes bind to the surface of such "knobbed" erythrocytes by a mechanism similar to that of cytoadherence further compromising microcirculatory flow.
    - On account of anchorage to the endothelium through cytoadherence the infected red cells are prevented from being washed into the spleen where these may be sequestrated.

## Syndromes of "Serious" Types of Malaria

Because of the predilection of the mature forms of *P. falciparum* for almost all the deep organs, *falciparum infection* is often a *multisystem disease*. It is to be noted that while "serious" cases of malaria most often result from *falciparum* infection, an increasing number of such cases is being reported even with *P. vivax* infection. The organ(s) predominantly affected and the resulting clinical picture is given at **Table 8.2.** No age is immune, the disease being most common at extremes of ages (because of lower immunity), in pregnancy, in immunocompromised patients, and in those with splenectomy.

## Clinical Features

Symptoms of malaria usually begin 10–14 days after the infection. Initial symptoms are flu-like and nonspecific. These may include headache, fatigue, fever, shivering, vomiting, and joint pains. The fever occurs classically every 2 days *(tertian)* or every 3 days *(quartan fever)*. Fever in *falciparum* infection can be high *(even in hyperpyrexia! range)* and occurs every 36–48 hours, or it may be less pronounced and almost continuous in type. The duration of febrile symptoms is usually short in children, but in adults moderate to high fever with periodic spiking, shivering and sweating, may continue for several days. Other features common to all cases of *P. falciparum* infection are *rapidly developing anemia, jaundice, and clinical deterioration*. Some of the important

## Table 8.2: Clinical syndromes of falciparum malaria.

| Organ affected | Clinical state |
| --- | --- |
| Brain | Cerebral malaria |
| Kidneys | Renal failure |
| Lungs | • Acute respiratory distress syndrome<br>• Pulmonary edema |
| Hepatic | • Hepatitis<br>• Hepatic coma (rarely) |
| Blood and cardiovascular system | • Rapidly developing severe anemia<br>• Hemoglobinuria<br>• Disseminated intravascular coagulation<br>• Algid malaria (shock) |
| Miscellaneous | • Hyperpyrexia<br>• Hypoglycemia<br>• Lactic acidosis |

clinical syndromes/complications resulting from the disease (usually from *P. falciparum* infection) are described separately.

### Diagnosis and Investigations

There are no specific signs or symptoms of falciparum malaria. It may mimic any febrile illness and, compared to other types of malaria, is more often associated with nausea, vomiting, headache, delirium, and jaundice. The presence of hepatosplenomegaly and severe anemia can be strong collaborative evidence. The final confirmation comes from finding of malaria parasites in peripheral blood smear. Both thick and thin smears should be examined. *Thick smears may detect parasites even when their density is low. Thin smear is helpful in defining the species of malaria parasite.*

The detection of malarial parasites in blood films requires a certain amount of expertise not generally available. This huge problem in clinical practice has been overcome by the antigen-based *rapid diagnostic tests (RDT) for detection of malarial antigens, both against vivax and falciparum malaria*. The test has a very high degree of sensitivity and specificity.

Other laboratory parameters, which should be monitored, include complete blood count, blood sugar, renal and hepatic function tests, and when indicated, prothrombin time, partial thromboplastin time, and platelet count. A routine chest X-ray and electrocardiogram are also desirable.

It should however, be kept in mind that detection of malarial parasites (other than *P. falciparum*) does not prove that malaria is the cause of patient's illness, since asymptomatic parasitemia is not uncommon in endemic areas. Whenever doubt persists regarding possibility of severe malaria, it may be worthwhile to give a *therapeutic test with artesunate for 3–4 days*.

## Management

"Severe" malaria should be regarded as a medical emergency requiring immediate hospitalization and administration of rapidly effective antimalarial drugs. The urgency of treatment cannot be overemphasized since, after a certain stage irreversible damage occurs and then even the best antimalarial therapy may fail.

### Specific Measures

**Antimalarials:** Uncomplicated malaria may be treated with oral medications. Four drugs are available: chloroquine phosphate, quinine dihydrochloride (seldom used now), mefloquine hydrochloride, and artesunate.

- **Chloroquine** is the drug of choice in both chemoprophylaxis as well as treatment of most of the uncomplicated cases of malaria. It is given in a dose of two tablets twice a day (each containing 150 mg active base) for two days and then one tablet twice a day for next 3 days. When chloroquine-resistance is suspected, artesunate should be used.
- **Mefloquine** is a rapidly acting erythrocytic schizonticide with mechanism of action similar to quinine. It is used for oral prophylaxis and treatment of chloroquine-resistant malaria. Mefloquine is not available in parenteral formulation, and therefore it should not be used as the sole drug for severe malaria.

  Oral absorption is good and effective blood concentration is reached within 6 hours. The drug is metabolized in the liver, and is generally well-tolerated though some patients may develop nausea, vomiting, abdominal discomfort, vertigo, postural hypotension, and self-limited bradycardia. It should not be used in children less than 15 kg in weight. The drug is safe in pregnancy but may be avoided in the first trimester. *Mefloquine is contraindicated* in the presence of hepatic impairment, cardiac conduction defects, or a history of psychiatric or neurologic disorder including epilepsy.

  In uncomplicated cases the drug is given orally (15–20 mg/kg) as a single dose or in two equal divided doses 4–6 hours apart. When used in patients already receiving quinine, it should not be given earlier than 8 hours after the last quinine dose in order to avoid cardiovascular toxicity.
- **Artesunate:** This is a water-soluble hemisuccinate derivative of artemisinin (Qinghaosu) and is the *most rapidly acting antimalarial agent*. Both in severe malaria (including cerebral malaria) and chloroquine-resistant malaria, the drug provides faster relief of fever and considerably faster clearance of parasites than other antimalarial agents including quinine. For severe malaria, artesunate is superior to quinine in both children and adults. Artesunate is a potent schizonticidal agent, has a rapid bioavailability after IV injection, and is also rapidly absorbed after oral or

IM administration. It acts early in the asexual parasite development cycle by destroying early ring forms.

In severe malarial infections the drug is administered IV, 120 mg on the first day followed by 60 mg daily for next 4 days. It is constituted by mixing artesunate powder (60 mg) with 1 mL of 5% sodium bicarbonate, shaking it for 2–3 minutes, and after the solution becomes clear, diluting it further for IV injection by 5 mL of D5W or normal saline (2 mL for IM use). The final concentration of the drug should be 10 mg/mL for IV use (administered slowly over two minutes) and 20 mg/mL for IM use. It is free from any serious adverse reactions and has been reported to be quite safe in pregnancy, except the first trimester. The only shortcoming is that it has a short action, and hence may not eliminate all parasites. *It should therefore always be followed by adjuvant therapy (vide infra).*

*Resistance to artesunate* has been reported from South-Eastern countries, and occasionally even from India. In such cases treatment of "severe" forms of malaria which are largely due to *P. falciparum* is becoming difficult. Recourse will have to be taken to use of *quinine dihydrochloride*. It is administered in a dose of 10 mg/kg (maximum 600 mg) diluted in 200 mL normal saline given over 2–4 hours, every 8 hours. **Quinine should never be administered as IV bolus injection.** IV quinine dihydrochloride should be continued for 7 days but the dosage can be reduced after 48–72 hours (when peak blood levels are reached) by one-half.

❖ **Other drugs:** *Fansidar* and *Halofantrine* alone are no longer recommended either in the treatment or prophylaxis of malaria.

## *Adjuvant Therapy*

In all cases of severe malaria (especially those acquired in Southeast Asia and presumed to be chloroquine-resistant), artesunate should be combined with one of the following drugs to *ensure elimination of any residual strains* and prevent resistance to any single drug component:

❖ Tetracycline 250 mg four times a day for 7 days, **OR**
❖ Doxycycline 100 mg twice a day for 7 days, **OR**
❖ Mefloquine 15 mg/kg (maximum 1.5 g) orally in single or two divided doses, **OR**
❖ Fansidar (sulfadoxine 500 mg and pyrimethamine 25 mg) 1–3 tablets according to patient's weight.

## *General Measures*

If the patient is unconscious, usual measures as described in the section on "The Unconscious Patient" (Chapter 4) should be adopted. In any severe form of malaria, fluid balance should be carefully regulated by recording central venous pressure, which should be kept 7–8 cm $H_2O$ to prevent pulmonary overloading. Rectal temperature should be recorded frequently and kept below 39°C.

Since severe **hypoglycemia** is common, blood sugar should be monitored frequently and when less than 60 mg%, treated with IV dextrose. Severe anemia often develops, sometimes rapidly, and should be treated judiciously with transfusions of whole blood or packed red blood cells.

## Prognosis

With prompt and appropriate antimalarial therapy patients usually become afebrile and show clinical improvement within 48–72 hours. Parasitemia starts decreasing in about 24 hours and should be reduced by 75% within 48 hours. If the response is inadequate after 72 hours of initiation of treatment or there is deterioration, *inappropriate therapy, high-grade drug resistance, or development of serious complications should be suspected. Following parameters indicate poor prognosis in "severe" cases of malaria.*

### Clinical

- Age less than 5 years or over 60 years
- Deep coma
- Convulsions within a few hours of onset, and features of decerebration
- Associated pregnancy (especially primigravida), history of splenectomy
- Delayed treatment

### Laboratory Indices

- Hyperparasitemia (>5% erythrocytes parasitized)
- Peripheral schizontemia
- Leukocytosis (>12,000/mm$^3$)
- High CSF lactate and low CSF glucose
- Blood urea nitrogen >60 mg% and serum creatinine >3 mg%
- Hemoglobin <7 g or PCV <20%
- Blood glucose <70 mg%
- More than threefold increase in serum enzymes (aspartate and alanine aminotransferases)

## Complications

Several complications can occur in cases with **"severe malaria"** (Table 8.2), largely due to *P. falciparum infection*. Each of these will require appropriate treatment according to severity of the complication. The most serious complication is "cerebral malaria", which is described here under.

## ■ CEREBRAL MALARIA

This is the most serious form of severe malaria (usually falciparum infection), and is characterized by a *diffuse symmetric encephalopathy* resulting from microcirculatory and metabolic disturbances in the brain.

## Clinical Features

Cerebral malaria is characterized by impaired consciousness, which may range from confusion and delirium to coma. The onset is acute or subacute, and marked by *fever*, which is initially irregular or even continuous. *Headache* is invariable and may be either diffuse or localized to the occipital or temporal region. *Seizures* commonly accompany the altered state of consciousness but may precede other features. Neurologically, cerebral malaria is characterized by diffuse encephalopathy. *Focal neurological signs are unusual* but there may be abnormalities in pupillary size, conjugate vision, muscle tone, and body posturing. Hyper-reflexia and bilateral extensor plantar reflexes are common. Occasionally, spastic hemiplegia and paraplegia occur but papilledema and signs of meningeal irritation are rare. *Convulsions,* which are usually generalized, occur in about half of the cases in adults and more often in children.

*Cerebrospinal fluid* pressure may be increased but is otherwise normal though a mild increase in protein level and cell count has been reported. Glucose content is always normal; if low, systemic hypoglycemia should be excluded. With successful treatment, recovery is complete except in children who may have some residual neurologic deficit. **Bad prognostic signs** include infection of more than 5% of red blood cells, deepening coma, hypoglycemia, advent of renal impairment, and acute pulmonary insufficiency (acute respiratory distress syndrome). Rarely, bleeding tendency develops with evidence of disseminated intravascular coagulation. Hematemesis may also occur due to acute (stress) ulcers.

## Diagnosis

Cerebral malaria may need to be differentiated from acute meningitis, encephalitis, heat hyperpyrexia, and even acute cerebrovascular catastrophes. Presence of leukopenia and a near normal CSF coupled with demonstration of parasites in blood smear, or positive antigen-based rapid diagnostic test (RDT) confirm the diagnosis. Whenever feasible a CT scan of the brain should be done. It is usually normal but may show diffuse or local cerebral edema or even infarction if patient is in coma and has focal neurological deficit. Its main role is to exclude alternative diagnosis.

## Treatment

Specific treatment with IV artesunate should be started immediately and supplemented with one of the adjuvant drugs already described (preferably mefloquine). Clinical improvement is expected within 48–72 hours of starting the treatment. Corticosteroids, routinely recommended earlier to reduce cerebral edema, have been found to be unhelpful, and even deleterious. Likewise, mannitol and glycerol are not useful. Prophylactic anticonvulsant therapy is also without proven benefit.

**General measures** pertaining to such cases (vide supra) should not be ignored.

## Falciparum Malaria in Pregnancy

Pregnant women, especially primigravida, developing falciparum infection are particularly vulnerable to hyperparasitemia, anemia, hypoglycemia, and pulmonary edema. Since placenta is a site for preferential parasite development and sequestration, transplacental delivery of nutrients to fetus is compromised resulting in low birth weight, premature labor, miscarriage, or abortion. Rarely, congenital malaria occurs in the newborn when mother is infected, and is related to parasite density in the placenta.

## Treatment

*Artesunate is quite effective but should be avoided in the first trimester.* Intravenous quinine is an alternative since it is safe in all stages of pregnancy.

## Prevention

Chemoprophylaxis for malaria is required for travelers to endemic areas, in pregnant women, children below 5 years of age, immunocompromised patients, and in individuals with abnormal hemoglobins. Drugs available for this purpose include pyrimethamine-sulfadoxine *(Fansidar), chloroquine, and mefloquine.* Fansidar is generally not recommended because of the high risk of side effects. The dosage of chloroquine phosphate is 500 mg (active base 300 mg) for adults (for children, 5 mg/kg), and of mefloquine 250 mg (for children, 5 mg/kg, maximum dose 250 mg), administered once per week. The latter should be preferred for individuals traveling to areas known for chloroquine-resistant malaria. Chemoprophylaxis should be started 1 week before the projected travel, and continued during stay in the malarial region, and for 4 weeks after leaving the area.

Complete protection is not obtained with any of these drugs. When symptoms of malaria develop while a person is receiving chloroquine chemoprophylaxis, a single therapeutic dose of Fansidar is recommended (for treatment of presumptive chloroquine resistant *P. falciparum* if immediate medical help is not available). Mefloquine 1.5 mg/kg (maximum 1.5 g) orally in single or two divided doses would be even better.

## New Malaria Vaccine

*Very recently (July 2015) Glaxo Smith Kline launched a vaccine "MOSQUIREX" which has received positive opinion from European regulators for the prevention of malaria in young children in sub-Saharan Africa caused by P. falciparum. This infection caused in 2013 around 500,000 deaths in children mostly under the age of 5 years in sub-Saharan Africa.*

## Summary

- ❖ Malarial infection should be considered severe or complicated, if it is associated with any of the complications defined by WHO (vide supra).

- Artesunate is the preferred drug in all cases of *falciparum malaria* because of simpler and shorter regimen (than quinine); IV quinine should be considered for complicated cases of *P. falciparum* infection with multisystem involvement especially since resistance to artesunate has been reported.
- Specific antimalarial therapy must be started at the first suspicion of *falciparum malaria* since serious complications can develop with dramatic suddenness, and fatalities are known to occur within 24 hours.
- Blood sugar, electrolytes, urea, creatinine, hemoglobin, and bilirubin levels (and when possible acid-base balance) should be closely monitored.
- With effective treatment asexual parasitemia should decrease and disappear by fifth day; otherwise suspect drug resistance. Gametocytes of *P. falciparum*, because of their insensitivity, may, however, persist for several days until their natural death.

## AMEBIASIS

Amebiasis is a worldwide disease but is most prevalent in the tropical and subtropical countries. It is caused by *Entamoeba histolytica* (EH), and is one of the most common disorders encountered in general practice all over the country. The disease **(dysenteric colitis)** exists in a chronic form, principally involving cecum, ascending colon and sigmoid colon (dependent parts of the large gut). Not infrequently, **amebic liver abscess (ALA) occurs** and can present as a medical emergency.

### Specific Measures

- **Metronidazole:** The drug and its related compounds are highly *effective against all forms of amebiasis, at all sites, and in all age groups*. Such drugs are easy to administer, and are free of serious side effects. The dose of metronidazole varies from 400 to 800 mg three times a day for 5–7 days, depending upon the severity of disease. In cases with severe toxemia, the drug may be given initially by IV route, 500 mg every 8 hours for 3–4 days. It has greatly simplified the treatment of amebiasis, and is usually well-tolerated though some patients develop distressing nausea and vomiting.
- **Emetine/dehydroemetine (DHE):** This is a powerful amebicidal drug *effective against trophozoites* in all tissues (intestinal and extraintestinal) but is ineffective against luminal amoebae. It has long been the mainstay of treatment in severe amebiasis. However, it is a relatively toxic drug and is now seldom used (since the availability of metronidazole). Anyway its use in general practice is not recommended.

## AMEBIC LIVER ABSCESS

Amebic liver abscess (ALA) is the most common extraintestinal form of amebiasis and results from invasion of liver by the trophozoites of EH.

Concurrent intestinal symptoms are not common; in fact many cases may not be able to even recall having suffered from intestinal symptoms.

## Site

Majority of the cases of ALA have a single abscess usually located in the posterior and superior parts of the right lobe of liver. This accounts for the frequent involvement of the diaphragmatic pleura and base of the right lung. However, an amebic abscess may be located anywhere in the liver, and accordingly, it will have a variable predilection to involve different adjacent organs such as:
- An abscess in the left lobe may extend into pericardium or left pleura.
- Amebic liver abscess situated far laterally in the right lobe will tend to spread forward toward right lower chest wall in front or in axilla.
- Occasionally, an abscess deep in the center of the liver may be virtually silent without producing any significant enlargement of liver, and present itself only as a case of pyrexia of uncertain origin.

## Clinical Features

The clinical picture thus, can be extremely variable, and symptoms may start suddenly or gradually. In initial stages, patient only has discomfort in the liver area, a vague dyspepsia, and slight fever. The liver is enlarged, firm and tender. As the abscess enlarges, toxemia and pain in the hepatic region increase, and pain may be referred to the right or left shoulder, depending upon the location of the abscess. At this stage the patient may be gravely ill and have swinging high temperature, profuse perspiration, dry cough, and marked tenderness on deep pressure in the right hypochondrium and lower chest. The liver is often greatly enlarged, soft to firm and extremely tender.

In untreated or neglected cases, a localized soft bulge may appear in the area of the liver where abscess is located. Boggy edema of the lower chest wall may appear, if the abscess is in the right lobe and enlarges toward the parities. Rarely, on reaching the periphery abscess may even erode into any of the surrounding tissues such as peritoneal cavity, lesser sac, or through the diaphragm into the pericardial cavity or the pleura and lung. In the last event, a spontaneous drainage may be established, sometimes providing considerable relief to the patient. Some degree of pleural reaction with fluid formation is not uncommon.

## Diagnosis

The diagnosis is quite easy in advanced stage of the disease. However, ALA has an enormous potential for protein manifestations and the only way to avoid mistakes is to constantly keep the condition in mind. In the early stages, the patient may present with only *pyrexia of uncertain origin.*

"**Point tenderness**" in the posterolateral portion of a right lower intercostal space is a valuable sign in such cases, and is often observed in the absence of diffuse liver pain. Jaundice is unusual except in advanced cases.

**Ultrasonography** is the investigation of choice and clearly defines the location, size of the abscess, and also the nature of the contents. *Serologic tests* are now seldom carried out. *Liver function tests* are usually normal or only mildly disturbed. Elevation in serum liver enzymes is minor and nonspecific. Some degree of increase in serum alkaline phosphatase and reduction of serum albumin are common. Other suggestive investigations include moderate polymorphonuclear leukocytosis and a raised immobile right diaphragm. Stool examination is of no particular value. Differentiation from pyogenic liver abscess may be sometimes difficult. In such cases aspiration of the abscess (under ultrasonic guidance) and its laboratory examination will clear the issue.

## Management

- ❖ **Drug therapy:** All cases in which ALA is diagnosed should be hospitalized. In most of the cases metronidazole alone will suffice, but many cases will require concurrent or sequential use of chloroquine as additional drug (chloroquine is concentrated 500 times in liver tissue and is therefore quite effective in hepatic amebiasis).
  Metronidazole can be administered orally, 600–800 mg three times a day for 5–7 days, but it may be preferable to give it IV (500 mg 8 hourly) for the first few days especially if there is marked toxemia or symptoms of gastric upset. This should be supplemented with chloroquine therapy, two tablets (300 mg active base) twice daily for 2 days and then one tablet twice a day for next 3–4 weeks.
- ❖ **Antibiotics:** Ciprofloxacin 500 mg twice a day (IV in serious cases) or ampicillin 500 mg four times a day for 7–10 days can be valuable adjuncts even though amebic pus is usually bacteriologically sterile.
- ❖ **Aspiration:** Most of the cases of ALA respond adequately to drug treatment. However, under certain conditions aspiration of abscess cavity becomes desirable. These are:
  - A large abscess threatening to rupture
  - A large abscess in the left lobe which is often associated with higher rate of serious complications
  - Cases who respond inadequately to 3 days of drug therapy, and
  - Nature of liver abscess needs evaluation

Repeated aspirations should be avoided as this increases the risk of secondary bacterial infection, bleeding, and peritoneal spillage. If required a self-retaining catheter can be placed in the abscess cavity percutaneously under ultrasonic guidance for *continuous drainage* for a few days.

# CORONAVIRUS DISEASE (COVID-2019)

COVID-19 is a novel disease which results from infection with CORONAVIRUS 2 (SARS-CoV-2). It is primarily transmitted from person-to-person through close. Contact (approximately 6 ft) by respiratory droplets. The disease is highly contagious with sustained spread. Other sources of transmission include contaminated surfaces or fomites with subsequent contact with the eyes, nose, or mouth.

COVID-19 spread rapidly throughout the world, and the World Health Organization (WHO) declared it as a pandemic on March 11, 2020. The virus has infected and killed millions of people around the world, severely affected global economy, and unprecedented numbers of individuals under travel restrictions or quarantine.

## Symptoms

These are like other viral upper respiratory illnesses. The disease can take three major trajectories:
1. Mild disease with upper respiratory symptoms
2. Non-severe pneumonia
3. Severe pneumonia complicated by acute respiratory distress syndrome (ARDS).

Other complications of COVID-19 include secondary bacterial infection, septic shock, acute kidney injury, ventilator-associated pneumonia, and myocarditis. Emergencies and hospitalizations arise only in the last type.

Most of the patients are 30 to 79 years of age, and about 80% of cases are mild with a low fatality rate (2–3%). Highest case mortality occurs in those over 80 years of age. Contributory factors include burden of heart and metabolic diseases, especially diabetes and obesity which impair the body's immune response. This may be one reason why COVID-19 causes more harm in people with these underlying conditions.

## Treatment

Only supportive treatment, preferably with acetaminophen, is required in most of the cases. Special consideration should be given to those at the extremes of ages, the immunocompromised, or pregnant women. All seriously ill patients will have features of respiratory insufficiency and desperately need oxygen supplementation to maintain an oxygen saturation of 90%. Since no specific medicine against COVID-19 is yet available, certain drugs have been tried empirically. These are Remdesivir, Lopinavir, Chloroquine, Hydroxychloroquine, and Azithromycin. Immunoglobulins, and convalescent serum have also been used with varying success. More recently, however, availability of specific vaccine has virtually taken the sting out of the disease.

# 9 Acute Poisoning

## INTRODUCTION

Acute poisoning can be a serious medical emergency requiring prompt and effective treatment. Its nature can usually be diagnosed by historical details and circumstantial evidence. Acute poisoning should be considered in any acute obscure illness and in any comatose patient without lateralizing features. A careful *physical examination* can be rewarding since poisoning by many drugs often results in one of the following four syndromes.

1. **Sympathomimetic syndrome:** This is usually seen in cases of poisoning by ephedrine, cocaine, and amphetamines. Both blood pressure and pulse rate are increased, temperature is elevated and tongue is dry.
2. **Sympatholytic syndrome:** Poisoning by barbiturates, benzodiazepines, **opioids, clonidine, and ethanol** are good examples. The **clinical** features are **opposite** of those described above. In some cases consciousness may **also** be impaired.
3. **Cholinergic syndrome:** Poisons such as organophosphates, carbamates, and physostigmine result in stimulation of muscarine receptors resulting in sweating, bradycardia, miosis, and hyperperistalsis. Salivary and bronchial secretions are also increased, and bronchospasm may be present.
4. **Anticholinergic syndrome:** Classical example is *atropine poisoning* but similar features may also be seen in over dosage with tricyclic antidepressants, and antihistamines. Patients may have agitated delirium and abnormal movements such as myoclonus or athetosis. Body temperature is often elevated (even hyperthermia may occur), skin is flushed and dry, pupils are widely dilated, and pulse rate and blood pressure are invariably increased. Peristalsis is decreased and urinary retention may become a problem.

## PRINCIPLES OF MANAGEMENT

Maintenance of vital functions should be the top priority. Various steps required are easily remembered by the mnemonic *ABCD* (Airways, Breathing, Circulation, and Drugs).

## Maintenance of Vital Functions

- **Airways:** Oral cavity should be cleared of any foreign body, and secretions removed. The patient should be made to lie on one side to *prevent the tongue falling back and an anesthetic airway inserted*. Some cases in deep coma may require even endotracheal intubation.
- **Breathing:** If respiration is depressed, assisted ventilation should be provided as required and supplemental oxygen given. Oxygen status is best determined (quickly) by pulse oximetry.
- **Circulation:** Circulation should be assessed by pulse and blood pressure, and *tissue perfusion* by urine output, and skin turgor. When possible, blood gases and arterial pH should be studied. ECG monitoring is also desirable. In hypotensive patients, *central venous pressure (CVP) monitoring* can be valuable in regulating fluid therapy.
- **Drugs:** Hypoglycemia may be present, and should be quickly determined by glucometer. If blood sugar is <70 mg/dL, IV infusion of D5W or D10W should be given until blood sugar reaches 110 mg. If alcohol intoxication is suspected, thiamine 100 mg IM is recommended.
- **Antidotes:** Poisons, which have specific antidotes, are given at **Table 9.1**. However, these should be used keeping in mind the patient's clinical condition. In cases with heavy metal poisoning, a rather broad-spectrum antidote is British Anti- Lewsite (BAL). It is given deep intramuscularly in a dose of 4 mg/kg 4 hourly on the first day, 6 hourly for the next 2 days, and then thrice daily for up to 7 days. BAL has proved most valuable in the treatment of mercury and arsenic poisoning, but may also be used in cases of poisoning by cobalt, copper, gold, nickel, and zinc compounds. It should be remembered that antidotes by themselves can have serious adverse effects, and therefore should not be used indiscriminately.

**Table 9.1:** Some poisons which have specific antidotes.

| Poisons | Specific antidote |
| --- | --- |
| Acetaminophen | Acetylcysteine |
| Anticholinergics | Physostigmine |
| Benzodiazepines | Flumazenil |
| Beta-blockers | Glucagon |
| Calcium channel blockers | Calcium |
| Carbon monoxide | 100% oxygen |
| Cyanide | Sodium nitrite, Sodium thiosulfate |
| Digoxin | Digoxin-specific antibodies |
| Heavy metals | Chelating agents |
| Isoniazide | Pyridoxine (vitamin $B_6$) |
| Narcotics | Naloxone |
| Tricyclic antidepressants | Sodium bicarbonate |

## Removal of Poison

- **Unabsorbed poison:** Poisoning can occur through ingestion, inhalation, or absorption through skin. If the poison is noncorrosive and has been taken within the last 4 hours, vomiting should be induced (only in conscious patients) by stimulating the pharynx with fingers or making the patient drink a glassful of saline water. Use of *apomorphine IM for inducing vomiting is not recommended.*

  If poisoning has occurred in the preceding 8–12 hours, a **gastric lavage** must be done (except when contraindicated), irrespective of whether vomiting has occurred or not. In unconscious patients gastric lavage should be done only after endotracheal intubation to prevent aspiration. Except in certain specific poisoning, plain water, slightly warm, should be satisfactory for stomach wash. A specimen of stomach wash (and also of the vomitus, if any) should be preserved for *medicolegal purpose.*

  When poisoning is *through inhalation,* the patient should be removed immediately from the contaminated environment. When poisoning is by *absorption through skin,* the soiled clothing should be removed and the contaminated area washed thoroughly with plain water.

- **Systemically absorbed poison:** Varying amount of poison would have been absorbed depending upon the time that has elapsed since its ingestion. The excretion of the poison can be accelerated by **diuresis,** by **alkalinization of urine,** repeated doses of **activated charcoal** orally or through gastric tube (20–30 g every 3–4 hours), and **dialysis.** A list of the dialyzable toxic agents is given at **Table 9.2**. Dialysis is doubly indicated if acute renal failure sets in.

**Table 9.2:** Toxic agents for which dialysis is beneficial.

| Sedative-Hypnotics | Halides |
|---|---|
| • Alcohols<br>• Chloral hydrate<br>• Ethyl alcohol (ethanol)<br>• Barbiturates<br>• Carbamates | • Bromides<br>• Fluorides<br>• Iodides<br>• Alkaloids<br>• Quinidine<br>• Quinine |
| **Non-narcotic Agents** | **Miscellaneous** |
| • Acetaminophen<br>• Aspirin<br>• Phenacetin<br>• Metals<br>• Arsenic (after dimercaprol)<br>• Iron (after deferoxamine)<br>• Lead (after edetate)<br>• Mercury (after dimercaprol)<br>• Calcium<br>• Lithium<br>• Potassium | • Amphetamines<br>• Boric acid<br>• Carbon tetrachloride<br>• Phenytoin<br>• Sulfonamides<br>• Thiocyanates |

## Fluid and Electrolyte Balance

Daily fluid requirement comprises imperceptible water loss (10–15 mL/kg) plus the quantity lost daily in urine, stools, sweat, and gastric aspiration. Fluid deficit and replacement should be monitored by CVR

Electrolyte imbalance can occur from vomiting, diarrhea, sweating, or renal malfunction. The management is easy if kidney functions are normal, but when renal functions are impaired, serum electrolytes and blood gases should be studied and properly regulated (for further details *see* section on "Clinical fluid, Electrolyte and Acid-Base Abnormalities, Chapter 5).

## ■ SEDATIVE-HYPNOTIC TOXICITY

Sedative-hypnotics include several classes of drugs used in the treatment of anxiety and insomnia, most common being *benzodiazepines,* and *Zolpidem.* All these drugs can induce tolerance, and can cause a withdrawal syndrome resembling ethanol withdrawal. The drugs vary in their absorption, distribution, and elimination. Their toxicity is generally related to central nervous system depression similar to that caused by ethanol.

Since benzodiazepines are one of the most highly prescribed classes of drugs, these are also the most commonly employed agents in self-poisoning by drug overdose (replacing barbiturate of the earlier era).

### Signs and Symptoms

Benzodiazepines have a wide therapeutic index and taken alone in overdose rarely cause severe complications. Most of the patients who inadvertently take more than the prescribed dose will simply feel drowsy and fall asleep for a few hours. However, when (even ordinary doses of benzodiazepines) are consumed along with alcohol or other drugs such as antidepressants, heroin, opioids, and even antihistamines, symptoms may assume alarming proportion ending in coma and death.

Following an *acute overdose* of benzodiazepines with suicidal intent, symptoms develop rapidly, usually between 4 and 6 hours. Initial signs and symptoms include nystagmus, ophthalmoplegia, ataxia, dysarthria, lethargy, and somnolence. Memory impairment is common and this is more marked in elderly and heavy alcohol drinkers. A peculiar symptom of benzodiazepine toxicity is *"lapses in memory"* and *"amnesic episodes".* During such episodes the subject is unaware of his actions, may indulge in antisocial acts (may be charged with shoplifting, etc.), and even homicide.

Cases of *severe overdose* display prolonged deep coma, respiratory depression, hypoxemia, hypotension, hypothermia, severe bradycardia, pulmonary aspiration, with the possibility of death. The duration of symptoms following overdose is usually between 12 and 36 hours in majority of cases.

Occasionally *paradoxical reactions* such as anxiety, delirium, insomnia, nightmares, aggressive behavior, and hostility may manifest resulting in attacks of rage and violent behavior. Such reactions are particularly common with *triazolam* especially when given in high doses (0.5–1 mg).

### Diagnosis

The diagnosis of benzodiazepine overdose is based on clinical presentation of the patient along with a history of overdose. Estimation of benzodiazepine blood concentrations can be useful in diagnosis in patients presenting with CNS depression or coma of unknown origin. However, serum levels may be misleading, and do not appear to be related to any toxicological effect nor are predictive of clinical outcome.

### Treatment

Careful observation and supportive measures are the mainstay of treatment of benzodiazepine overdose. *Gastrointestinal decontamination* with activated charcoal, gastric lavage or whole bowel irrigation is without proven benefit in pure benzodiazepine overdose, but may be useful when benzodiazepines have been taken along with other drugs. Likewise, hemodialysis, hemoperfusion, or forced diuresis is unlikely to be beneficial as these procedures have little effect on the clearance of benzodiazepines (due to their large volume of distribution and lipid solubility).

**Supportive measures** include observation of vital signs and degree of coma [according to Glasgow Coma Scale (*see* Chapter 4)]. Airway patency should be ensured; mechanical ventilation may be required, if respiratory depression or pulmonary aspiration occurs.

Hypotension should be corrected with fluid replacement (under CVP monitoring), but some cases may also need catecholamines. Comatose patients should be in *intensive care units* with continuous cardiac monitoring and frequent oxygen estimation by pulse oximetry.

### Antidote

*Flumazenil* is a benzodiazepine antagonist but should be used with extreme caution since it can have serious side effects such as seizures, adverse cardiac effects, and even death. The dose is 0.2 mg IV slowly repeated every 5-10 minutes up to a maximum of 3-5 mg. *Contraindications* to flumazenil include known seizure disorder, benzodiazepine addiction, and tricyclic antidepressant overdose. The drug is not required in most of the cases with benzodiazepine overdose, and general and intensive supportive care usually suffices.

## SALICYLATE POISONING

This usually takes the form of over-ingestion of aspirin tablets. Salicylates increase body metabolism and also directly stimulate the respiratory center. The resulting hyperventilation leads to *respiratory alkalosis* which persists despite excessive metabolism. When consumed in large quantity, salicylates depress respiratory center and displace several milliequivalents of bicarbonate, thereby producing grave *metabolic acidosis,* which may prove fatal. In addition, salicylates may impair *carbohydrate metabolism* and result in accumulation of acetoacetic, lactic and pyruvic acids *(increased anion gap).*

## Clinical Features

Symptoms and signs usually appear several hours after consuming an overdose of salicylates, and since the patient is nearly always conscious, a good clinical history should be revealing. The patient has severe tinnitus, dimness of vision, is restless, and has excessive sweating, and rapid deep breathing. There may be hyperpyrexia and features of gastric irritation such as epigastric pain, vomiting and even hematemesis. Large doses may also produce *hypoprothrombinemia* with hemorrhages in the skin and mucus membranes.

Moderate to severe dehydration often complicates clinical picture with resulting hypotension and *impairment of renal functions.* The latter may also be due to shedding of the epithelial cells in the renal tubules with consequent blockage of the tubules. Massive over dosage may result in agitation, impaired consciousness, seizures, and pulmonary edema. Death may occur from renal or cardiorespiratory failure.

## Diagnosis

This is usually clear from historical details. When relevant history is not available, a combination of *hyperpnea, perspiration, and hypotension* should suggest the correct diagnosis. It can be confirmed by a positive ferric chloride test (appearance of violet color on addition of a few drops of ferric chloride solution to 5 mL of boiled and acidified urine containing salicylates). The severity of poisoning can be assessed by *blood salicylate levels.* Serious poisoning usually occurs at blood levels greater than 100 mg%. Levels above 50 mg% suggest subacute intoxication. Arterial blood gas analysis usually reveals respiratory alkalosis with an underlying metabolic acidosis.

## Management

- ❖ **Activated charcoal** is recommended for prompt adsorption of aspirin. However, this may not be readily available. A more practical alternative is *gastric lavage.* This should be done irrespective of the time elapsed since the drug was ingested as salicylates often induce pylorospasm thereby delaying absorption. Antacids in gel form may be given every 2-3 hours to counteract gastric irritation caused by salicylates.
- ❖ **Alkalinization and forced alkaline diuresis** should help since salicylates are excreted chiefly through the kidneys.
    - *Alkalinization of urine* when combined with forced diuresis can increase renal excretion of the drug 8-10 times. The urinary pH should be increased till it gives a definite red color with phenol red indicator

(pH = 8.4). This can be achieved by infusion of 100 mEq of sodium bicarbonate in 1L of D5W over 5-6 hours. If oliguria is not a problem, 20 mEq of potassium should be added to this infusion.
- *Forced diuresis* Details of the regime are as follows:
  - D5NS infusion should be given IV at a rate of 1 L during the first hour and 500 mL every 1-2 *hours till free urine outflow is established*
  - Furosemide 60-100 mg IV should be given at the start and repeated after 2 hours, if required
  - 300 mL of 20% mannitol infusion may also be given.

ote

> These measures may produce enormous diuresis, even 8–10 L in 24 hours. A close watch should therefore be kept on fluid and electrolyte balance.

- ❖ **Fluid, electrolyte and acid-base balance:** Severe dehydration may occur, and as much as 2 L of fluid per hour may be required for the first 2-3 hours. In children, the rate of infusion should be 20-30 mL/kg/hr. D5W and normal saline solutions are quite appropriate fluids and should be used in a ratio of 2:1. Once free diuresis has started, potassium supplements should also be given IV (20-40 mEq over 4-6 hours) keeping a watch on serum levels.
- ❖ **Dialysis:** Hemodialysis can be life saving. It is especially indicated in patients with severe metabolic acidosis, altered mental status, or when there is threatened renal failure.
- ❖ **Miscellaneous measures:** All supportive measures as outlined in the earlier part of this chapter should be instituted. Vitamin K 20 mg IM should be given if there is significant hypoprothrombinemia. Respiratory depression may require artificial ventilation. Convulsions should be treated with diazepam.

## Complications

- ❖ Severe disturbance in acid-base equilibrium
- ❖ Hyperthermia
- ❖ Acute renal failure.

## ACUTE OPIATE POISONING

This is rather uncommon medical emergency, and is encountered mostly in opium addicts. Not infrequently, it results from abuse of the drug in crude form, either alone or mixed with "dhatura", or is due to overdose of one of its several related narcotic preparations (morphine, pethidine, heroin, codeine, fentanyl).

### Clinical Features

All these compounds act on *"opiate receptors"* in the brain, thereby decreasing central nervous system activity and sympathetic outflow. Consciousness is impaired, pupils are constricted, respiration is slow and shallow and may be periodic, pulse is slow, and there may be hypothermia. The addition of *"dhatura"* (a belladonna-like compound) modifies many of these clinical features. Instead of hypothermia the skin may be hot and flushed, and the pupils rather dilated. In the most severe cases of opium poisoning there is deepening coma and cyanosis with progressive respiratory depression, and finally cardiorespiratory arrest. The pupils may dilate terminally due to severe brain anoxia.

## Management

**Emergency measures** include hospitalization, protection of the airway, and assisted ventilation. If the drug has been taken orally, gastric lavage should be done and stomach washed with a weak (1:5,000) solution of potassium permanganate till the color of the returning fluid remains unchanged. This should be done irrespective of the time elapsed since the drug was ingested as opiates induce pylorospasm thereby delaying gastric emptying.

**Specific antidote** for opioid intoxication is *naloxone,* which acts as a competitive antagonist and rapidly reverses signs of narcotic over-dosage. It however, has a short duration of action (2–3 hours) and therefore repeated doses may be required. The usual dose is 0.4–2 mg IV, repeated as required (every 30–60 min) to awaken the patient and restore adequate respiration. However, the total dose should not exceed 40 mg since, in large doses naloxone itself can cause respiratory depression.

**General measures** include maintenance of respiration and other vital functions, and institution of other supportive measures already described in this chapter.

## Complication

Acute pancreatitis.

## CARBON MONOXIDE POISONING

Poisoning by carbon monoxide (CO) is usually the result of accidental or suicidal exposure to the gas, and may occur from automobile exhaust with closed doors and windows, during combustion of coal in an improvised furnace placed in a closed room for heating purposes, or from smoke inhalation in a fire. In industry CO is produced in many situations such as blast furnaces, tunnels, and coal mines. *The cooking gas supplied in gas cylinders does not contain carbon monoxide.*

Carbon monoxide poisoning *results in severe tissue hypoxia* since it has affinity for hemoglobin 200 times more than that for oxygen. Further, carboxyhemoglobin (COHB) also interferes with release of oxygen from oxyhemoglobin, which results in reduced oxygen delivery. Poisoning is more serious in men at work than at rest (because of the greater volume of gas respired), and in children than in adults (because of lesser amount of hemoglobin). Anemia, alcohol, barbiturates, old age, and general debility worsen the prognosis.

### Clinical Features

The symptoms and signs depend upon concentration of the gas in the inspired air, the duration of exposure, and the individual's state of activity. With minimal exposure (CO <0.01% in inspired air) the COHB concentration is <10% and the individual has no symptoms or only minimal headache. Following exposure to 0.05% for 1-2 hours and during moderate activity, the CO saturation may reach 30-50%. At this stage there may be shortness of breath and throbbing headache followed by blurred vision, confusion, and dizziness, nausea, vomiting and fainting. As the level of COHB reaches over 50%, convulsions, coma and respiratory failure occur, rapidly ending in death.

With more acute poisoning, consciousness may be lost suddenly and without warning. The skin and mucosa are of cherry red color (because of bright red COHB), tendon reflexes are increased, and the pupils become dilated. Severe tissue anoxia, especially in older people, may compromise cerebral and coronary circulation and result in cerebral stroke or myocardial infarction.

### Diagnosis

This is usually obvious from the circumstantial evidence and from *cherry red color of the skin and mucous membranes which is characteristic of CO poisoning*. Patient will complain of severe headache and may have altered mental status. Diagnosis is confirmed by estimation of arterial or venous COHB saturation. However, a simple test carried out by adding 1 mL of 5% sodium hydroxide to 1 mL of patient's blood diluted with 10 mL water may be helpful. An oxyhemoglobin solution will turn brown, but if significant amount of COHB is present the solution will turn straw yellow (COHB < 20%) or will remain pink (COHB >20%). Pulse oximetry or arterial blood gas estimation is misleading.

### Management

The treatment of CO poisoning essentially requires effective ventilation with high oxygen concentration. If the patient is unconscious, he should be removed from his environment as quickly as possible by dragging him out by the heels. However, the rescuer should take precautions not to get trapped himself.

Thereafter, resuscitation should be started immediately, initially by mouth-to-mouth breathing. As soon as facilities permit, 100% oxygen should be administered preferably by a well-fitting oronasal mask. Some cases may need mechanical ventilation. Administration of hyperbaric oxygen (at two atmosphere pressure) results in speedier dissociation of COHB, and hence quicker recovery, but the necessary equipment is seldom available.

Prolonged coma should raise suspicion of cerebral edema, which may occur due to capillary endothelial damage resulting from severe hypoxemia. This should be treated with diuretics and corticosteroids.

General measures comprise loosening of all clothing, careful control of blood pressure, fluid and electrolyte balance, and other steps already described for care of comatose patient.

## Complications
- Cerebral stroke
- Myocardial ischemia or actual infarction
- Psychotic behavior and parkinsonism (late complications).

## ACUTE ALCOHOLIC (ETHANOL) INTOXICATION

### Clinical Features

Alcohol is primarily a *central nervous system depressant*. Following a single dose, peak level is reached in about 1 hour, persists for 2 hours, and then declines gradually. After consuming appreciable quantity (tolerance varies markedly from person to person) there is *initially a release of inhibitions* resulting in a state of exhilaration and euphoria. Further doses of alcohol produce progressively, dizziness, slurred speech, ataxia, tremors, confusion, nausea, vomiting, and increasing impairment of mental faculties until stupor and coma supervene.

Physical examination at this stage reveals the skin to be hot and flushed or pale and sweating, deep reflexes are exaggerated with bilateral extensor plantars, pupils are dilated, breathing is stertorous, and pulse MI and bounding. Death can occur from respiratory or circulatory failure, but is uncommon. A scale-relating blood alcohol levels to signs and symptoms of acute alcoholic intoxication in non-habituated persons is given at **Table 9.3**.

Occasionally, acute alcoholic intoxication manifests in **atypical patterns**. These include: (i) *"acute excitation"*, which may take the form of sudden and unprovoked outburst of anger with even assaultive and destructive behavior, and (ii) *"black outs"* in the form of episodes of transient amnesia that accompany heavy intoxication.

**Table 9.3:** Blood level and clinical features of alcohol intoxication.

| Blood level | Clinical features |
|---|---|
| 30 mg% | Mild euphoria |
| 50 mg% | Dizziness, mild incoordination |
| 100 mg% | Ataxia, slurred speech |
| 200 mg% | Confusion, drowsiness, blurred vision |
| 300 mg% | Stupor, and later progressively increasing coma |

## Diagnosis

In the presence of a flushed face, semi-coma or coma and the odor of alcohol, the diagnosis of alcohol intoxication is easy. However, when confronted with a comatose patient, it is advisable not to ascribe the loss of consciousness to alcohol per se (even though the patient smells of alcohol) until all other possible causes of coma have been ruled out. When coma persists for more than 24 hours, possibility of mixed poisoning, complicating head injury, subdural hematoma or cerebral stroke should be strongly considered.

## Management

Most of the patients with mild to moderate degree of intoxication usually sleep it off and requires no special treatment. When stupor or coma has supervened, the stomach should be lavaged with tap water to remove unabsorbed alcohol. **Forced diuresis** may also prove useful in such cases (see, section on "Salicylate Poisoning"). **Dialysis** is indicated if: (i) patient is in deep coma, (ii) blood alcohol level is extremely high (over 400 mg%) especially if accompanied by acidosis, and (iii) there is possibility of concurrent ingestion of methanol or barbiturates. Administration of insulin and glucose or analeptic drugs is of little practical value.

Supportive measures should be applied as described in the section on "Barbiturate Poisoning". Violent delirium, if present, should be controlled with injection diazepam *(not barbiturates because of their synergistic effect with alcohol)*.

## Complications

- ❖ Acute hepatic failure
- ❖ Gastrointestinal bleeding
- ❖ Cardiac decompensation (alcoholic cardiomyopathy)
- ❖ Associated head injury.

## ACUTE WITHDRAWAL (ABSTINENCE) SYNDROME

### Clinical Features

Sudden withdrawal of alcohol in a chronic alcoholic can result in acute and frightening symptoms in the form of confusion, irritability, tremulousness, nausea and vomiting, insomnia, hallucinations, psychosis and convulsive seizures *(rum fits)*. The most severe form of withdrawal syndrome results in *"delirium tremens"* characterized by confusion, hallucinations and delusions, coarse tremors, agitation and sleeplessness. The patient has a flushed face and features of autonomic over-activity such as dilated pupils, tachycardia, raised temperature, and excessive sweating. In severe cases death may occur from hyperpyrexia or peripheral circulatory failure.

## Management

With mild withdrawal symptoms, all that is required is rest and sleep with the help of tranquilizers. When classical delirium tremens has developed, it is an emergency and therefore the patient should be hospitalized immediately.

* **Control of agitation:** *Agitation* is best controlled by long-acting benzodiazepines (to avoid rapid changes in blood levels) such as diazepam. An average patient requires 40-60 mg diazepam on first day, administered in four divided doses. This should alleviate most of the symptoms of withdrawal. The dose is then reduced by 20% on successive days over a 3-5 days period. It is important to remember that in cases with associated liver disease long-acting benzodiazepines may prove hazardous, and in such patients drugs with short half-life should only be used, e.g., oxazepam.
* **Other measures:** Proper fluid and electrolyte balance should be maintained, and large doses of vitamins administered especially vitamin B1 since glucose infusions may utilize last available stores of thiamine, and precipitate Wernicke's encephalopathy.

# METHYL ALCOHOL (METHANOL) POISONING

Methyl alcohol is usually consumed as a cheap substitute for (ethyl) alcohol but may be ingested as methylated spirit accidentally or with suicidal intent. The so called *"country-liqor"* is often contaminated with methyl alcohol and accounts for localized outbreaks of methanol poisoning. The toxic dose is quite variable. Death may occur after just 20 mL, but even 200 mL has been ingested with survival. Permanent blindness is a great risk.

## Clinical Features

Methyl alcohol is less inebriating than ethyl alcohol but is more toxic because it is *oxidized in the body to formaldehyde and formic acid with consequent metabolic acidosis.* It may persist in the body for several days, its rate of metabolism being only 50% that of ethyl alcohol.

The toxic effects of methanol are entirely because of its metabolites, especially *formaldehyde*. Since these take time to accumulate, the symptoms of methanol poisoning may be delayed up to 12-24 hours after ingestion. Usual manifestations include epigastric pain, vomiting, headache, dizziness, delirium, and visual disturbances ranging from blurred vision to blindness (due to *retrobulbar neuritis and optic atrophy)* which may be permanent. In more severe poisoning *metabolic acidosis* occurs, and death may result from respiratory or circulatory failure.

## Management

* **Gastric lavage:** When the patient is seen within the first 2-4 hours of methanol ingestion, the stomach should be washed out with plain water.

- **Administration of ethyl alcohol:** This acts by blocking the metabolism of methanol as it competes for the same oxidative enzyme (alcohol dehydrogenase). Treatment with ethanol is indicated when poisoning is severe or blood level is very high (over 20 mg%). In such cases ethyl alcohol is given IV 1 g/kg body weight in D5W over 30 minutes (as loading dose) followed by 7-8 g/hour so as to maintain blood ethanol level at about 100 mg%.
- **Fluid and electrolyte balance** should be carefully monitored. Acidosis, if significant, is treated by 50-100 mL of 7.5% sodium bicarbonate IV. Large amounts of IV glucose and B vitamins should also be given.
- **Diuretics and dialysis:** Mannitol diuresis should be induced whenever methanol poisoning is associated with more than minimal signs and symptoms. In severe poisoning, besides ethanol therapy, hemodialysis should be considered especially if there is visual impairment.

## CORROSIVE POISONING

This usually results from accidental splashing of strong acids, alkalis or phenolic compounds in industry, or from throwing of such corrosives on a victim with homicidal intent. Occasionally, such substances are ingested in suicidal attempt.

### Clinical Features

The toxic effects of strong corrosives are almost entirely due to irritation, local edema, and destruction of tissues. At the site of contact chemical burns are produced which may result in serious damage if vital areas like face or eyes are involved. When such compounds are ingested there is often severe pain in mouth, pharynx, chest and upper abdomen. Swallowing becomes intensely painful and greyish white ulcers may be seen on the inner side of lips, tongue and buccal mucosa. In severe cases shock, asphyxia (due to edema and spasm of the glottis), and circulatory collapse may occur.

### Management

- **General measures:**
  - In the case of *skin contamination,* the area should be immediately and thoroughly washed with plain water followed by suitable antiseptic dressings. When there is *risk to the eyes* the head of the patient should be held under a running tap and patient asked to blink his eyes repeatedly. Thereafter, the eyes should be washed thoroughly with normal saline solution, 1% homatropine drops instilled, a light bandage applied, and patient referred to the nearest ophthalmic center.
  - In cases where the *corrosive has been ingested* the patient should be hospitalized at the earliest. Pain should be controlled with parenteral analgesics, adequate nutrition, fluid and electrolyte balance maintained,

and antibiotics administered prophylactically. Impending shock should be managed on usual lines but corticosteroids are contraindicated at this stage for fear of causing rupture of the esophagus/stomach.
- **Use of antidote:** In case of **acids,** a thick paste of magnesia or aluminum hydroxide gel should be given orally to dilute and neutralize the ingested acid. White of eggs and milk are also suitable antidotes especially if doubt exists as to the type of corrosive ingested. *Sodium bicarbonate is contraindicated because it will produce effervescence and may rupture esophagus or stomach.* In case of poisoning by **alkalis,** the poison should be neutralized by large amount of water, fruit juices or 10% vinegar. *Gastric lavage is contraindicated in all types of corrosive poisoning.*
- **Delayed effects:** These include esophageal stricture and rupture of corroded viscous. For the former a thoracic surgeon should be consulted, and small doses of corticosteroids may be used cautiously. The latter may occur unexpectedly at any time during convalescence and result in mediastinitis, peritonitis, or sudden death.

## SNAKE BITE POISONING

Snakes are widely distributed in tropical and subtropical countries, mostly in rural areas and in jungles. Most of such snakes are, however, non-poisonous. The poisonous snakes belong to five families: *(1) Elapidae* (cobras, kraits, mombas and tiger snakes), *(2) Viperidae* (vipers), *(3) Hydrophidae* (sea snakes), *(4) Crotalidae* (pit vipers), and *(5) Colubridae* (bird snakes). In India most of the cases of snake bite poisoning are due to *Elapidae* group including common cobra *(Naja naja)* and king cobra, or *Viperidae* group including *Russell's* viper and pit viper.

The *differentiation between poisonous and nonpoisonous snakes* is important and can be made by the presence, in the former, of broad ventral scales, which cover the belly completely, and two fangs through which the venom is injected. Nonpoisonous snakes, on the other hand, usually have a blunt tail, solid teeth, semicircular scales, and absence of fangs. Snake bite is usually associated with one or more of the following features:
- **Intense fright and fear:** Intense autonomic over activity may result after bite by a snake, whether poisonous or non-poisonous, and may result in immediate syncope.
- **Secondary infection:** This may result from the presence of various bacteria in the mouth of the snake or on the skin of the victim.
- **Effect of injected venom:** Snake venom consists of several toxic proteins and enzymes with varied pharmacological effects such as neurotoxic, cardiotoxic, curare-like, hemolytic and hemorrhagic. However, *cobra and sea snake bites are predominantly neurotoxic and cardiotoxic, whereas viper bites have chiefly cytolytic effects* resulting in tissue destruction through hemolysis and destruction of the endothelial lining of the blood vessels.

### Factors Affecting Severity of Snake Bite Poisoning

- **Amount of venom injected:** This depends chiefly upon the species and size of the snake and the amount of the poison in the glands at the time of the bite. If the latter have recently discharged their contents, little or no venom may be injected *(dry bite)*. Further, if the bite has been through a layer of clothing, the amount of venom injected and thereby the toxic effects may be greatly reduced. On the other hand repeated strikes by the snake may result in more severe poisoning since snake's entire supply of venom may not be exhausted by the initial bite.
- **Host factor:** Snake bite poisoning is likely to be more serious in children (small size), in old age, and in debilitated subjects.
- **Location of bite:** Bites on extremities are less dangerous than those on the face and trunk.
- **Physical activity after bite:** Physical exertion such as running immediately after the bite, speeds up absorption of poison, and hence increases the severity of poisoning.

### Clinical Features

Both cobra and viper bites usually show clear marks of two fangs set about an inch apart, and are accompanied within 20 minutes by severe local pain, numbness or weakness and local edema. The *systemic effects of poisoning usually appear within 15 minutes to 12 hours of the snake bite.* If the subject is completely well after 12 hours of the bite, it was in all probability by a non-poisonous snake.

**Cobra and sea-snake bites** typically produce *paralytic features* manifesting as increasing weakness of limbs, ataxia and multiple cranial nerve palsies. There may be excessive salivation, slurred speech, dysphagia, and occasionally nausea and vomiting. In severe poisoning respiratory paralysis develops, convulsions may follow, and death occurs within a few hours. If the patient survives for 24 hours after the bite, all paralytic symptoms quickly recover, almost completely.

**Cardiotoxic symptoms** appear more abruptly, usually within 2 hours, and comprise sudden hypotension, cardiac arrhythmias, and cardiac arrest.

The bites by **viper snakes,** on the other hand, produce predominantly a *disturbance in the hemostatic system, particularly in capillary endothelium.* This may result in a severe hemorrhagic state with bleeding into the skin, various mucous membranes, and retroperitoneal tissues. In fact the appearance of a local hemorrhagic area with uncontrollable bleeding at the site of the bite is the earliest and often diagnostic feature of viper bite. Local ischemic necrosis may ultimately develop and progress over weeks presenting as dry gangrene.

Hemorrhagic manifestations may appear soon after the bite or be delayed for as long as 24 hours. Severe hemolysis can occur with appearance of jaundice and anemia. Acute circulatory failure may result partly from such hemorrhages and hemolysis and partly from extravasations of serum in the bitten area. Death may occur within a few hours of the bite from spontaneous hemorrhage into a vital organ especially the brain, from circulatory failure and shock or renal failure. Not infrequently, paralytic and hemotoxic features exist in the same patient.

## Management

### *Immediate (Prehospital) Measures*

The patient should be reassured and kept as much inactive as possible to prevent the spread of the poison. The *bitten area* and the related extremity should be lightly wrapped with an elastic crepe bandage starting from distal towards bitten site. The bandage pressure should be just enough to permit one finger to be easily introduced between the bandage and the skin. Thereafter the limb should be splinted so as to *immobilize* it in a neutral position. Further, the bitten part should be kept below the heart level. *Very tight pressure-immobilization should be avoided* since by restricting venom to the site of bite it may worsen local tissue necrosis though systemic toxicity may be lessened to some extent. *Never apply ice or occlusive tourniquet that may cut off arterial supply.* Do not give beverages or stimulants.

*Local incisions* should not be given by unskilled people as these may result in trauma to underlying structures. The value of *local suction* commonly employed in the field management of snake bite is unproven, especially if applied *after* the first few minutes of the snake bite. Very little venom may be extracted from the depot at the site of bite, and prolonged suction (more than 20–30 minutes) may actually be detrimental.

### *Subsequent Treatment*

- ❖ **Care of the wound:** The wound should be washed and cleaned with a weak solution of potassium permanganate but crystals of permanganate should never be applied. Surgical debridement of the wound is best postponed till about the end of the first week following the bite. Hemorrhage in the area of bite, if prolonged, should be controlled **by** local hemostatics as described in the section on "Hemophilia" (Chapter 6).
- ❖ **Antivenin:** Immunotherapy with anti-snake venom *(ASV-Antiveniri)* is the only specific therapy available for snake-bite poisoning. The exact dose varies but generally 100 mL of ASV diluted in 500 mL of normal saline should be given IV over 2–4 hours in all cases of snake bite without waiting for signs of poisoning to appear. If and when such signs appear, a further dose of 50 mL ASV may be given IV slowly over 12 hours. It should, however, be realized that **therapy with antivenin is effective against only the circulating toxin,** and therefore it must be given as early as possible after the bite. Antivenin has no action against the toxins already absorbed since the venom gets attached to target organs such as neuromuscular receptors, platelets, red blood cells, renal tubules, and myocardium.

The ASV infusion should be started very slowly under close supervision and discontinued immediately if acute reaction occurs. After the first

20-30 minutes, if there is no reaction, the infusion rate may be increased. *Skin testing* with AVS is not reliable. It is therefore safer to administer prophylactically *pheniramine maleate (Avil) 45 mg (2 mL) and ranitidine 50 mg IV to minimize acute reactions* following ASV infusion. Additionally, *epinephrine and hydrocortisone injections* should always be available. Serum sickness reactions occurring 5-10 days after serum administration usually respond well to prednisolone.

❖ **Analgesics and sedatives:** Severe pain may be present and should be relieved **by** norphine/tramadol/diazepam. These drugs will also help allay associated anxiety which may be intense.

❖ **Corticosteroids:** These are indicated when blood dyscrasias (hemorrhages/hemolysis) occur or when shock is impending. For the former, 40-60 mg prednisolone is given daily in divided doses for 3-4 days. Much bigger doses are required for treatment of shock (*see* Chapters 1 and 11).

❖ **Treatment of paralytic complications:** Some of the cobra venom toxins compete with acetylcholine for receptors in the neuromuscular junction and lead to curare-like paralysis. This should be treated with IV neostigmine 1 mg slowly followed **by** neostigmine infusion in a dose of 25 g/kg/hour. The infusion may be continued for 12-24 hours and flow rate adjusted according to the state of neurological recovery. To avoid undue bradycardia, neostigmine should be preceded **by** 0.6 mg atropine intravenously. When respiratory paralysis is threatened mechanical ventilation will be required.

❖ **Treatment of hemorrhagic manifestations:** Antivenin therapy, blood transfusions and corticosteroids are the mainstay in the treatment in such cases. Transfusion of fresh plasma during the first 24 hours is also beneficial.

### General Measures

Every case should be given tetanus toxoid, and suitable antibiotics to ward off secondary infection. In patients who develop hemorrhagic tendency IM injections should be avoided to prevent risk of deep seated hematomas.

Severe hemorrhages will require blood transfusions. Appearance of oliguria is ominous, and should be managed with adequate hydration, 20% mannitol infusions, and IV furosemide. In severe cases dialysis may be required.

### Complications

❖ Acute renal failure
❖ Shock

## INSECTICIDE (PESTICIDE) POISONING

The widespread use of insecticides/pesticides in agriculture and vector control during the past few decades has been associated with a large number of cases of acute poisoning from such compounds. This may be due to occupational exposure to these chemicals, accidental misuse, or (mostly) with suicidal intent (because of their easy availability). In fact, this has become one of the most common poisoning in large parts of India and other developing countries dependent on rural economy.

## Classification

Three groups of insecticides/pesticides are commonly used in agriculture:
1. **Organochlorine insecticides (OCI):** These include: (a) chlorinated ethane derivatives of which DDT (chlorophenothane) is the best known, (b) chlorinated cyclodienes, which include compounds like aldrin, chlordane, dieldrin, and endrin, and (c) other hydrocarbons such as BHC, mirex, and toxaphene.
2. **Organophosphorus insecticides (OPI):** These are the most common types of insecticides used and are *primarily Cholinesterase inhibitors.* Some of the better known OPI are parathion, methyl parathion, DALF (fenthion), Nitrox 80, demeton (Systox), EPN, TEPP, OMPA, Diazinon, Dipterex, Tugon, Symtox (TIK-20), malathion, DEF, chlorthion, and methyl demeton (Meta-Systox). Of these the first seven are more dangerous. A complete classification of all such chemical agents according to their degree of toxicity has been provided by WHO (1975).
3. **Carbamates:** These include Carbaryl, Sevin, and Baygon. Their mode of action is qualitatively similar to that of OPI, and therefore, the two are discussed as a group.

### Organochlorine Poisoning

*Mode of action*

Organochlorine insecticides (OCI) are highly soluble in lipid and organic solvents but not in water. When appropriately dissolved these may enter the body through the skin, lungs or gastrointestinal tract. Their toxicity varies considerably, and may be modified to a great extent by the properties of the dissolving agent.

OCI have a wide margin of safety and are generally less toxic than OPI. Their *main site of action is brain where these compounds produce initial stimulation followed by paralysis.*

*Clinical features*

Toxic reactions to these compounds usually follow their accidental or suicidal ingestion. The initial symptoms therefore are gastrointestinal (nausea and vomiting), followed by headache, dizziness, paresthesia of the tongue, lips and face, irritability, delirium, tremors and tonic/clonic convulsions. Later, there is *progressive depression of CNS resulting in paralysis, coma, and death.* Rarely, severe hepatotoxicity and ventricular fibrillation may occur.

*Treatment*

The treatment is entirely symptomatic since there is *no specific antidote*. Necessary supportive measures should be adopted to maintain vital life functions. Emergency measures include attempts to induce vomiting, and gastric lavage if the toxin has been ingested within last 3-4 hours. When poisoning is suspected through skin, it should be scrubbed with soap and water to remove any traces of intoxicant.

A rather specific antidote is *cholestyramine,* which interrupts the enterohepatic circulation of organochlorines, and should therefore be administered in all symptomatic patients (4 g every 4-6 hours). Hyperreactivity and convulsions should be controlled with diazepam or barbiturates. *Stimulants such as epinephrine should never be used since these may induce ventricular fibrillation.* Prognosis is good except when convulsions are severe and protracted.

### *Organophosphate and Carbamate Poisoning*

*Mode of action*

OPI and carbamates *inhibit the enzyme, acetyl cholinesterase,* which inactivates acetylcholine wherever released. While *OPI bind firmly and irreversibly* to action sites of the enzyme, the *inhibition with carbamates is reversible.* Consequently, there is accumulation of acetylcholine at both sympathetic and parasympathetic synaptic junctions (cholinergic nerve endings) throughout the body. The action of acetylcholine at the cholinergic receptors is very short lived and is normally terminated (in a flash-like manner) by Cholinesterase. The consequent **overabundance of acetylcholine** initially stimulates and subsequently disrupts impulse transmission in both the peripheral and central nervous systems.

*Pathophysiology*

Cholinergic fibers are present in central nervous system, autonomic ganglia, somatic nerves, parasympathetic nerve endings, neuromuscular junctions, and even in some sympathetic nerve endings such as sweat glands.

- **Autonomic effecter cell** *(post-ganglionic parasympathetic fibers):* Their stimulation is associated with *muscarine effect* such as Diarrhea, Carnation, Miosis, Bronchoconstriction, tmesis, Lacrimation, and Sweating *(DUMBELS).*
- **Autonomic ganglion cell** *(pre-ganglionic sympathetic and parasympathetic) and striated muscles.* These are *nicotine receptors,* and their stimulation results in features like tachycardia, hypertension, muscle weakness, cramps, and fasciculation.
- **Central nervous system neurons:** Cholinergic receptors in CNS neurons are predominantly either nicotinic (spinal cord) or muscarinic (thalamus, cerebral cortex). Over-stimulation of these receptors results in impairment of nerve impulse transmission. The common symptoms include severe

headache, generalized weakness, restlessness, convulsions, confusion, coma, and later cardiorespiratory depression.

*Clinical features*

Most OPI are lipid-soluble and well-absorbed from the skin, conjunctivae, oral mucous membrane, and gastrointestinal tract. Because of the widespread distribution of cholinergic nerve endings in the body (vide supra), a diversity of clinical features is encountered in such cases (**Table 9.4**).

Intoxication may occur by *inhalation, ingestion, or percutaneous absorption of the OPI* and the nature of the initial symptoms will vary according to the portal of entry. Local effects on the eye and respiratory tract may be the earliest symptoms, if the exposure is in the form of dust and vapors, or follows their inhalation. These include miosis, conjunctival congestion, watery nasal discharge, wheezing respiration and tightness in the chest due both to intense bronchoconstriction and increased bronchial secretions. When OPI are absorbed through the skin, muscular fasciculation and localized sweating in the immediate vicinity are the usual early symptoms. Following ingestion, gastrointestinal symptoms occur earliest and include anorexia, nausea, vomiting, abdominal cramps, and diarrhea.

The onset and intensity of symptoms in organophosphate poisoning (OPP) is determined by its type, degree and rate of exposure, by the nature

**Table 9.4:** Clinical features of organophosphate poisoning.

| Site of action | Clinical effect |
|---|---|
| **Muscarinic manifestations** | |
| • Bronchial tree | Increased bronchial secretions, bronchoconstriction, dyspnea, cyanosis, even pulmonary edema |
| • Sweat glands | Increased sweating |
| • Salivary glands | Increase in salivation |
| • Lactimal glands | Increase in lacrimation |
| • Gastrointestinal | Nausea, anorexia, vomiting, abdominal cramps, tenesmus, diarrhea, fecal incontinence |
| • Cardiovascular | Bradycardia, hypotension, arrhythmias |
| • Ocular | Miosis, may be unequal, blurred vision |
| • Bladder | Frequency, even urinary incontinence |
| **Nicotinic manifestations** | |
| • Striated muscle | Fasciculations, cramps, weakness including that of muscles of respiration |
| • Sympathetic ganglia | Pallor, tachycardia, hypertension |
| **Central nervous system manifestations** | Anxiety, restlessness, impaired consciousness, cogwheel rigidity and tremor, slurred speech, ataxia, convulsions, bilateral pyramidal signs, paralytic signs including respiratory paralysis |

of the particular compound, by its lipid solubility, and rate of metabolic degradation. Onset is most rapid following inhalation, and least rapid following percutaneous absorption. The **latent interval** (time between exposure and appearance of symptoms) may be as short as 5 minutes after massive ingestion, but is usually less than 12 hours. Further, highly lipid-soluble agents (e.g., fenthion) may produce symptoms and signs of cholinergic over activity over an extended period of time (several days and even weeks) because of subcutaneous lipid storage and subsequent slow release. Such compounds may also result in repeated relapses after apparent successful management. Once symptoms appear, these usually progress for up six hours.

*Late onset signs*

Occasionally, manifestations of OPP may be delayed by as much as 12–20 hours after ingestion of the compound. Usually confined to the CNS, such features appear after the muscarinic signs, and represent nicotinic effect (hence do not respond to atropine). These have been labeled as type II signs of OPP or **"intermediate syndrome",** and comprise weakness of neck and trunk followed by bulbar palsy, facial and proximal muscle weakness, ophthalmoparesis, and respiratory paralysis. If the patient survives the acute phase, these symptoms and signs clear completely in 4–7 days.

*Cause of death*

In most of the patients of OPP death is due to respiratory failure attributable to all the three pharmacological actions of organophosphates: muscarinic (bronchospasm and increased bronchial secretions), nicotinic (generalized muscular weakness including weakness of intercostals and diaphragm), and central nervous effects (depression of respiratory center). Contributory factors include tachycardia, fall in blood pressure and arrhythmias due both to hypoxemia and **toxic myocarditis.**

## CARBAMATE INSECTICIDES

These compounds also combine with **Cholinesterase,** but this **combination is reversible** with time. Therefore, if symptoms develop, these do not persist for more than 8–12 hours.

### Diagnosis

This does not offer much problem and is based on history of exposure, typical clinical features (most helpful being miosis, muscular **fasciculation,** weakness, and excessive sweating), and response to atropine and pralidoxime. In doubtful cases estimation of RBC or plasma **Cholinesterase** activity is very helpful, the latter being easier to measure. In severe cases, assessment of myocardial function (echocardiography), and serial arterial blood gas estimation is also recommended.

## Management

Organic insecticides are one of the most lethal chemical agents. Immediate and energetic treatment should be instituted covering three aspects: (1) *maintenance of vital life functions,* (2) *removal of unabsorbed material,* and (3) *specific therapy.* All the three measures must be adopted concurrently.

- **Maintenance of vital life functions:** Airway patency should be ensured including endotracheal aspiration if required, and oxygen should be administered at high flow rates. Some cases may require mechanical ventilation. Hypotension or convulsions, if present, should be treated appropriately.
- **Removal of unabsorbed material:** Where intoxication has occurred by mouth, gastric lavage must be done immediately, and cathartics administered to eliminate as much of the intoxicant from the gastrointestinal tract as possible. If the clothing is contaminated it should be removed and the skin washed thoroughly with soap and water. Contamination of the eyes should be treated by irrigation of conjunctiva with water for 10 minutes.
- **Specific therapy:** Two drugs, **atropine and pralidoxime** (PAM), are available as specific antidotes for OPI intoxication. Atropine is effective against the muscarinic and central nervous effects of organophosphates but has no action against their nicotinic manifestations. On the contrary, PAM is ineffective against the muscarinic effects of OPI. The two drugs are therefore, complementary to each other. The two drugs also act differently in respect of their antidote properties. While atropine only blocks the effects of excessive acetylcholine, PAM actually helps in restoring acetylcholinesterase by reversing the phosphate ester bond, both in blood and tissues. It is worth noting that the ***process of irreversible binding of Cholinesterase to OPI occurs only gradually,*** and therefore treatment with PAM is most effective if started early.
    - **Atropine:** This is a symptomatic treatment for muscarinic signs. Large doses may be required starting with 1-2 mg IV (0.5 mg in children) followed by repeated doses of 2-4 mg until signs of atropinization occur (i.e., flushing, mydriasis, dryness of secretions, and tachycardia). Use of up to 50 mg in 24 hours may be required. Thereafter, atropine therapy in appropriate dosage should be continued for at least 72 hours, since symptoms may recur and prove fatal, if untreated. The drug should therefore be withdrawn only gradually and judiciously.
    Atropine crosses the blood-brain barrier, and may cause severe toxic effects such as confusion, delirium, convulsions, and even coma. Since these features may be indistinguishable from acute OPP, careful observation and monitoring of atropine doses is necessary.
    - **Oximes** (Pralidoxime, Obidoxime): These drugs competitively inhibit binding of organophosphates to acetylcholinesterase. This action can occur only shortly after OPP after which the bond becomes quite firm

and cannot be reversed by oximes. To be effective therefore, oximes should be given as early as possible, *preferably within 6 hours of poisoning*. However, beneficial response may occur even when oxime therapy is delayed for as long as 24 hours.

The usual adult dose of PAM is 1 g (or Obidoxime 250 mg) in saline IV slowly over 5-10 minutes. This dose may be repeated every 6-8 hours for next 24 hours. PAM is not indicated in poisoning by carbamates since the bond between these agents and cholinesterase is reversible and short lived.

ote

- Mouth-to-mouth respiration should be avoided when OPP is by ingestion, since the vomited material may contain dangerous amount of toxic substances.
- Sympathomimetic drugs should be avoided in poisoning by organochlorine insecticides since these compounds increase susceptibility to ventricular fibrillation.

## ALUMINUM PHOSPHIDE POISONING

Aluminum phosphide (ALP) poisoning is used as a **fumigant** in grain (especially wheat) storage and preservation and is marketed as "Celphos" "Quickphos", "Alphos", "Synfume", etc. All of these are highly toxic to man.

Ingestion of ALP is one of the most common types of poisoning (suicidal or accidental) in this country especially in the wheat producing belt in Northern India. The compound is widely used (by fumigation) and is marketed as tablets or pellets (Celphos, Quickphos, Alphos, Synfume, etc.), each weighing 3 g and containing 57% ALP and about 40% ammonium carbonate. On exposure to moisture phosphine gas (PH3) is liberated (besides small amounts of ammonia and carbon dioxide), which is highly reactive and poisonous.

$$ALP + 3 H_2O = AL(OH)_3 + PH_3 \text{ (gas)}$$

This reaction is accelerated by the presence of hydrochloric acid in the stomach. Ordinarily, 3 g of compound generate 1 g of phosphine. The toxic effects are dose related, and ingestion of three or more tablets is nearly always fatal.

### Pathophysiology

Phosphine gas is a powerful *inhibitor of cytochrome oxidase* (like cyanide). Its *inhalation* in human beings causes severe pulmonary edema. Following *ingestion* of ALP, phosphine gas is liberated in the stomach which is rapidly absorbed and diffuses throughout the body. Extensive capillary damage occurs with widespread congestion, hemorrhages, and peripheral capillary leakage, resulting in *severe hypovolemia* and hemoconcentration.

The cellular damage involves almost all organs notably the heart, lungs and kidneys. Myocardium shows vacuolation, interstitial edema and diffuse (but sparse) polymorphonuclear cell infiltration suggestive of **toxic myocarditis**.

Severe myocardial depression occurs which coupled with hypovolemia results in vascular collapse. The situation is made worse by pulmonary changes which may comprise pulmonary edema, aspiration and often acute respiratory distress syndrome **(ARDS)**. Severe hypoxemia occurs and **metabolic acidosis** is common, probably due to lactic acidosis caused by blocking of oxidative phosphorylation (similar to cyanide toxicity).

## Clinical Features (Table 9.5)

Immediately after swallowing the tablets, there is retrosternal and epigastric pain which may be extremely severe. This is often accompanied by profuse vomiting (and occasionally diarrhea), restlessness, headache, and vertigo. The most prominent feature is **severe hypotension** which sets in early and is due both to marked decrease in cardiac output and hypovolemia (due to extensive capillary leakage). In fact the patient very often presents in a state of **shock** with thready or imperceptible pulse, profuse perspiration, cold extremities, and complaining of thirst. Orientation is preserved initially but impairment of consciousness soon develops (due to persistent hypotension).

Many patients who survive 12-24 hours develop respiratory distress with medium to coarse crackles all over the chest. Persistent severe hypotension (especially recurrence of hypotension after initial stabilization), progressive oliguria and development of coma are ominous. Most of the cases die within 24-48 hours especially if three or more tablets of ALP have been consumed.

**Prognosis** is better if less than one, or if pre-exposed tablets have been consumed since much of PEL would have already been liberated on exposure to atmospheric moisture.

## Investigations

Routine investigations including blood chemistry do not reveal any characteristic change. Serum CPK-MB is elevated in nearly all cases especially if tested early. Metabolic acidosis, hypokalemia and hemoconcentration are prominent features.

| Table 9.5: Salient features of ALP poisoning. | |
|---|---|
| Gastrointestinal | Retrosternal and epigastric pain, vomiting |
| Cardiovascular | Severe hypotension and shock, supraventricular and ventricular arrhythmias (both tachy- and bradyarrhythmias) |
| **Hepatic** | |
| Metabolic | Severe acidosis (elevated lactates) |
| Electrolytes | Hypokalemia, hypocalcemia, hypomagnesemia |
| Pulmonary | Pulmonary edema, ARDS (late feature, if patient survives) |
| Miscellaneous | Vascular collapse, progressive oliguria, coma |

*Electrocardiogram* shows characteristic changes comprising bizarre wide QRS-T complexes (resembling ventricular tachycardia), ST segment elevation or depression with inverted T waves, and a variety of rhythm disturbances such as atrial fibrillation, multiple supraventricular ectopics, supraventricular tachycardia, and ventricular tachycardia. Echocardiography reveals global hypokinesia, and provides valuable information regarding the extent of myocardial dysfunction.

## Management

In the absence of any specific antidote, treatment of ALP poisoning has to be largely symptomatic and supportive keeping in view the pathophysiology described above.

- **Gastric lavage:** Any patient suspected of ALP poisoning should have a stomach wash with a mild oxidizing agent (such as potassium permanganate). This should be followed by a copious lavage with sodium bicarbonate solution since this may help to reduce systemic acidosis without causing fluid overload.
- **Control of hypovolemia:** Massive fluid therapy (3-10 L) is required during the first 12-24 hours guided by central venous pressure (CVP) maintained near 10-12 cm of water. Overloading of circulation should be avoided as there is serious risk of pulmonary edema. If CVP is found to be elevated at any stage, IV furosemide should be used.
  Usual fluids employed are D5W and normal saline. These should be supplemented with potassium chloride and/or sodium bicarbonate according to serum electrolyte and blood gas results.
- **Control of hypotension:** Hypotension is due both to hypovolemia and severe myocardial depression, and therefore fluid replacement should be supplemented with dopamine so as to keep systolic pressure above 90 mm Hg. Occasionally dobutamine/noradrenalin infuse ion may also be required.
- **Control of cardiac arrhythmias:** Specific therapy varies according to the type of arrhythmia encountered. *Hypomagnesemia* has been observed in many of these cases, and this constitutes the basis of therapy with magnesium sulfate ($MgSO_4$). Relatively large doses are recommended, beginning with 1 g $MgSO_4$ every hour for 4 hours followed by 1 g every 6 hours. Therapy should be monitored by frequent estimation of serum magnesium. Severe *hypocalcemia,* if present, should be treated with IV calcium gluconate. Marked tachycardia (heart rate >140/min) sometimes occurs, and may by itself be a factor in the genesis of hypotension. Use of *beta-blockers* in such cases is a double-edged weapon, but may be worth a trial beginning with short-acting esmolol. Occasionally, severe bradycardia is the overwhelming response even when the patient is in shock. Such cases should be treated with IV atropine.
- **Other measures:** Oxygen tension is invariably low in these cases, initially because of shock, and later due to ARDS (which is a frequent complication).

Continuous oxygen at high flow rates should therefore be administered to all cases. When ARDS supervenes, suitable ventilatory support should be provided (*see* section on ARDS, Chapter 2). Corticosteroids and antibiotics have only a limited role.

## LESS COMMON TYPES OF POISONING

The common types of poisoning met in general practice have been described above. However, any chemical or therapeutic agent may be abused occasionally, either accidentally or with suicidal intent. The salient clinical features and specific measures for treatment of poisoning by some such agents are summarized in **Table 9.6**. General supportive measures to preserve vital life functions, control of convulsions, and maintenance of proper fluid and electrolyte balance are extremely important in every case of poisoning. These are not detailed separately for individual poisoning.

**Table 9.6:** Important clinical features and treatment of less common types of poisoning.

| Poison | Clinical features | Treatment |
|---|---|---|
| Acetaminophen (paracetamol) | Nausea, vomiting, drowsiness, confusion, hypotension, cardiac arrhythmias, liver tenderness/jaundice and acute renal failure. Hepatic toxicity increased by alcohol. Fatal dose: 1 g/kg | • Gastric lavage (preferably within 4 hours<br>• Saline catharsis<br>• N-acetylcysterine (mucocyst) 140 mg/kg (20%) every 4 hours for 3 days (Antidote)<br>• **General:** IV dextrose for first 48 hours; vitamin K, if prothrombin time much prolonged; blood transfusion may be necessary |
| Amphetamine | Restlessness, excitement, tremors, flushing, hallucination, insomnia, tachycardia, convulsions | • Gastric lavage<br>• Sedate with chlorpromazine 0.5–1 mg/kg every 30 minutes as needed<br>• Maintain high urine output and acidic urine<br>• **General:** Control convulsions with diazepam |
| Antidepressants-tricyclic | Dryness of mouth, psychosis, fits, progressive loss of consciousness, hypothermia, dilated pupils, increased reflexes, cardiac arrhythmias, respiratory depression, hypotension and urinary | • Gastric lavage<br>• Control convulsions<br>• Forced diuresis (dialysis not effective)<br>• **General:** Monitor cardiac rhythm; avoid vasoconstrictor agents; maintain BP by giving fluids. |

*Contd...*

Contd...

| Poison | Clinical features | Treatment |
|---|---|---|
| Antihistamines | Lethargy, drowsiness, ataxia, hallucinations, stupor and coma. Occasionally, agitation, fever, tachycardia, tremors, fits, hyper-reflexia | • Gastric lavage<br>• Control convulsions<br>• General supportive measures<br>• Avoid stimulants |
| Aresenic compounds | Severe abdominal pain, vomiting, diarrhea, muscle cramps, confusion and circulatory collapse | • Gastric lavage<br>• Replace fluids and control diarrhea<br>• Give injections of BAL (dimercaprol)—4 mg/kg body weight every 4 hours on first day, 6 hourly for next 2 days and then thrice daily for 1 week (antidote)<br>• Treat anuria; consider hemodialysis |
| Barium* (carbonate, chloride, hydroxide) | Vomiting, diarrhea, abdominal pain, tremors, cardiac arrhythmias, breathing difficulty, convulsions, and death from cardiac and respiratory failure | • Give soluble sulfates† orally (antidote)—30 g sodium or magnesium sulfate in 250 mL water, orally or by Ryle's tube; repeat in 1 hour<br>• Induce forced alkaline diuresis<br>• Monitor serum $K^+$; control cardiac arrhythmias and respiratory abnormality |
| Belladonna alkaloids | Dry mouth, flushed dry skin, thirst, blurred vision, dilated pupils, tachycardia, fever, delirium and stupor | • Gastric lavage followed by saline catharsis<br>• Prostigmine 0.5–1.0 mg IM every 7 hours till symptoms abate or up to a maximum of 6 mg (antidote)<br>• Sedate with diazepam, avoid morphine<br>• **General:** Control convulsions; monitor rectal temperature; ensure adequate urine output by IV fluids |
| Copper salts (copper sulfate-blue vitriol) | Nausea, vomiting, diarrhea, abdominal pain, tachycardia, dehydration and collapse. | • Gastric lavage with 1% solution of potassium ferrocyanide followed by demulcents<br>• Replace fluids; control diarrhea<br>• General supportive measures |
| Cyanides (hydrocyanic acid) | Quickest acting poison. Odor of bitter almonds, pink color of skin and mucosae, rapid onset of unconsciousness, convulsions, circulatory collapse, dilated pupils. No cyanosis | • Immediate inhalation of amyl nitrite (antidote) one ampoule (0.2 mL) every 5 minutes<br>• 10 mL of 3% sodium nitrite IV in 3–5 minutes<br>• Sodium thiosulfate 50%, 25 mL IV in 3–5 minutes<br>• General supportive measures |

Contd...

Contd...

| Poison | Clinical features | Treatment |
|---|---|---|
| Formaldehyde (formaline) | Severe abdominal pain, vomiting, diarrhea, metabolic acidosis, collapse and anuria | • Dilute, inactivate or adsorb ingested formaldehyde by giving milk, activated charcoal or tap water. Do not use gastric lavage or emetics<br>• Give sodium bicarbonate IV to correct acidosis (monitor pH)<br>• Treat shock and anuria |
| Iodine tincture | Oral mucosa stained brown and edematous; burning epigastric pain, vomiting, bloody diarrhea; shock, severe edema of glottis, delirium, stupor and renal failure. Like corrosives, esophageal stricture may follow | • Give milk or white of eggs beaten in milk as demulcent. Avoid gastric lavage in the presence of esophageal injury<br>• Absorb iodine with starch solution (one heaped tablespoonful of cornstarch or flour added to 500 mL water)<br>• Administer sodium sulfate 5% 100 mL orally and 10% 10 mL IV every 4–6 hours<br>• Maintain patent airways and respiration; watch for anaphylaxis, and treat, if required with epinephrine, antihistamines and corticosteroids |
| Iron preparations | Nausea, vomiting, diarrhea, hematemesis/melena, collapse and encephalopathy | • Perform gastric lavage and leave in the stomach 5 g deferoxamine-Desferal (antidote) in 100 mL of water<br>• Desferal 2 g IM<br>• Desferal 7–10 mg/kg/hour IV in saline up to a maximum of 80 mg/kg in 24 hours<br>• General measures |
| Lysergide (LSD) | Excitement, auditory and visual hallucinations, confusion, psychosis, fits and dilated pupils | • Chlorpromazine 25–50 mg IM every 4–6 hours<br>• General supportive measures |
| Mercury | • Metallic taste, burning pain in throat, thirst, acute vomiting, and diarrhea with collapse<br>• Acute renal failure (tubular necrosis) may occur | • Dimercaprol by injections as for arsenic poisoning<br>• **General:** Treat anuria and shock |
| Naphthalene (naphthalene balls) | Nausea, vomiting, diarrhea, headache, confusion, convulsions, hepatic and renal damage with acute renal failure | • Gastric lavage<br>• Cathartics<br>• Alkalinize urine; give fluids upto 15 mg/kg/hour with furosemide 1 mg/kg to produce maximum diuresis and reduce injury to kidney. Hemodialysis, if required<br>• Consider corticosteroids to limit naphthalene hemolysis |

Contd...

*Contd...*

| Poison | Clinical features | Treatment |
|---|---|---|
| Nitrates and Nitrites | Headache, dizziness, flushing of skin, weakness and dyspnea (because of methemoglobinemia), vomiting, marked fall in blood pressure, collapse, cyanosis, convulsions, coma and respiratory paralysis | • Gastric lavage<br>• Maintain BP<br>• Methemoglobinemia (over 30% or when as associated with dyspnea) should be treated with methylene blue, 1% solution, 0.1 mL/kg IV over a 10-minute period. If methylene blue is not available, give ascorbic acid, 1 g slowly<br>• **General:** Oxygen therapy |
| Petroleum distillates and paraffin (kerosene, petrol, diesel oil, paint thinner, etc.) | Burning sensation in mouth and throat, vomiting, diarrhea and pallor; bronchopneumonia may develop | • Avoid gastric lavage because of risk of aspiration and consequent severe bronchopneumonia, or (preferably) gastric lavage with activated charcoal and a cuffed endotracheal tube to prevent aspiration<br>• Saline cathartics<br>• Broad-spectrum antibiotics<br>• General measures |
| Phenol (carbolic acid, cresol, creosote, lysol, tannic acid) | Burning in lips, mouth and throat with corroded ulcers draw-white in appearance; vomiting, bloody diarrhea, epigastric pain, acidosis, stupor, fits, coma, pulmonary edema and shock. Hepatic and renal failure may occur | • Cautious gastric lavage; contraindicated in the presence of esophageal injury; avoid vomiting<br>• Administer 60 mL castor oil (or olive oil) which dissolves phenol, retards its absorption, and hastens its removal<br>• Correct acidosis; maintain respiration; control convulsions |
| Phenothiazines (chlorpromazine and related drugs) | Drowsiness, hypotension, hypothermia, tachycardia, dryness of mouth, nausea, anorexia, ataxia, tremor, fever, blurred vision, stiffness of muscles, urinary retention, and coma. ECG may show prolonged QT and a widened QRS complex. Death may occur from hypotension and ventricular arrhythmias Toxicity enhanced by antihistamines, alcohol, barbiturates and morphine. Fatal dose: 15–50 mg/kg. | • Gastric lavage<br>• Diphenhydramine (Benadryl), 1–5 mg/kg IV will reverse extrapyramidal signs (antidote)<br>• Treat ventricular arrhythmias with phenytoin, amiodarone; lidocaine is contraindicated<br>• Treat hypotension, but avoid norepinephrine; control convulsions with phenytoin or phénobarbital; avoid diazepam |

*Contd...*

Contd...

| Poison | Clinical features | Treatment |
|---|---|---|
| Phosphorus inorganic (yellow phosphorus), rat paste, fireworks, matches, etc. | Garlic taste, burning pain in stomach, gastroenteritis, jaundice, hypotension, oliguria, convulsions, collapse | • Gastric lavage thoroughly with potassium permanganate solution (1:2,000); repeat half-hourly 3–4 times<br>• Saline cathartics<br>• Demulcents<br>• **General:** Treat pulmonary edema, shock; administer calcium gluconate IV to maintain calcium level; liberal IV glucose solutions |
| Potassium permanganate | Brown discoloration and edema of mucous membrane of mouth and pharynx, cough, laryngeal edema and stridor, necrosis of oral and pharyngeal mucosa, slow pulse, vascular collapse, hypotension and shock. Jaundice and oliguria or anuria may appear | • Remove poison from mucous membranes by washing repeatedly with tap water; avoid gastric lavage<br>• Treat shock and anuria<br>• Maintain ventilation |
| Silver salts (photographic developers, silver nitrate) | Blackening of skin and/or mucosa, pain in mouth and throat, nausea, vomiting of black material, salivation, diarrhea, convulsions, anuria, collapse, shock and death | • Give water containing sodium chloride (1%)-repeatedly, to dilute and precipitate silver ion as silver chloride<br>• Cathartics with added sodium chloride to precipitate and remove silver from intestines<br>• Administer demulcents, e.g., milk<br>• **General:** Look for and treat, if required, shock and methemoglobinemia |
| Volatile oils (turpentine oil, citronella oil, eucalyptus oil, menthol) | Nausea, vomiting, diarrhea, abdominal colic, delirium, convulsions, respiratory depression, acute tubular necrosis with anuria and finally coma | • Gastric lavage should be done carefully to prevent aspiration<br>• Control convulsions<br>• Dialysis may be required for renal failure<br>• General supportive measures |

*The sulfate salt is innocuous, and is used as a radiopaque contrast medium.

†Do not administer sulfates IV since barium sulfate may be precipitated in kidneys leading to renal failure. In very severe cases give 10 mL of 10% sodium sulfate slowly IV while maintaining maximum diuresis.

# Iatrogenic Emergencies

## INTRODUCTION

Certain clinical procedures and intravenous (IV) administration of drugs and fluids are an integral part of practice of critical care medicine. These may be associated with a variety of untoward reactions (**iatrogenic**) which may vary from minor to life-threatening. It is essential that every medical practitioner should have a good knowledge of all such reactions.

## PROCEDURE-RELATED EMERGENCIES

A certain degree of morbidity and even a small mortality, though undesirable, may nevertheless, have to be accepted as part of the price for *therapeutic intervention/procedure* in patients with serious illness. However, when serious complications follow a *diagnostic procedure* these are especially loathsome, and are a matter of concern both for the doctor and the patient. The risks and merits of the procedure should therefore be properly assessed, discussed with the patient and his relatives, and necessary precautions taken to lessen the chances of complications.

### Lumbar Puncture

Lumbar puncture (LP) may be required for diagnostic studies, and for injection of anesthetic agents and antibiotics. Two conditions warrant an emergent LP: (1) suspected central nervous system (CNS) infection, and (2) a strong suspicion of subarachnoid hemorrhage, when brain scan does not reveal any bleed. *Contraindications* include infection in the tissues near the puncture site, and increased intracranial pressure from a space occupying lesion. Following major complications may occur during or soon after an LP:

- ❖ **Headache:** This is by far the most common complication after LP. The headache begins within 48 hours of the procedure, is usually dull or throbbing, and lasts for 1–2 days but may continue up to 7 days. It is most marked in cervical and suboccipital regions and is probably due to leakage of cerebrospinal fluid (CSF) through the dural puncture site at a rate faster than it is formed in the choroid plexus.
  *Prevention and treatment:*
    - Recumbency (without pillows) for 24 hours after LP prevents headache. Use of a small-bore LP needle also decreases risk of headache.

- Mild to moderate headache often subsides spontaneously in a couple of days. If headache is incapacitating, besides analgesics, one liter of D5W should be infused IV.
- Caffeine is also recommended to assist with termination of LP-associated headache.

❖ **"Coning":** This implies herniation of the midbrain or medulla oblongata through the tentorium cerebelli or foramen magnum, respectively. It is likely to occur in patients with intracranial space occupying lesions, especially supratentorial, since such cases may have large pressure gradients between cranial and lumbar compartments. The complication may supervene immediately following LP or several hours thereafter, and can be recognized by respiratory depression and impairment of consciousness suddenly or gradually over 12 hours. Evidence of papilledema on funduscopy is a useful warning sign but this is present in only about half of the cases who may develop "Coning" following LP.

*Prevention and treatment:* Before carrying out LP, *funduscopy* must be done to detect papilledema which contraindicates LP. Even in its absence, caution should be observed if there is history of headache associated with progressive mental changes and/or localizing neurological signs. In such cases a CT brain should be done prior to LP. If bacterial meningitis is suspected, blood cultures should be obtained and antibiotics administered even before CSF is obtained to avoid delay in treatment (*see* section on "Acute Bacterial Meningitis", Chapter 4). In high-risk cases, following precautions should be observed:
- A unit of **mannitol** (300 mL 20%) should be infused rapidly in about 1 hour followed by furosemide 40 mg, 2 hours before planned LP.
- *A fine bore LP needle* (No. 22 or 24) should be used, minimal amount of fluid removed, and the procedure made as brief as possible. *Manometry and Queckenstedt test should never be performed.*
- If the patient collapses during LP and before the needle is withdrawn, normal saline should be injected through the LP needle equal in volume to the amount of fluid removed. If the needle has already been withdrawn, foot end of the bed should be raised, dexamethasone 8 mg IV administered, and 20% mannitol infusion started. Artificial respiration may be required, and the help of neurosurgeon obtained for urgent ventricular decompression.

❖ **Infection:** The risk of infection during LP is inversely proportional to the degree of asepsis observed. Spinal puncture is absolutely contraindicated in the presence of local infection at the puncture site. *Lumbar puncture-induced meningitis usually manifests 48 hours after the procedure.* The organisms should be isolated and the condition treated appropriately (*see* section on "Acute Bacterial Meningitis", Chapter 4).

## Gastric Intubation

Gastric intubation may be required for gastric lavage (in poisonings), gastric aspiration (in intestinal obstruction, etc.), or oral feeding (in comatose patient).

While performing gastric lavage, not more than 250 mL fluid should be used per wash (10 mL/kg in children). Larger amounts have the potential to force the gastric contents through the pylorus into the small intestine where more rapid absorption may result in fluid and electrolyte imbalance. Further, *in stuporous or comatose patients gastric lavage should be done only after the patient is intubated* (to prevent pulmonary aspiration). The chief complication of gastric intubation is aspiration pneumonia.

- **Aspiration pneumonia:** This can be a serious complication especially when it occurs in an already compromised patient. It may occur while the tube is being introduced, but more often takes place during feeding. Sometimes an asthma-like condition and even pulmonary edema may occur due to regurgitation of fluid into lungs.
  *Prevention and treatment: (a) Position of the tube should be checked* (by hearing injected air enter the stomach) before feeding is started. Not more than six ounces of feed should be given at one time, and unless there are contraindications (e.g., hypotension), the head of the patient should be elevated on pillows by 6-9″ (to prevent regurgitation), *(b) If aspiration has occurred,* attempts should be made to clear it by electric suction or bronchoscopic aspiration as the situation warrants. Broad spectrum antibiotics should also be given.

## Pleural Tapping (Thoracentesis)

This may be required for diagnostic or therapeutic purposes. The possible major complications are as follows:

- **Pneumothorax:** This is the most frequent complication of thoracentesis and may result from: (a) laceration of lung underneath, and (b) introduction of air from outside due to improper technique or drainage system. The resulting pneumothorax is usually small.
  *Prevention and treatment:* Use of proper technique and drainage system will greatly reduce the risk of pneumothorax. Small pneumothorax does not require any special treatment, but if it becomes large or tension pneumothorax supervenes, it should be managed as described in the section on "Pneumothorax" (Chapter 2).
- **Air embolism:** This occurs due to air entering into one of the radicles of pulmonary vein. The air reaches the left side of heart, and further symptoms depend upon the route taken by the air. Air embolism of the coronary arteries can prove rapidly fatal. More often, the air enters the cerebral arteries and may result in focal neurological signs depending upon the site of impaction of embolus.
  *Treatment:* The procedure should be discontinued at once, patient put in supine position, and head end the bed lowered. Oxygen therapy should be instituted, and any respiratory depressant avoided.
- **Pleural shock:** This is a type of vagal syncope but may also result from air embolism.
  *Treatment:* (a) Morphine 7.5-15 mg or norphin 1.5-3 mg should be given IV unless respiration is already depressed. Alternatively, atropine 1 mg

and promethazine 25 mg IM may be given to cut off vagal influences and allay apprehension, (b) If cardiorespiratory arrest occurs, immediate resuscitative measures should be adopted as described in the section on "Cardiac Arrest" (Chapter 1).

❖ **Acute mediastinal shift:** This can occur whenever a large quantity of fluid (over one liter) is removed rapidly at one time. There may be resultant acute pulmonary edema (often unilateral), or syncope.
*Treatment:* This is mainly preventive. When pulmonary edema does occur, it should be treated on the lines already described (*see* section on "Acute Left Heart Failure", Chapter 1).

❖ **Other complications:** These include introduction of *infection into pleural space,* and *post-thoracentesis hypoxia.* The latter is not uncommon and is due to ventilation/perfusion mismatch (with perfusion of atelectatic lung), or areas of localized pulmonary edema. Such complications should be managed along conventional lines.

## Pericardial Tapping

This must always be done in a well-equipped hospital, preferably intensive care unit, and under echocardiographic (or at least ultrasonic) guidance (*see* also section on "Cardiac Tamponade", Chapter 1). Serious complications include intercostal/internal mammary artery hemorrhage, injury to the myocardium, cardiac arrhythmias, and shock. All these are greatly reduced if the pericardial tapping is done by experienced personnel, and premedication is given with atropine and promethazine.

## INTRAVENOUS INFUSION RELATED EMERGENCIES

### Transfusion of Glucose/Saline

Intravenous infusion of any fluid may result in following complications:
❖ **Febrile reaction:** A variable degree of pyrexia, often associated with chills, is not uncommon during or soon after an infusion, and is usually due to the presence in the infusate of proteins to which the recipient is allergic. Occasionally, full blown anaphylactic reaction may occur.
*Treatment:* The transfusion should be temporarily discontinued, and restarted after a few hours at a slower speed. Preferably a new bottle of infusate and a new transfusion set and needle should be used. Hydrocortisone 100 mg IV and pheniramine maléate *(Avil)* 25 mg IM should be given if the reaction is more than mild. Observance of strict asepsis, use of good quality transfusion fluid, and gamma ray irradiated transfusion sets will, to a great extent, diminish the risk of such a reaction.
❖ **Circulatory overload:** Administration of large amount of fluids rapidly may precipitate acute left heart failure and pulmonary edema (*see* also Chapter 1). This is especially likely to occur in older subjects who often

| Table 10.1: Types of transfusion reactions. | |
|---|---|
| **Acute (within 48 hours)** | **Delayed (after 48 hours)** |
| **Immunologically mediated** | |
| Acute hemolytic transfusion reaction | Delayed hemolytic transfusion reaction |
| Febrile reaction (nonhemolytic) | Post-transfusion purpura |
| Allergic reactions | Graft-versus-host disease |
| **Nonimmunological** | |
| Circulatory overload | Infections (viral and others) |
| Bacterial contamination | Siderosis |
| Air and fat embolism | Thrombophlebitis |
| Metabolic shock | |
| Transfusion coagulopathy | |

have borderline cardiac reserve, or in patients with severe anemia, or overt heart disease.

*Prevention and treatment:* Unless special indications exist (e.g., dehydration) IV fluids *should not be given at a speed >1 mL/lb body weight/ hour.* If features of volume overload do appear, 40 mg furosemide should be administered IV, and other measures implemented as described earlier.

## Blood Transfusion

Whole blood or its components are transfused in a number of conditions, sometimes as a life-saving measure. About 5% of such transfusions are associated with adverse reactions which may vary from mild fever to life-threatening complications. These can be classified as *acute reactions* (occurring within minutes to a few hours of starting transfusion, and *delayed reactions* (occurring more than 48 hours after transfusion). Most of these reactions are immunologically mediated **(Table 10.1)**.

❖ **Hemolytic reaction:** This is usually due to the administration of mismatched blood. Consequently, *the red cells of the donor blood are agglutinated and hemolyzed. The recipient red cells are rarely if ever, hemolyzed* since the plasma portion of the donor blood is immediately diluted by the plasma of the recipient thereby diluting the titer of the infused agglutinins to a level too low to cause agglutination. Hemolysis may occur instantaneously (intravascular) as in the case of ABO incompatibility, or more gradually over several hours when incompatibility involves some other blood systems (such as Rh, Kell, Duffy, and Kidd systems). In the latter, red cell destruction occurs mostly in the reticuloendothelial tissues (extravascular), and these are usually minor reactions.

*Clinical features:* With major (ABO) incompatibility, symptoms start early and include burning sensation at infusion site and a feeling of vague uneasiness. Very soon, however, classical features of acute hemolysis develop comprising fever with chills, headache, lumbar pain, tachycardia, hypotension, and in severe cases, tightness in the chest or throat, respiratory distress, renal failure and even diffuse microvascular bleeding. The morbidity is chiefly due to renal failure (acute tubular necrosis) and/or bleeding.

*Diagnosis:* Acute hemolysis can be rapidly diagnosed by centrifugation of an anticoagulated blood sample and examining plasma by naked eye for free hemoglobin. After a few hours, methemoglobin appears (imparting a brown color to the serum) and this may persist for several days. When red colored urine is passed **(hemoglobinuria) the diagnosis is all too obvious. Hemolysis is also confirmed by a** *positive direct Coombs* test unless immune destruction is so rapid that no donor cells remain. In severe reactions, *coagulation tests* (prothrombin time, partial thromboplastin time, and fibrinogen level and fibrinogen degradation products) should also be done *to detect evidence of disseminated intravascular coagulation (DIC)*. With minor reactions, the only evidence of hemolysis may be an increase in bilirubin level, best detected within 24 hours of transfusion.

*Prevention and treatment:* Careful cross-matching and labeling will greatly decrease the risk of hemolytic transfusion reaction. A relatively slow infusion during first 10–15 minutes is helpful in detecting such reactions at a very early stage. When hemolysis is suspected the transfusion should be discontinued immediately, and suitable measures adopted according to the nature of the symptoms. Adequate blood pressure and urine flow should be maintained, if necessary by IV saline infusions and vasopressors. Mannitol infusion and/or IV furosemide may be required for oliguria. If acute renal failure or DIC set in, these should be managed as described in earlier sections.

❖ **Febrile reaction:** Fever with chills following blood transfusion (BT) is usually due to (nonhemolytic) febrile reaction, other causes being hemolytic transfusion reaction and bacterial infection. It is usually an *immunological response to white blood cells in the blood transfusion.* The leukoagglutinating antibodies interact with leukocytes and release an endogenous pyrogen (interleukin I). Accordingly, it is *more likely to occur in patients who receive whole blood transfusion(s),* or who are pregnant and therefore, have pre-existing antibodies.

Typically, febrile reaction develops toward the end of BT or within 2 hours post-transfusion, and is characterized by chills, headache and an abrupt rise in temperature. Generally mild and self-limited, it can sometimes be very severe and result in shock. The intensity of febrile response depends, to some extent, on the rate of transfusion.

*Prevention and treatment:* When correction of anemia is the primary aim, transfusion of *packed red cells should be preferred over whole blood.* Use of disposable syringes and needles and gamma-ray irradiated transfusion sets will decrease the risk of febrile reaction due to exogenous pyrogens.

If the reaction is mild, transfusion should be discontinued for a few hours, and then restarted at a slower rate (using a new transfusion set and needle) after ensuring there is no hemolysis. Pyrexia should be treated symptomatically. Administration of hydrocortisone 100 mg IV and *Avil* 25 mg IM before starting BT is helpful in reducing the frequency/severity of such reactions.

❖ **Allergic reactions:** These are *related to plasma component in the transfusion* and are therefore, more common with infusion of fresh frozen plasma, especially if given rapidly. *Symptoms usually arise within minutes of transfusion.* Minor skin reactions are quite common and comprise urticaria, erythema and itching, without any associated pyrexia. Very rarely, anaphylactoid reaction may occur and result in life-threatening situation. This is usually seen in some IgA deficient individuals who are transfused with blood products containing IgA. The symptoms are often dramatic, starting with flushing and uneasy feeling, and rapidly progress to abdominal cramping, vomiting, diarrhea, wheezing, bronchospasm, hypotension and collapse. Fever does not occur.

*Prevention and treatment:* Minor reactions usually settle down with slowing of the transfusion, or may require at most an antihistamine injection. Anaphylactic reaction need emergent resuscitative and supportive measures including administration of adrenaline, antihistamines and hydrocortisone (*see* section on "Critical Allergic Reaction", Chapter 11).

❖ **Infection:** Bacterial contamination of the transfused blood is rare, but when it does occur the reactions produced are very severe. High level of *endotoxin produced by contaminating gram-negative organisms can, within minutes of transfusion, result in shock syndrome* characterized by high fever with chills, hypotension, renal failure and circulatory collapse. When *symptoms are due to bacterial growth these are slower in onset* (1-3 days) and result from septicemia or DIC.

Another problem related to infections concerns *transmission of viral diseases* such as viral hepatitis type B/type C, and HIV, and other communicable diseases (e.g., malaria, syphilis, brucellosis, cytomegalovirus infection). The illness will be a delayed reaction, its time of occurrence depending upon the incubation period of the disease.

*Prevention and treatment:* Strict aseptic technique should be observed during collection and transfusion of blood. When acute bacterial reaction is suspected, BT should be stopped immediately and emergent resuscitative and supportive measures instituted. Appropriate antibiotics should be administered urgently without waiting for results of culture and sensitivity on the donor blood.

Screening tests on donor blood for hepatitis B and C virus, HIV, and syphilis are now a routine, and must be ensured. Storage of blood at 4-6°C for 48 hours is a very important measure in eliminating risk of transfusion syphilis. Malaria is still endemic in India, and *malarial parasites of all species can remain viable in stored blood for 1-2 weeks.* Possibility of

malaria should therefore, be considered in any patient who develops fever with chills within a few days of BT.
- ❖ **Circulatory overload:** This is a serious but entirely preventable complication which may follow too rapid infusion of blood in patients with severe anemia or cardiac and/or renal insufficiency. Clinical features resemble acute left heart failure and pulmonary edema, and usually develop toward the end of the transfusion or within 24 hours post-transfusion.
  *Prevention and treatment:* Limiting the rate of infusion to less than 2 mL/kg/hour, use of packed red cells, keeping the patient in semirecumbent position, and administering 10–20 mg furosemide IV before starting BT will almost eliminate the risk of circulatory overload.
- ❖ **Other reactions:** Some uncommon complications that may follow BT include potassium intoxication, transfusion coagulopathy (with transfusion of more than 10 units of blood within 24 hours which may result in dilutional thrombocytopenia and deficiency of factors V and VIII which are labile in stored blood), citrate intoxication (with clinical features of hypocalcemia) and transfusion hemosiderosis (with large and repeated blood transfusions). Such complications seldom present as medical emergency and can usually be managed on symptomatic lines.

## DRUG INTERACTIONS AND DRUG-INDUCED EMERGENCIES

### Drug Interactions (Table 10.2)

These are not uncommon, and can result even from an apparently innocuous combination of medicines. These are more common under following circumstances:
- ❖ In elderly patients who often have decreased glomerular filtration rate and reduced hepatic clearance resulting in impaired drug metabolism.
- ❖ In the presence of multiple comorbidities requiring a large number of drugs to be prescribed (**polypharmacy**).
- ❖ When a patient is being treated simultaneously by more than one service provider (for problems involving different systems) which is not uncommon in the current "specialist era". Each physician/consultant may hand over his own prescription without knowledge of the medicines already prescribed by another physician. Thus it is not uncommon to see a patient consuming more than one nonsteroidal anti-inflammatory drug (NSAID), or multiple vitamin/mineral supplements, or even multiple antibiotics. Further, multiple prescriptions may lead to certain combination of medications which are very likely to result in drug-drug interactions (e.g., oral anticoagulants and antibiotics; NSAIDs and angiotensin-converting enzyme inhibitors).
- ❖ The presenting symptoms may be the result of a drug(s) patient has been taking recently but are thought to be some new medical condition. A common example is administration of benzodiazepines with antiallergic

**Table 10.2:** Important drug interactions (commonly used interacting drugs or those associated with serious consequences are set in color print).

| | Primary drug | Interacting drugs | Potential effects |
|---|---|---|---|
| 1. | **Alcohol** | • Analgesics, antidepressants, antianxiety drugs, hypnotics, antipsychotics | • Increased CNS depression if consumed with alcohol |
| | | • Biguanides (e.g., metformin) | • Hyperactive academia Disulfiram-like reaction |
| | | • Sulfonylurea antidiabetics<br>• Prokinetics (e.g., metoclopramide, mosapride) | • Faster absorption of alcohol with early peak in blood level |
| | | • Metronidazole, ketoconazole | • Disulfiram-like reaction |
| 2. | **Analgesics** | Alcohol, corticosteroids | Increase in risk of gastric mucosal damage, and upper gastrointestinal (GI) bleed |
| | Aspirin, NSAIDs, salicylates Paracetamol | Alcohol (chronic use), barbiturates, isoniazid | Increase in risk of acute hepatic necrosis with large cases of paracetamol |
| 3. | **Anthelmintics** | | |
| | Praziquantel | Carbamazepine, phenytoin | Marked decrease in bioavailability of praziquantel |
| 4. | **Antianxiety drugs** | | |
| | *Alprazolam, benzodiazepine* | Dextropropoxyphene, fluoxetine | Increased sedative effect of antianxiety drugs |
| 5. | **Antiarrhythmic drugs** | | |
| | Adenosine | Beta-blockers, digoxin, diltiazem, verapamil | Potentiation of cardiovascular (CV) effect of adenosine |
| | | Caffeine, theophylline | Reduced CV effect of adenosine |
| | *Amiodarone* | Beta-blockers | Bradycardia, possible cardiac arrest |
| | | Diltiazem, verapamil | Bradycardia, decreased cardiac output |
| 6. | **Antibacterial drugs** | | |
| | Ampicillin, amoxicillin | Allopurinol | Higher risk of antibiotic related skin rash |
| | *Aminoglycosides* | • Amphotericin B | Increased risk of nephrotoxicity |
| | | • Vancomycin "Loop" diuretics | Increased risk of ototoxicity in cases with renal failure |
| | | • NSAIDs | Increased risk of nephrotoxicity, especially in elderly |
| | *Fluoroquinolones* | Antacids, sucralfate, ferrous sulfate | Decreased absorption and bioavailability of quinolones |

*Contd...*

Contd...

| | Primary drug | Interacting drugs | Potential effects |
|---|---|---|---|
| 7. | **Anticoagulants (Coumarins)** | | |
| | a. Drugs that *potentiate* anticoagulant effect | Acute alcohol ingestion Chronic alcoholic liver disease | Warfarin effect may be much increased |
| | b. Drugs that *inhibit* anticoagulant effect | Amiodarone, NSAIDs, aspirin, heparin, broad-spectrum antibiotics, gemfibrozil, lovastatin, dextropropoxyphene + paracetamol, fluoxetine, metronidazole, quinine, chloroquine, quinidine, tamoxifen, thyroid hormones | |
| | | Barbiturates, primidone, carbamazepine, phenytoin, sucralfate, etretinate, estrogens, rifampicin | |
| 8. | **Antidepressants** | | |
| | *Selective serotinin reuptake inhibitors (SSRIs)* | Carbamazepine, lithium, selegiline | "Serotonergic syndrome" (abdomen cramps, myoclonus, contusion, tachycardia, hypertension, sweating, cerebellar signs) |
| | Tricyclic antidepressants | Alcohol Antiparkinsonian drugs, amantadine, anticholinergics | Increased antidepressant effect Increased risk of troublesome anticholinergic effects, especially in elderly |
| | | SSRIs | Marked increase in risk of tricyclics clinical toxicity |
| 9. | **Antiemetic/prokinetic drugs** | | |
| | Cisapride (CP) | Ketoconazole, itraconazole | Increased plasma level of CP, with prolongation of QT interval and risk of ventricular arrhythmias |
| | *Metoclopramide* | Ranitidine | Increased chances of akathisia |
| 10. | **Antiepileptic drugs** | | |
| | Carbamazepine | Fluoxetine | Risk of extrapyramidal symptoms, and serotonergic syndrome |
| | Phenytoin | Alcohol, amiodarone, fluoxetine | Moderate to marked increase in plasma concentration of phenytoin |

*Contd...*

*Contd...*

| Primary drug | Interacting drugs | Potential effects |
|---|---|---|
| | Rifampicin | Moderate to marked decrease in plasma phenytoin concentration |
| Valproic acid | Barbiturates, carbamazepine, phenytoin | Decreased plasma concentration of valproic acid by up to 50% |
| **11. Antihypertensive agents** | | |
| ACE inhibitors | NSAIDs | Possible loss of hypotensive effect |
| | Potassium supplements potassium-sparing diuretics | Increased risk of hyperkalemia, especially in presence of renal impairment |
| Beta-blockers | Diltiazem, verapamil | Increased risk of myocardial depression, and AV blocks |
| | Digitalis glycosides | Risk of bradycardia and AV block |
| All antihypertensive agents | Sympathomimetics, bronchodilators, NSAIDs, oral contraceptives | Control of hypertension may become more difficult |
| **12. Antitubercular drugs** | | |
| Isoniazid | Aluminum hydroxide gel | Decreased absorption of isoniazid |
| Rifampicin | • Antacids, antifungals | • Decreased absorption of rifampicin |
| | • Phénobarbital | • Marked decrease in rifampicin levels |
| **13. Digitalis glycosides** | | |
| (e.g., digoxin) | • Alprazolam | • Increased plasma digitalis levels |
| | • Amiodarone, quinidine | • Marked increase in digitalis levels |
| | • Diuretics | • Hypokalemia with increase in risk of digitalis toxicity |
| | • Diltiazem, verapamil | • Increased risk of AV blocks |
| | • NSAIDs | • Increase in plasma digoxin levels |
| **14. Diuretics** | | |
| Potassium sparing diuretics | ACE inhibitors | Risk of hyperkalemia, especially in cases with azotemia |
| "Loop" diuretics | Aminoglycosides | Combination increases risk of ototoxicity in cases of renal failure |

*Contd...*

Contd...

| | Primary drug | Interacting drugs | Potential effects |
|---|---|---|---|
| 15. | **Endocrine drugs** | | |
| | *Thyroid hormones* | • Carbamazepine | • Increased hormone requirement in hypothyroid patients |
| | | • Ketamine | • Severe hypertension and tachycardia |
| 16. | ***Potassium supplements*** | ACE inhibitors, amiloride, spironolactone, triamterene | Risk of hyperkalemia increases in elderly and azotemic patients |

**Note:** This is not an all-comprehensive list of possible drug interactions.
(ACE: angiotensin-converting enzyme; MAOI: monoamine oxidase inhibitor; NSAIDs: nonsteroidal anti-inflammatory drugs)

drugs and some antidepressants, especially if consumed over a prolonged period. Frightening episodes of confusion and lapses of memory may occur even resulting in antisocial acts. Accordingly, more medications may be prescribed leading to a **"prescribing cascade".**

It is, therefore a good clinical habit *to ask the patient to bring at each visit all medications currently being consumed.* These should be scrutinized for their dosage and frequency of administration, as well as possible side effects, and only then a new set of medicines prescribed.

**Mechanism of drug interactions:** Theoretically, *whenever the pharmacokinetic or pharmacodynamic behavior of one drug is altered by another drug,* it can result in a certain type of drug interaction. In clinical practice however, such reactions become important only when the alteration reaches a threshold where the changed toxicity of the drug is significant. This will of course vary from person to person, and hence *predictability becomes difficult.* Nevertheless, practicing physicians should be aware of important drug interactions which are likely to be of clinical significance, and involving medicines used commonly in one's practice.

It may be pointed out that **drug interactions are not uncommon,** and have been reported to account for as much as 10% of the medical emergencies, or patients' new symptoms, especially if the number of medicines prescribed exceeds 10, and the patient is elderly. The list of drug interactions given at **Table 10.2** is not comprehensive, and is limited to drug-interactions of major clinical significance. It is advised that these serious/life-threatening interactions should be committed to memory (and better still written and displayed on the physician's desk), especially if these involve medicines prescribed commonly by the physician. Drug-induced emergencies can be ascribed to a number of mechanisms:

### *Toxicity*

Such reactions are generally due to either (a) *overdosage* or (b) *prescription errors.*

*Overdosage*

Intentional drug overdose by an individual comprises attempt at suicide. More often, overdosage is unintentional, a common example being digitalis toxicity which may occur in certain situations even when an apparently normal dose is administered. Such instances will include elderly people, associated hypokalemia, or when diuretics are administered simultaneously. In all such cases, the dosage of digitalis needs to be reduced appropriately.

*Prescription/medication errors*

- ❖ A very common cause of wrong medication is *"telephonic prescribing".* This may prove detrimental to the patient in several ways:
    - A medicine pronounced on telephone may be wrongly interpreted by the patient or his relative, or even the nurse. A grave error often quoted in literature was the administration of chloroquine intravenously instead of (intended) chloramphenicol. Not surprisingly the patient died of toxic myocarditis. Another example (which resulted in terrible consequences for the physician) was the advice on telephone to administer an IV antibiotic which was given by the nurse without performing sensitivity test (a standard practice, but not instructed on telephone, or ignored), resulting in severe anaphylactic reaction and death of the patient.
    - An even more common error with *telephonic prescribing* is underrating the gravity of illness, or wrong interpretation of a symptom, with consequent advice of an inappropriate and sometimes dangerous drug, e.g., suggesting NSAID when myalgias are due to dengue fever, or prescribing a sedative when agitation is due to impending hepatic failure, or advising aspirin or some other simple analgesic when acute headache may be the first symptom of a grave illness such as meningitis.
- ❖ Failure to adjust the dose appropriately in patients in whom drug metabolism and elimination are impaired because of *hepatic and/or renal disease* **(Tables 10.3 and 10.4)**. Likewise, medication errors may occur while treating pregnant or lactating mothers. Important drugs which should be avoided or prescribed with caution in such patients are listed in **Table 10.5**.
- ❖ Inappropriate use of the drug may create complications, e.g., beta-blockers or sedatives prescribed to patients of asthma or chronic obstructive pulmonary disease may precipitate respiratory failure; likewise sedatives/tranquilizers advised in hepatic disease may precipitate encephalopathy.
- ❖ Administration of the drug by the *wrong route*, e.g., adrenaline, unless very dilute (1:50,000), may cause death from ventricular fibrillation if given IV, or carbachol given IV may cause collapse; likewise chloroquine given IV (undiluted) is likely to result in cardiac arrest.
- ❖ Poorly written prescriptions which may not be legible/clear to the duty nurse or dispensing chemist, e.g., dispensing quinine in place of quinidine. *It is always a good practice to write name of the medicine in CAPITAL letters.*

## Chapter 10: Iatrogenic Emergencies

**Table 10.3:** Drugs to be avoided/used cautiously in patients with hepatic disease.

| Analgesics | Chemotherapeutic agents |
|---|---|
| • Propoxyphene<br>• ASA/salicylates | • Cotrimoxazole<br>• Erythromycin<br>• Ketoconazole |
| **Antiepileptics**<br>• Carbamazepine<br>• Phenytoin<br>• Valproic acid | • Nitrofurantoin<br>• Sulfonamides<br>• Tetracycline |
| **Antituberculars**<br>• Ethionamide<br>• Isoniazid<br>• Pyrazinamide<br>• Rifampin | **Miscellaneous**<br>• Allopurinol<br>• Benzodiazepines<br>• Gold salts<br>• Methimazole<br>• Phenothiazines |
| **Cardiac**<br>• Amiodarone<br>• Methyldopa<br>• Nifedipine<br>• Perhexiline<br>• Verapamil | |

**Table 10.4:** Drug therapy in renal disease (serum creatinine >2.5 mg%).

| Name of drug | Elimination and metabolization | Half-life (hours) | Dose adjustment |
|---|---|---|---|
| **ACE inhibitors** | | | |
| Captopril | R/H | 2.2.4 ± 0.5 | |
| Enalapril | H | 11.0 | Avoid |
| Lisinopril | R | 12.36 | |
| **Antiarrhythmic agents** | | | |
| Amiodarone | H | 53 ± 24 d | NR |
| Disopyramide | R/H | 6.0 ± 1.0 | Req |
| Lidocaine | H/R | 1.8 ± 0.4 | NR |
| Procainamide | R/H | 3.0 ±0.6 | Req |
| Quinidine | H/R | 6.2 ± 1.8 | NR |
| **Antibiotics** | | | |
| Aminoglycosides | R | 2.3 ± 0.5 | Req |
| Amoxicillin | R | 1.7 ± 0.3 | Req |
| Ampicillin | R | 1.3 ± 0.2 | Req |
| Azithromycin | H/R | 40 | NR |
| Cephalosporins | R/H | 1.0 ± 0.50 | Req |
| Chloramphenicol | H/R | 4.0 ± 2.0 | Req |
| Doxycycline | H | 16 ± 6 | NR |
| Erythromycin | H/R | 1.6 ± 0.7 | NR |
| Imipenem/piperacillin | R | 0.9 ± 0.1 | Req |

*Contd...*

*Contd...*

| Name of drug | Elimination and metabolization | Half-life (hours) | Dose adjustment |
|---|---|---|---|
| Penicillin | R/H | 0.5 ± 0.1 | Req |
| Quinolones | R# | 5.0 ± 1.0## | NR* |
| Tetracycline | R/H | 10 ± 1.5 | a |
| Vancomycin | R/H | 5.6 ± 1.8 | Req |
| **Antiepileptics** | | | |
| Carbamazepine | H/R | 15 ± 5 | NR |
| Phenytoin | H/R | 6–24 d | NR |
| Valproic acid | H/R | 14±3 | NR |
| **Antihypertensives** | | | |
| Clonidine | R | 12 ± 7 | NR** |
| Hydralazine | H/nonrenal | 0.9 ± 0.28 | NR** |
| Methyldopa | R/H | 1.8 ± 0.2 | NR** |
| Prazosin | H/R | 2.9 ± 0.8 | NR |
| Reserpine | H | 4.0–5 | Avoid |
| Calcium channel blockers | H | 1.0–4.04 | NR |
| **Antimalarials** | | | |
| Chloroquine | R/H | 41 ± 14 d | NR |
| Quinine | H/R | 11 ± 2 | NR |
| Mefloquine | Fecal | 20 ± 4 d | NR |
| Artesunate | H | 0.5 (IV route) | NR |
| **Antituberculars** | | | |
| Ethambutol | R/H | 3.1 ± 0.4 | Req |
| Isoniazid | R | 2.1 ± 0.6 | Req |
| Rifampin | H | 4.9 ± 2.0 | NR |
| Pyrazinamide | E | 2–3 | Req |
| **Beta-blockers** | | | |
| Atenolol | R | 6.1 ± 2.0 | Req |
| Labetalol | H | 4.9 ± 2.0 | Req |
| Metoprolol | H | 3.2 ± 0.2*** | NR |
| Propranolol | H | 3.9 ± 0.4*** | NR |
| Sotalol | R | 5–8 | Req |
| **Other drugs** | | | |
| Ciprofloxacin | R/H# | 4.1± 0.9## | NR1 |
| Dexamethasone | H/R | 3.0 ± 0.8 | NR |
| Digoxin | R/nonrenal | 39 ± 13 | Req |
| Dobutamine | H/R | 2.4 ± 0.7 min | NR |
| Dopamine | H/R | 1–2 min | NR |
| Famotidine | R | 2.6 ± 1.0 | Req |
| Isosorbide dinitrate | H | 0.8 ± 0.4 | NR |

*Contd...*

Contd...

| Name of drug | Elimination and metabolization | Half-life (hours) | Dose adjustment |
|---|---|---|---|
| Metronidazole | H/R | 8.5 ± 2.9 | NR** |
| Norfloxacin | R/H | 5.0 ± 0.7 | NR** |
| Norfloxacin | R/H | 5.0 ± 0.7 | NR** |
| Pentazocine | H | 4.6 ± 1.0 | NR |
| Pentoxifylline (oral) | H | 1.6 ± 0.8 | NR |
| Prednisolone | H/R | 2.2 ± 0.5 | NR |
| Ranitidine | R | 2.1 ± 0.2 | Req |

(a: numerator is the principle organ involved; b: dose adjustment according to severity of renal failure; d: days; H: hepatic; NR: not required; R: renal; Req: required; CI: contraindicated)
*Half-life (in hours, unless stated otherwise);
**Except in severe renal failure;
***Increased in hepatic diseases;
¢ Except Ceftriaxone (½ life 8 hours);
# Excretion of Pefloxacin mostly nonrenal (CI in hepatic failure)
##~1/2 life much longer with pefloxacin and lomefloxacin

❖ Failure to prescribe tablet strength, e.g., acitrom dispensed as 4 mg instead of 1 mg tablet may result in serious and even fatal hemorrhage; on the other hand, lower dose tablet than desired may predispose to thromboembolic episodes.

A sound knowledge of the subject and good prescribing habits will help in avoiding most of such medication errors. Besides, *the physician should personally check the medicines periodically* to see there is no discrepancy between the medicines prescribed and actually being consumed by the patient.

## Side Effects (of drugs)

Almost every drug has potential side effect(s). Usually minor and nonconsequential, these can sometimes be serious, and may present as emergencies. Every medical practitioner should therefore be aware of the possible adverse reactions of medicines prescribed, especially when employing less familiar drugs. Some common examples of emergency situations directly attributable to medication include massive gastric bleed following NSAIDs, hypoglycemic coma due to antidiabetic agents, bone marrow depression induced by drugs such as chloramphenicol, butazolidine, amidopyrine, thiouracils, hydantoins, and anticancer drugs, intracerebral hemorrhage following anticoagulants, and renal failure precipitated by aminoglycosides.

## Allergy and Anaphylaxis

Immunologic or allergic reactions may be precipitated by blood products, antisera, radio contrast agents, or a variety of drugs to which the patient may be sensitive. Often temporary and of minor nature (such as urticaria,

**Table 10.5:** Medication in pregnancy.

| Type of medication | Quite safe | Relatively safe | Some risk associated | Contraindicated |
|---|---|---|---|---|
| Analgesics | • Acetaminophen<br>• Codeine*<br>• Meperidine*<br>• Morphine* | | • Salicylates<br>• Indomethacin | |
| Antibiotics | • Ampicillin<br>• Erythromycin<br>• Miconazole<br>• Penicillin | • Amoxicillin<br>• Cephalosporins<br>• Newer penicillins | • Metronidazole<br>• Nitrofurantoin<br>• Streptomycin<br>• Sulfonamides<br>• Trimethoprim | • Aminoglycosides<br>• Chloramphenicol<br>• Tetracycline |
| Anticoagulants | Heparin | Dipyridamole | • Warfarin<br>• Dicoumarol | |
| Antiepileptics | Barbiturates** | Ethosuximide | • Phenytoin<br>• Primidone<br>• Valproic acid | |
| Antihypertensives | • Hydralazine<br>• Methyldopa<br>• Alpha-blockers | • Beta-blockers<br>• Diuretics | • ACE inhibitors<br>• Nifedipine | • Reserpine<br>• Nitroprusside |
| Antimalarials | • Chloroquine<br>• Quinine | • Artesunate**<br>• Mefloquine ** | | |
| Antituberculars | • Ethambutol<br>• Isoniazid<br>• Pyrazinamide | | Rifampin | |
| Bronchodilators | • Aminophylline<br>• Ephedrine | • Beclomethasone<br>• Salbutamol***<br>• Terbutaline*** | Cromolyn sodium | |

*Contd...*

## Chapter 10: Iatrogenic Emergencies

*Contd...*

**Table 10.5:** Medication in pregnancy.

| Cardiac drugs | • Atropine<br>• Digoxin<br>• Lidocaine | • Procainamide<br>• Quinidine<br>• Verapamil | • Diltiazem<br>• Disopyramide<br>• Nifedipine |
|---|---|---|---|
| Diuretics | | • Ethacrynic acid<br>• Furosemide<br>• Hydrochlorothiazide | Bumetanide | Acetazolamide |
| Hypoglycemics | Use only insulin for optimal control; oral hypoglycemics not indicated | | | • Chlorpropamide<br>• Tolbutamide |
| Sedatives | | • Diazepam<br>• Nitrazepam | | • Alprazolam<br>• Chlordiazepoxide |
| Thyroid preparations | Thyroxin | • Methimazole<br>• Propylthiouracil | | Iodide |
| Other drugs | • Ferrous sulfate<br>• Probenecid<br>• Vaccines (polio, tetanus, rabies, influenza) | • Allopurinol<br>• Antacids<br>• Clofibrate<br>• H₂ antagonists | • Clonazepam<br>• Corticosteroids<br>• EDTA<br>• Haloperidol<br>• Lithium<br>• Penicillamine<br>• Phenothiazines<br>• Tricyclic antidepressants | • Antineoplastic drugs<br>• Bromocriptine<br>• Disulfiram<br>• Estrogens<br>• Isotretinoin<br>• Vaccines (rubella, mumps, measles, smallpox) |

\* Avoid prolonged use
\*\*Risk of congenital anomalies is uncertain in first trimester
\*\*\*Quite safe when given by nebulizer/inhaler

(ACE: angiotensin-converting enzyme; EDTA: ethylenediaminetetraacetic acid)

rashes, fever, arthralgias), these may be anaphylactic in type and produce life-threatening emergencies with frightening speed. Exposure to such agents releases a large number of primary and secondary mediators (such as histamine, leukotrienes, prostaglandins, platelet-activating factor, plasminogen, lysosomal enzymes, vasoactive amines), and activates various physiological cascades (such as coagulation cascade, fibrinolytic pathway and kinin system). The result is widespread changes in muscle tone, a leaky vasculature, and tissue edema.

Clinical manifestations will comprise hypotension (due to severe vasodilatation), respiratory distress (due to bronchospasm and upper airway edema), and even noncardiogenic pulmonary edema. Such a clinical picture developing within a few minutes of exposure to the offending drug is classical of anaphylactic reaction. Occasionally, however, these symptoms may be delayed up to 12 hours after administration of the offending drug. For further details, *see* section on "Critical Allergic Reactions", Chapter 11.

A special pattern of drug allergy manifests predominantly as **"vasculitis"**, and is exemplified by clinical syndromes resembling polyarteritis nodosa and systemic lupus erythematosus (SLE). Many drugs have been implicated notably antibiotics, hydralazine, isoniazid and procainamide. Allergic reactions may follow almost any medicament but are more common with parenteral than with oral therapy (e.g., iron therapy), and in patients with allergic diathesis (history of urticaria, asthma, eczema, etc.). Anaphylactic reaction may occur with the very first injection of the drug but is more likely in patients who have already received the offending drug sometimes in the past. The following drugs are particularly likely to produce allergic reaction: sulfonamides, penicillin and other related antibiotics, barbiturates, aspirin, amidopyrine, and some vitamin preparations.

*Prevention and treatment:* Always inquire meticulously about past history of adverse reaction to any drug (and especially about the one to be prescribed), or a history of allergic diathesis. If present, this should be noted prominently on the patient's case file.

*A skin test* (0.2 mL intradermally) must be performed in all patients before starting penicillin (or any other antibiotic parenterally), or any kind of serum therapy, or conducting radiological studies with iodinated compounds. However, it is important to remember that occasionally serious reactions may follow even when skin test is negative. Since anaphylactic reaction may be rapidly fatal, an **emergency tray** containing the following medicines must be readily available whenever injections are to be given intravenously *(especially in domiciliary practice):* (i) a syringe loaded with 1 mL of 1:1,000 dilution of adrenaline hydrochloride, (ii) hydrocortisone hemisuccinate 100 mg, and (iii) pheniramine maleate (Avil) 50 mg. For details, *see* section on "Critical Allergic Reactions", Chapter 11".

## Idiosyncrasy

This implies unusual susceptibility to the pharmacological or even smaller doses of a drug. There may be associated features suggestive of an allergic reaction such as fever and eosinophilia, e.g., fever resulting from antibiotic(s) itself which are being administered to treat pyrexia of uncertain origin *(antibiotic fever)*. Genetic factors may be involved accounting for toxicity from a metabolite that is produced only in such predisposed individuals. Many drugs can cause such idiosyncratic (toxic) reactions including aspirin, amiodarone, chloramphenicol, duloxetine, halothane, streptomycin, oxacillin, isoniazid, pyrazinamide, lamotrigine, carbamazepine, phenytoin, ketoconazole, methyldopa, quinidine, rofecoxib and troglitazone, etc.

# 11 CHAPTER

# Shock Syndrome and Critical Allergic Reactions

## SHOCK SYNDROME

"Shock syndrome" is a clinicopathological state characterized by circulatory failure. Such a degree of decreased perfusion leads to *decreased cellular oxygen delivery and utilization, as well as decreased removal of waste products of metabolism*. Consequently, widespread tissue hypoxia occurs, and functional and structural changes develop in multiple organs. While initially reversible, if identified quickly, with passage of time the risk for pervasive tissue damage increases and mortality is extremely high.

### Pathophysiology

Effective circulation and adequate tissue perfusion is maintained by several factors:
- **Intravascular volume:** Main reservoir of intravascular volume is the *venous capacitance bed,* which extends from medium-sized veins to the vena cava. This reservoir moderates effective circulating volume and venous return *(preload).*
- **Myocardial contractility** along with *cardiac rate and rhythm.*
- **Systemic vascular resistance bed,** *chiefly arterioles,* where vascular smooth-muscle tone (and some other variables) regulate *afterload.*
- **Vast capillary bed** where exchange of fluid and metabolites occurs between the intravascular and extravascular compartments. Significant and characteristic alterations occur in these compartments in different clinical states marked by acute hypotension **(Fig. 11.1)**.

In order to understand the mechanism of "hypotension" in various "shock states", it is desirable to know the *normal physiological determinants of blood pressure (BP):*
- **BP** = cardiac output (CO) × systemic vascular resistance (SVR)
- **CO** = Heart rate × stroke volume (SV)
- **SV** = End diastolic volume – end systolic volume (EDV – ESV). *EDV is linked to venous return (preload) while ESV is related to myocardial contractility.* Normally EDV is about 100 mL in adults while ESV averages 40 mL.

*Blood pressure is thus normally determined by four variables:* (1) SVR, (2) HR, (3) preload (EDV), and (4) myocardial contractility. All types of "shock syndrome" are governed by derangement in one or more of these variables. Initial derangements, which can precipitate a state of shock, are:

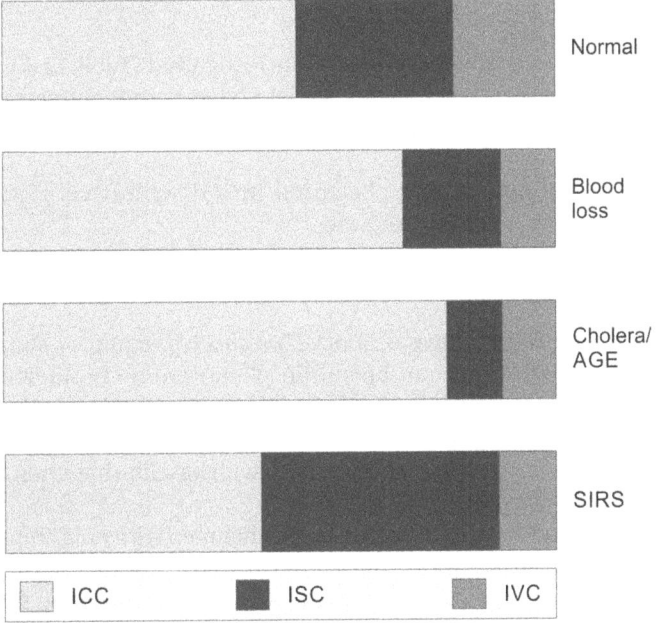

**Fig. 11.1:** Effect of different disease states on size of fluid compartments.
(AGE: acute gastroenteritis; ICC: intracellular compartment; ISC: interstitial compartment; IVC: intravascular compartment; SIRS: systemic inflammatory response syndrome).

- *Vasodilatation* causing a decreased SVR as seen in sepsis, anaphylaxis, neurogenic shock, adrenal crisis, and overdose or overuse of certain vasodilator drugs such as beta-blockers and calcium-channel blockers.
- Severe *brady-or-tachyarrhythmias*
- *Loss of preload volume* with decrease in EDV (from blood or fluid loss)
- *Decreased myocardial contractility* (heart failure) leading to increased ESV.

Initial compensatory mechanisms evoked by above mentioned derangements are as follows:

- Compensatory *tachycardia* in response to vasodilatation with decreased of SVR. Consequently, despite tissue hypoxemia, the skin remains perfused and warm initially.
- *Increase in SVR* following blood or fluid loss (preload) results in increased diastolic BP (narrow pulse pressure), increased sympathetic cholinergic perspiration associated with pallor, thirst, and cool extremities. Further volume loss leads to tachycardia and hypotension.
- *SVR also increases* in response to decreased myocardial contractility resulting in similar symptoms.

If the causative pathology of "shock" continues unabated, these compensatory mechanisms fail leading to irreversible cell death, microcirculation plugging, free radical generation, and eventual death.

## Etiology

Many causes/types of "shock syndrome" are recognized (**Table 11.1**). However, it is important to remember that these various types are not mutually exclusive, and on occasions, more than one factor may be contributing toward the shock syndrome.

Clinically, shock can be classified into distributive, cardiogenic, obstructive, or hypovolemic categories.

## Clinical Presentation

The recognition of early stages of shock *("preshock")* requires a sharp clinical acumen since symptoms can be subtle. There are no biological tests to determine shock, and compensatory mechanisms start to function early. Hypotension is usually the first clinical sign but an anxious patient may maintain blood pressure initially, or patients with baseline hypertension could present as normotensive.

Bedside indicators of low cardiac output include: (i) a feeble/imperceptible pulse suggestive of narrow pulse pressure (which reflects poor stroke volume), (ii) cold extremities; and (iii) delayed capillary refill. On the other hand, *when decrease in SVR is the chief component of shock,* it is often associated with increased cardiac output manifested by wide pulse pressure (chiefly due to reduced diastolic pressure), a full pulse, warm extremities, and rapid capillary refill.

During *early or preshock state,* skin is cool, moist, and pale reflecting elevated SVR seen in cardiogenic and hypovolemic shock. Blood pressure narrows with a slight drop in systolic pressure and rise in diastolic pressure,

**Table 11.1:** Causes (types) of shock.

| Hypovolemic shock | Cardiogenic shock |
|---|---|
| • **Blood loss**<br>➤ Traumatic hemorrhage<br>➤ Non-traumatic hemorrhage (e.g., GI bleed)<br>• **Volume loss**<br>➤ Burns<br>➤ Vomiting/diarrhea<br>➤ Diabetic ketoacidosis<br>➤ Decreased fluid intake | • Dysrhythmia<br>➤ Bradycardias and blocks<br>➤ Tachycardias<br>• Cardiomyopathy<br>• Mechanical |
| | **Distributive**<br>• Anaphylactic shock<br>• Septic shock<br>• Neurogenic shock<br>• Adrenocortical insufficiency |
| **Obstructive shock**<br>• Tension pneumothorax<br>• Pericardial disease<br>➤ Pericardial tamponade<br>➤ Constrictive pericarditis<br>• Massive pulmonary embolism | |

and the patient looks anxious. At this stage blood is shunted preferentially from nonessential sites [skin and gastrointestinal (GI) tract] to heart and brain. After about 25% volume loss in hypovolemic shock, heart rate increases, and renal blood flow decreases resulting in diminished urine output. Patients in cardiogenic shock may develop left heart failure and pulmonary edema. This may be followed by right-sided heart failure with its characteristic features of elevated jugular venous pressure and peripheral edema.

In *full blown shock,* patients become initially agitated and finally apathetic with mental confusion. The patient has hypotension, tachycardia, and tachypnea. Finally *respiratory failure* occurs and *metabolic acidosis* develops due to accumulation of lactic acid from anaerobic metabolism. At the cellular level, tissue oxygen extraction is maximal and is reflected in decreased mixed venous oxygen saturation. Terminally, multiple organ failure develops, and irreversible shock follows unless treatment is aggressive in a well-equipped intensive care unit.

Laboratory studies may show an elevated lactic acid level. This study is a measure of tissue hypoperfusion. If a central line has been placed already, the mixed venous oxygen saturation levels can be used to help differentiate between distributive shock and the other etiologies. In distributive shock, the mixed venous oxygen saturation will be high; whereas, in cardiogenic or hypovolemic shock, the mixed venous oxygen saturation will be low.

## Management

Although possible cause(s) of shock are being explored, the priority should be to maintain vital functions. Patency of airway should be ensured and oxygen administered at high flow rates. If hypoxemia persists, endotracheal intubation, and mechanical ventilation may be required. Varying degree of hypovolemia is common, even in some cases of cardiogenic shock, and *should be suspected as a major contributory factor if central venous pressure (CVP) is less than 8 cm of water.*

In all cases with severe shock, multiple IV access lines should be established and crystalloid infusion of normal saline or lactated Ringer's solution started 30 cc/kg given rapidly over the first 2 hours of presentation. Administration of colloids or albumin has not shown any advantage over crystalloid solutions, which have the benefit of cost and availability. Volume replacement should be guided by CVP maintained in the range of 12-15 cm of water. Bedside diagnostic maneuvers such as the straight leg raise or ultrasound visualization of IVC compressibility are useful markers of the patient's fluid responsiveness and can be used to guide further resuscitation efforts. *Hemorrhagic shock* should be treated with whole blood infusions. Further, appropriate measures must be adopted to achieve rapid hemostasis. *Hypotonic fluids and glucose-containing solutions should be avoided as these diffuse more readily into the interstitial space.*

*Vasopressors* are recommended to improve perfusion pressures and should be delivered through a central access line, rather than a peripheral IV. For most types of shock, including cardiogenic shock, norepinephrine is the first line vasopressor of choice. In cardiogenic shock, dobutamine may be added as an additional inotropic agent.

## Types of Shock

- ❖ Cardiogenic shock (*see* Chapter 1)
- ❖ Hypovolemic shock

This is the most common type of shock met with in general practice and is primarily due to loss of large amount of blood (comprising both red cell mass and plasma) or plasma volume alone due to large extravascular fluid loss as in acute gastroenteritis, diabetic ketoacidosis, burns, pancreatitis, anaphylaxis, etc. Consequently, *circulating blood volume becomes inadequate* resulting in reduced cardiac output, and impairment of tissue perfusion often associated with lactic acidosis.

## Clinical Features

Significant signs and symptoms occur only when circulating volume is reduced by 15–25%. Compensations result in generalized vasoconstriction, and there is *redistribution of blood* with relative ischemia of skin, kidneys, and gut. As shock develops, the closely autoregulated *cerebral circulation is among the first to be affected,* resulting in confusion and restlessness. This is associated with marked sympathetic overactivity with consequent tachycardia, pallor, pale and cold distal extremities, profuse perspiration, and oliguria. *Gastrointestinal tract* is another area, which is affected early, resulting in impairment of mucosal integrity, and even ischemic gut necrosis. Hepatic ischemia is almost universal with elevation of liver enzymes.

 ote

> Though shock is usually diagnosed when systolic pressure falls to 80 mm Hg or less, what is important is both the degree and *rapidity* of drop in BP. Further, in hypertensive patients, a sudden fall in systolic pressure to levels even higher than 80 mm Hg may denote a state of shock.

## Management

First principle in the management of hypovolemic shock is to control the cause of fluid loss by appropriate means. General resuscitative measures should be provided, breathing, and circulation stabilized, and volume loss corrected by crystalloid infusions in the form of isotonic saline or lactated Ringer's solution. Large amount of fluids may be required, and administered guided by CVP. Vasopressors and inotropic agents have little role to play in classical hypovolemic shock. Likewise, corticosteroids are of no use in such cases (unless these are required for treatment of the underlying etiological disease).

# Chapter 11: Shock Syndrome and Critical Allergic Reactions

## Distributive (Vasodilator) Shock

*Reduction in SVR is the main component of hypotension* in this type of shock. Consequently, cardiac output decreases despite adequate circulatory volume. The classical example is *anaphylactoid shock,* which is due to an antigen-antibody reaction and may be induced by any antigenic substance (most notably penicillin G, heterologous therapeutic sera, and iodinated contrast media). It may develop with dramatic suddenness, especially after intravenous administration of the offending agent. However, serious anaphylactic reaction may also follow their use by other routes such as intramuscular, subcutaneous, or even intradermal injection. In most of such cases the anaphylaxis is related to IgE. For further details, *see* section on "Critical Allergic Reactions" described later in this Chapter.

Other causes of distributive shock include **sepsis,** systemic inflammatory response syndrome **(SIRS)** encountered in cases of extensive burns, multiple trauma, severe pancreatitis, and acute adrenal insufficiency. Even "Neurogenic Shock" (vide infra) is physiologically a type of "distributive shock".

## Neurogenic Shock

Acute hypotension and shock can follow *high cervical spinal cord injury* (due to interruption of sympathetic input), but may also follow spinal anesthesia when the administered drugs inadvertently migrate toward cervical region. There is loss of vasomotor tone and *reduction in systemic vascular resistance with consequent hypotension.* Physiologically, both arteriolar and venodilatation occur the latter resulting in decrease in venous return and cardiac output. A characteristic feature is absence of compensatory tachycardia.

## Treatment

Other potential causes of traumatic shock must first be excluded by an aggressive clinical and investigative search. Volume status should be checked and a fluid challenge may be tried (as described already). Vasopressors (dopamine or noradrenalin) may be required, if BP remains unstable after fluid replacement. A reasonable endpoint is CVP 12–14 cm and a mean arterial pressure of 90 mm Hg.

## Obstructive Shock

This term includes cases of shock primarily due to decrease in preload impairing ventricular filling and cardiac output. Classical examples include tension pneumothorax, massive pulmonary embolism, and pericardial tamponade.

All these conditions have been described in earlier sections of the book, and should be managed urgently as already discussed.

## Sepsis and Septic Shock

A brief description of various terms related to "sepsis and septic shock" appears in order:

- ❖ **Bacteremia:** Invasion of blood stream by microbes from an infective source resulting in *positive blood cultures* is termed as bacteremia. *Transient bacteremia* often occurs in healthy people when anatomical mucosal barriers are injured, the classical example being dental extraction or dental scaling. These bacteremic episodes are often due to anaerobes (most common being *B. fragilis*), and are usually *without clinical significance in healthy people.*
  Unlike sepsis, bacteremia *(infection) is not usually associated with liberation of microbial toxins,* which evoke (septic) host response. However, in some cases with comorbid conditions, or in immunocompromised patients, blood stream invasion may result in extremely serious clinical picture with chills and hectic fever ranging up to 104–105°F (40.0–40.6°C). In such cases the differentiation between bacteremia and sepsis becomes blurred. This is especially likely when blood stream invasion is by aerobic gram-negative bacilli (e.g., *E. coli*).
- ❖ **Sepsis** is the conventional term used to describe a clinical state resulting from a *severe* infectious process when *body responses spread beyond the invaded tissue*. A consensus conference has *defined sepsis as "the systemic inflammatory response syndrome* (SIRS) *that occurs during infection".* It is associated with widespread release of inflammatory mediators, which evoke certain host responses associated with symptoms.
- ❖ **Severe sepsis:** This is a more severe form of "sepsis syndrome" in which the body defenses are overwhelmed, and homeostasis may fail. Clinically, *this is associated with dysfunction of one or more major organs.*
- ❖ **Septic shock** refers to a *subset of severe sepsis, which is dominated by hypotension* that persists despite adequate fluid resuscitation. This may or may not be accompanied by altered mental status, hypoxia and oliguria.
- ❖ **SIRS** is a *"sepsis-like" syndrome seen in response to both infectious and noninfectious conditions* such as burns, pancreatitis, or trauma. It is characterized by two or more of the following clinical manifestations: (1) body temperature >38°C or <36°C, (2) heart rate >90/min, (3) tachypnea (respiratory rate >20/min), $PaCO_2$ <32, and (4) white cell count >12,000/$mm^3$, or <4,000 $mm^3$.
- ❖ **Multisystem organ failure (MSOF)** implies progressive cumulative organ dysfunction occurring in critically-ill patients in whom *homeostasis cannot be maintained without outside intervention.* The condition often culminates in death.

# SEPTIC SHOCK

## Etiology

In a continuum of clinical states of "sepsis", "severe sepsis", and "SIRS", septic shock is at the extreme end, and the most serious of all these states. It is mostly associated with gram-negative infections but gram positive as well as fungi and

**Table 11.2:** Microbiology of septic shock (approximate frequency).

| Type of pathogen | Frequency |
|---|---|
| Gram negative | 30% |
| Gram positive | 20% |
| Mixed gram negative/positive | 20% |
| Fungal (Candida) only | 3% |
| Anaerobes | 2% |
| Unknown | 25% |
| **Gram-negative bacteria** | |
| *E. coli* | 25% |
| *Klebsiella* | 20% |
| *Pseudomonas aeruginosa* | 15% |
| *Enterobacter* spp. | 10% |
| *Proteus* spp. | 5% |
| Other gram-negative bacteria | 25% |
| **Gram-positive bacteria** | |
| *Staphylococcus aureus* | 35% |
| *Enterococcus* spp. | 20% |
| Coagulase-negative staphylococcus | 15% |
| *Streptococcus pneumoniae* | 10% |
| Other gram-positive bacteria | 20% |

certain other microorganisms (such as spirochetes) can also result in septic shock **(Table 11.2)**.

The *portal of entry* is usually respiratory or genitourinary tract, but skin, GI tract, and other intra-abdominal/pelvic pathologies are also important. A significant source of sepsis in ICU patients is intravascular catheters. *Approximately half of all cases of gram-negative bacteremia progress to frank septic shock.*

## Pathophysiology

The body's response to microbial invasion is controlled by certain regulatory mechanisms (not discussed here). Sepsis results when such mechanisms are overwhelmed by an *aggressive inflammatory response,* and infection spills over to affect normal, uninfected tissue. Yet, many infected patients with positive blood cultures do not develop sepsis suggesting *it is not infection per se that results in sepsis,* **but rather a combination of infection and host response.** The fact that a sepsis-like syndrome (SIRS) may develop even in response to noninfectious conditions (such as trauma, burns, and pancreatitis) further suggests that other factors, besides infection, play an important role in the pathogenesis of "sepsis syndrome".

The exact *mechanism of organ failure and death* in sepsis is not clear. Autopsy studies do not reveal widespread necrosis. It is likely that much of the organ dysfunction in such patients is the result of "cell hibernation" or "cell stunning" (as occurs during myocardial ischemia). This would explain how patients who survive "sepsis" ultimately make good recovery in baseline functions of the organs involved.

However, it has been observed that about 40% *of people who were treated in the hospital for severe sepsis and then discharged were rehospitalized within 90 days*. The cause of readmission in most of the patients was some preventable condition such as a second bout of infection, kidney failure, heart failure, and some other infections. Various risk factors associated with readmission included age, associated malignancy, one or more procedures during the index hospitalization, and low hemoglobin.

### Clinical Features

Sepsis is a clinical syndrome, and its **diagnosis should not be based on a single laboratory value or positive culture.** *Fever* is the most common clinical feature of sepsis syndrome, but it may be minimal or the absent in elderly, in cases of chronic renal failure, or in patients receiving corticosteroids or nonsteroidal anti-inflammatory drugs (NSAIDs). A few cases (about 10%) may even have *hypothermia.*

Other important features are *tachypnea and tachycardia.* The former is an early vital sign, and its absence coupled with lack of ABG abnormalities should raise questions about the very diagnosis of sepsis. Tachycardia (more than what can be accounted by fever) is also a cardinal sign of sepsis, unless patient has some intrinsic cardiac abnormality, or is receiving beta-blocker drugs.

The *blood pressure* is variable depending upon interplay of several factors. In the initial stage, despite decrease in total peripheral resistance (due to the opening of the precapillary sphincters of most vascular beds), and hypovolemia, the BP may be normal due to increase in cardiac output *(warm shock).* However, with worsening hypovolemia CO begins to fall resulting in hypotension and hypoperfusion of the tissues *(cool shock).* With continued decrease in CO (due to factors such as preload reduction, negative inotropism resulting from anaerobic metabolism, lactic academia, and possibly a circulating myocardial "depressant factor"), selective reduction of blood flow occurs in splanchnic viscera, myocardium, skeletal muscle, and skin, while blood flow to the brain and kidneys is preserved.

*Severe hypotension* (systolic BP <90, or a fall in BP >40 mm Hg) is present in about one-half of all the septic patients at the time of diagnosis, and develops in the remaining one-half during the next few days, if the pathology is not reversed in time. At this stage the skin becomes cold, pale, and moist *(cold shock),* central nervous system (CNS) functions decrease, oliguria develops, and there is *failure of GI functions* in the form of ileus, upper GI bleeding, and "shock liver" syndrome.

## Diagnosis

Frequent occult sites of infection include surgical or trauma wounds, biliary and urinary tracts, retroperitoneal, and perirectal areas. In menstruating women a picture like "toxic shock syndrome" may result from use of tampons. Severe sepsis and septic shock are diagnosed by a combination of some classical features, such as *fever, hypotension, tachypnea, hypoxemia, altered mental status,* and *white cell count >10,000/mm$^3$ or <4,000/mm$^3$.*

*There is no single classical symptom or sign nor a single laboratory test to diagnose severe sepsis. Investigative work should be broad-based, and aimed especially at assessing various vital organ functions.* Besides, complete blood count and routine laboratory studies, estimation of hepatic and renal functions, acid-base studies, and urine analysis, a chest skiagram, and ECG are required in all patients. In selected cases, echocardiography and appropriate CT studies can provide valuable information for locating the site of infection.

The second part of diagnostic exercise requires *identification of the site of infection,* and *causative pathogen(s)* by culture and sensitivity studies of appropriate specimens. As already stated, gram-negative bacilli are the chief cause of septic shock, but more and more cases are being identified with gram positive and fungal infections. Cultures may however, be negative in a large number of cases of sepsis.

## Management

Early recognition of sepsis is the key to the successful treatment of the "sepsis syndrome". Time is of critical value. Severe sepsis and septic shock are labor-intensive and financially costly. The first priority is stabilization of vital functions. Early intubation should be done to decrease the work of breathing and ensure oxygen delivery. CVP monitoring is mandatory to restore circulating volume. Vasopressors are invariably required (dopamine or noradrenalin) with an aim to achieve mean arterial pressure of 90 mm Hg. An arterial line should also be established and periodic arterial blood gases studied. Keys to successful therapy are aggressive volume resuscitation and early appropriate antibiotic usage.

After collecting appropriate samples for culture and sensitivity tests, antibiotics should be administered empirically at the earliest, depending upon possible site of pathology **(Table 11.3)**, and covering a broad spectrum of organisms. A third or fourth generation antibiotic with or without vancomycin is a reasonable choice. A macrolide may be added for chest infection. Additionally, newer generation quinolones and metrogyl should be administered IV, if infection with atypical organisms or anaerobic organisms, respectively, is suspected.

An equally important step is to promptly treat closed space infections (e.g., necrotic gut, deep-seated muscle necrosis, and pyonephrosis), even though surgery may be risky in such desperately ill patients. Dramatic recovery may

**Table 11.3:** Initial (empiric) antibacterial therapy in acutely ill hospitalized patients.

| | Initial clinical diagnosis | Likely pathogens | Preferred drugs |
|---|---|---|---|
| 1. | Intra-abdominal sepsis | Gram-negative bacteria, streptococci, anaerobic bacteria, *Clostridia* | Piperacillin-tazobactam, meropenem, or ticarcillin-clavulanate |
| 2. | Pyelonephritis/pyelonephrosis | *E. coli, Pseudomonas, Klebsiella, Enterobacter* | Ceftriaxone with quinolones |
| 3. | Pelvic inflammatory disease | Gram-negative bacteria, *N. gonorrhea*, anaerobes, *C. trachomatis* | Ceftriaxone with quinolones + metronidazole |
| 4. | Septic arthritis | *S. aureus, N. gonorrheae* | Ceftriaxone |
| 5. | Osteomyelitis | *S. aureus* | Ceftriaxone, cefazolin, nafcillin |
| 6. | Septic thrombophlebitis (e.g., IV tubing, IV shunts) | *S. aureus*, gram-negative aerobic bacteria | Vancomycin with ceftriaxone |
| 7. | Fever in neutropenic patient | *S. aureus, Klebsiella, Enterobacter, Pseudomonas* | Pipercillin-tazobactam or cefepime + vancomycin |

occur following surgical intervention in such cases. It is to be remembered that *unless the source of infection is contained/controlled, the patient cannot be cured of the infective process,* and that death will eventually ensue. Any associated comorbid conditions (especially diabetes, and hepatic and renal dysfunction) should also be properly controlled.

Administration of high doses of corticosteroids does not improve survival in patients with "sepsis syndrome", and may actually worsen prognosis by increasing frequency of secondary infections. *Recombinant human-activated protein C* though very costly, is recommended as an adjunctive treatment for very serious cases of septic shock. However, its use is associated with a significant risk of bleeding, and therefore it should not be used in patients with an elevated baseline risk of bleeding, and with a history of recent surgery or intracranial bleed. If hyperglycemia is present, it should be appropriately controlled with IV soluble insulin to maintain blood glucose level between 80 and 120 mg/dL.

## Prognosis

Many factors adversely affect prognosis in septic shock. These include patients with multiple traumas, extremes of ages, diabetes, and compromised immune status as in patients with cancer, renal failure, and on antimitotic drugs. *Hypothermia* also indicates a grave prognosis with mortality in three-fourths of cases.

## Complications

- Acute respiratory distress syndrome
- Acute renal failure
- Disseminated intravascular coagulation
- Multisystem organ failure

## Summary

- "Sepsis syndrome" represents systemic response to overwhelming infection. SIRS is a sepsis-like syndrome that occurs in response to both infectious and noninfectious conditions. In both, the body responses spread beyond the initial site of pathology.
- The lung and cardiovascular systems are most often involved and manifest features of dysfunction early in the septic process.
- Full blown renal failure requiring dialysis is rare, although oliguria is very common.
- Improving ventilation and oxygen delivery is vital, and often requires (besides supplemental oxygen), intubation and some type of ventilatory support.
- No specific therapy exists for "sepsis syndrome". Principles of management are:
  - An exhaustive search for infectious etiology
  - Drainage of closed-space infections
  - Appropriate antimicrobial therapy
  - Proper organ system support, especially improving hemodynamics and hypoxemia
  - Attention to avoid (i) nephrotoxic drugs, (ii) and nosocomial infections.

# CRITICAL ALLERGIC REACTIONS

Hypersensitivity reactions to various allergens are extremely common in day-to-day practice. While most often such reactions develop slowly and are of little consequence, they can sometimes develop with frightening speed, and present as grave medical emergency. Such reactions are usually acute systemic hypersensitivity reactions, and termed **"anaphylaxis"**. These are due to antigen-induced, *IgE-mediated* release, or formation of chemical mediators. The clinical syndrome results from target-organ involvement by the mediators.

A similar clinical syndrome can also result from *non-IgE-mediated reaction, and is termed* **"Anaphylactoid Reaction"**. Both types of reaction respond to similar emergency treatment.

## Etiopathogenesis

Anaphylaxis can follow IV or oral administration of almost any foreign substance, and are usually IgE-mediated **(Table 11.4)**. Anaphylaxis occurs in

| Table 11.4: Common areas involved in anaphylaxis with common symptoms. ||
|---|---|
| Organ involved | Signs and symptoms |
| 1. Skin | Itching or burning sensation, generalized hives, flushing, or swelling (angioedema) of the affected issues, running nose, and conjunctival swelling |
| 2. Respiratory | Shortness of breath, cough, wheezing, stridor, and hoarseness |
| 3. Cardiovascular | Fast or slow heart rate, myocardial infarction (coronary artery spasm), low BP, even shock |
| 4. Gastrointestinal | Abdominal cramps, vomiting, diarrhea |
| 5. CNS | Confusion, light-headedness, headache, loss of consciousness |
| 6. Miscellaneous | Pelvic pain, loss of bladder control |

individuals who are already sensitized by prior antigenic administration. On initial exposure, the allergen stimulates production of specific IgE antibodies, which bind to mast cells (and basophils). On re-exposure, these antibodies bind antigen and trigger mast cell degranulation with consequent release of several pharmacologically active chemical mediators. *The most prominent of such mediators is histamine* which promotes vascular permeability.

The *immediate effects of these chemical mediators* include capillary leakage, peripheral vasodilation, hypotension, angioedema (localized non-pitting edema), mucus hypersecretion, and bronchospasm. The incidence and severity of anaphylaxis is increased when: (a) allergen is administered parenterally, (b) exposure to allergens is frequent, (c) the patient is receiving beta-blocking drugs, and (d) in subjects with cardiac disease, bronchial asthma and atopy.

### Clinical Features

The *hallmark of anaphylaxis is appearance of manifestations of hypersensitivity in at least two organ systems within 5–30 minutes, if exposure is intravenous, and 2 hours for foods.* The most common areas affected (in descending order) are skin, respiratory, and gastrointestinal tracts, heart and vasculature, and central nervous system **(Table 11.4)**. Usually two or more areas are involved.

Early symptoms and signs include pruritus, cutaneous flushing, nausea, metallic taste, and change in voice. If carefully observed, these may warn of the impending catastrophe. When such nonspecific features are ignored, anaphylaxis may manifest through symptoms and signs in various organs **(Table 11.4)**, and in varying degrees, and combinations. Accordingly, prominent symptoms may include breathing difficulty with a feeling of tightness in the chest and audible wheeze (due to airway obstruction), hoarseness, or stridor (due to laryngeal edema), urticarial eruptions, angioedema, ocular itching, conjunctival injection, chemosis, eyelid edema, and sometimes, nausea, vomiting, abdominal cramping, and diarrhea. Severe cases may develop acute respiratory failure, profound hypotension, vascular collapse, coma, and even death. *The longer the time since the last exposure to the antigen in question, the lower the risk.*

## Diagnosis

The development of a full blown syndrome (vide supra) immediately following a possible triggering agent should at once suggest a diagnosis of anaphylaxis or anaphylactoid reaction. However, difficulty in diagnosis may arise when only a portion of the syndrome manifests, e.g., isolated urticaria, sudden bronchospasm in a known asthmatic patient, or unconsciousness following intravenous administration of an agent.

Several conditions will enter into differential diagnosis in these cases such as vasovagal syncope (bradycardia is a helpful differentiating feature), hypovolemic shock, anxiety reactions (e.g., hyperventilation, globus hystericus), hypovolemic shock, cerebrovascular accident, seizure disorder, etc. A quick relevant history covering questions regarding possible anaphylactic triggers, early symptoms observed, and previous major medical problems will invariably decide the issue. This should be supplemented with a brief physical examination of oropharynx, the skin, the lungs, the heart, and general assessment of vital signs so that suitable remedial measures can be adopted immediately.

## Management

### Emergency Treatment

Regardless of the cause, prompt treatment of anaphylactic and anaphylactoid reactions is mandatory, since death may occur within minutes or hours after the onset of first symptom. The specific drug for all such reactions is epinephrine. It prevents continued mast cell activation, reduces mast cell mediator release, and reverses action of mediators on target tissues. If the hypersensitivity is acute and generalized but not life-threatening (e.g., pruritus or urticaria, laryngeal edema, acute bronchospasm), 0.3–0.5 mL of 1:1,000 epinephrine should be given intramuscularly, well-diluted (IM route is preferable to subcutaneous administration because the latter may have delayed absorption). The injection may be repeated every 5–10 minutes, if the response is inadequate. However, a second injection is required in only about one-third of the cases. Even if the patient has cardiac ailment, he should receive prompt epinephrine treatment but at a reduced dosage, such as 0.1 mL of 1:1,000 solution diluted in 3 mL sterile water.

Minor adverse reactions following epinephrine include headache, palpitation, tremors, and anxiety. If the anaphylactic reaction is severe, with multiple organ system involvement, epinephrine may be given IV 0.3 mL *epinephrine diluted 1:50,000,* but this may be associated with arrhythmias and myocardial infarction.

The patient should simultaneously receive IV fluid resuscitation and be placed in the supine position to improve perfusion.

If there is evidence of respiratory compromise (wheeze, stridor, and hypoxia), the patient should be intubated and placed on a ventilator immediately.

### Adjuncts

*Antihistamines,* though commonly used and assumed to be effective, do not have any effect on bronchospasm or laryngeal edema. The role of *corticosteroids* in combating anaphylaxis is also suspect. However, both drugs may have some prophylactic effect. *Salbutamol* by nebulization may help to resolve bronchospasm that does not respond fully to epinephrine. Although commonly administered, there is little evidence to support the use of glucocorticoids in these patients.

### Subsequent Care

Once the patient's condition is stabilized, the incriminating drug or food or other known triggers should be avoided at all times. Subjects who had severe allergic reaction, and in whom re-exposure cannot be prevented, a course of *immunizing injections* with specific antigen should be recommended. Furthermore, patients in whom the cause of anaphylaxis is uncertain or unavoidable should learn self-administration of epinephrine and keep the injection kit absolutely handy.

# 12 CHAPTER

# Environmental Emergencies

## ACUTE HEAT REACTIONS

### INTRODUCTION

Human body temperature is normally maintained within a narrow range through certain thermoregulatory mechanisms, most important of which are—(a) sodium and water retention, (b) vasodilatation, and (c) increased sweat production facilitating heat dissipation. Acute heat related illness results when these physiological responses are no longer effective or are overwhelmed. A variety of clinical manifestations can occur which are often a continuum, and include (from relatively benign to more severe) "heat edema", "heat cramps", "heat syncope", "heat exhaustion", "hyperpyrexia", and "heat stroke".

Heat illnesses are particularly common in extremely young and old, obese, and those with chronic physical and mental impairments. Though each of these types can be clinically defined, there is often considerable overlap between them. These heat syndromes are particularly likely to occur during the first few days of a heat wave before the body gets acclimatized to the high environmental temperature.

*Hyperthermia of acute heat illness differs from fever of infection* in that the latter results from a resetting of the temperature set point in the hypothalamus. On the other hand, in hyperthermia of acute heat illness the homeostatic mechanism is essentially intact, and therefore antipyretics such as paracetamol are not effective in these cases.

### HEAT EDEMA

Swelling of the hands, feet and ankles may occur during the first few days of high environmental temperature when acclimatization has not yet set in. It is due to vasodilatation and venous stasis resulting in accumulation of interstitial fluid in the lower extremities. It is generally related with periods of prolonged sitting or standing, and is more common in women than men. The edema is not complicated by manifestations of congestive heart failure or lymphatic disease. The condition is purely temporary, and requires no treatment other than simple elevation of the lower limbs and reassurance.

## HEAT SYNCOPE

Fainting may occur suddenly after exertion in extreme heat. Cutaneous and muscular vasodilatation results in redistribution of intravascular volume to the periphery of the body leading to inadequate venous return. This is worsened by volume depletion and prolonged standing resulting in hypotension and inadequate cerebral hypoperfusion. The latter is characterized by dizziness, fainting and syncope. There is often history of engaging in vigorous activity a few hours before the episode. The patient's skin is cool and moist, and the pulse is weak. In general, core temperature is normal or mildly elevated.

**Treatment:** It comprises rest in recumbent position, cooling, and oral rehydration. However, elderly people who experience syncope should be evaluated for arrhythmias, hypoglycemia, and myocardial or cerebrovascular lesions.

## HEAT CRAMPS

Heat cramps are characterized by spasms of voluntary muscles of the abdomen and extremities on exposure to unusually high environmental temperature. There is invariably a history of vigorous physical activity preceding the onset of heat cramps, and the muscles involved are those most heavily used. Muscle fasciculation may be present. Profuse perspiration occurs, and often sweat losses are replaced with water alone. This results in ***dilutional hyponatremia*** and consequent painful muscle contractions. Dehydration is not an important accompaniment until very late stages, and hence, thirst is not a common feature of heat cramps. The core temperature may be normal or slightly increased, and the skin is moist and cool. Vital functions are stable. Laboratory data may reveal hemoconcentration, low sodium, and increased urea and creatinine.

**Treatment:** Heat cramps can be prevented by providing the susceptible subject ***abundant amount of common salt*** dissolved in either water or lemonade drinks. When cramps do develop, administration of salt either intravenous (IV **Normal** saline) or orally **(1/4 to 1/2** teaspoonful in a cup of water) will promptly relieve the symptoms. Supplementary potassium may also be required if hypokalemia is detected. The patient should also be advised rest in a cool environment. Further, continued dietary salt supplementation and physical rest for a couple of days is advisable before resuming strenuous activity.

## HEAT EXHAUSTION

Heat exhaustion is a type of acute heat reaction ***characterized by water depletion,*** heat cramps may coexist if there is associated salt deficiency.

It is also called heat prostration or heat collapse, this is the most common type of acute heat reaction. It is a premonitory syndrome that can rapidly evolve to heat stroke. It differs from heat cramps in that systemic symptoms are present.

Early symptoms are nonspecific and include headache, vertigo, nausea, apathy and fatigue due to dehydration and hypovolemia. Tachycardia, hypotension, and diaphoresis are common. If not immediately relieved, marked weakness and prostration set in as a result of excessive sweating and peripheral vasodilatation. Some cases may even develop cardiac insufficiency and syncope. Heat exhaustion may occur in both physically active and sedentary subjects. However, in contrast to heat stroke, body temperature is normal or only mildly elevated, and mental status is not impaired.

**Treatment:** Complete rest in a cool environment, preferably in recumbent position, and *oral administration of adequate fluids containing glucose and sodium* will provide relief to the patient. IV fluid therapy is required only in severe cases or when the patient is vomiting. Depending upon serum electrolyte values, N. or ½ Normal saline solution may be administered, initially at fast rates. After recovery, the subject should be advised to avoid heavy physical work for a few days.

## HEAT STROKE AND HEAT HYPERPYREXIA

### HEAT HYPERPYREXIA

Hyperthermia and heat stroke occur when *body's thermal regulatory system fails to dissipate adequate amount of heat.* Body temperature begins to rise and may reach levels (41-42°C) where heat stroke becomes imminent. Two broad types of hyperthermia are recognized—(1) *exertional hyperthermia,* and (2) *classic hyperthermia.*

- ❖ **Exertional hyperthermia** may occur sporadically in healthy young individuals engaged in strenuous and prolonged physical activity, especially in hot weather, e.g., marathon runners. In such cases *"sweating mechanism" is normal.*
- ❖ **Classic hyperthermia** can result from a large number of conditions **(Box 12.1)** including heat stroke. In this section, discussion is restricted to heat stroke resulting from protracted exposure to high atmospheric temperature. It is important to remember that heat stroke may occur after only a brief exposure to intensely high environmental temperature; direct exposure to sun is not essential.

The distinction between heat stroke and heat hyperthermia is largely arbitrary. Strictly speaking, the diagnosis of heat stroke should be made only in cases characterized by sudden and profound cerebral disturbances like convulsions or coma. In a tropical climate, however, all cases of heat "hyperthermia" are likely to develop into heat stroke unless quickly treated.

> Box 12.1: Causes of hyperthermia.

- **Disorders of excessive heat production**
  - Heat stroke (external high temperature)
  - Malignant hyperthermia of anesthesia
  - Neuroleptic malignant syndrome
  - Thyrotoxicosis
  - Pheochromocytoma
  - Salicylate intoxication
  - Cocaine, amphetamines, and other drugs of abuse
  - Delirium tremens
  - Status epilepticus
  - Generalized tetanus
- **Disorders of decreased heat dissipation**
  - Heat stroke
  - Occlusive dressings
  - Autonomic dysfunction
  - Anticholinergics
  - Neuroleptic malignant syndrome
- **Disorders of hypothalamic functions**
  - Neuroleptic malignant syndrome
  - Cerebrovascular accidents
  - Encephalitis, meningitis
  - Cerebral malaria
  - Trauma

# HEAT STROKE

Heat stroke results from an *acute breakdown of the normal thermoregulatory mechanism* so that the patient does not sweat normally. In fact, *complete cessation of sweating* (a major source of heat dissipation) occurs in many patients 24–48 hours before the onset of serious symptoms, and this ushers in the acute clinical attack. High humidity, heavy manual work in the presence of high temperature, dehydration, old age, any pre-existing chronic disease, and alcoholism are some of the predisposing factors.

## Pathogenesis

Very high temperatures result in *diffuse damage to endothelial cells in almost all organs,* especially brain, liver, kidneys, heart, lungs and muscles. The intensity of such changes is directly proportional to the duration of hyperthermia. Advanced cases (with prolonged hyperthermia) who may succumb to the illness often reveal features of *disseminated intravascular coagulation* and *acute respiratory distress syndrome.*

## Clinical Features

*High fever, cerebral dysfunction, and absence of sweating* comprise the classical triad of heat stroke. Patient may suddenly develop high fever 105°F

(41°C) or over, though many patients already have, for a couple of days or longer, temperatures of 100–102°F due to some infection or excessive heat. Early symptoms include headache, vertigo, abdominal discomfort, confusion, and fainting. If not promptly treated, the body temperature may suddenly and without any apparent reason shoot to 107°F (42°C) or even up to 110°F (43°C). The skin gets hot and dry, breathing becomes deep and sometimes irregular, marked tachycardia develops with pulse initially full and bounding, but later becoming small and irregular. Marked leukocytosis and albuminuria are frequent and electrocardiogram (ECG) may show significant alterations in ST-T complex.

*Neurological features characteristic of heat stroke develop* in more severe cases and comprise delirium, convulsions and rapid loss of consciousness. Focal neurological signs are unusual, and when present suggest some other acute neurological disorder. Occasionally, a bleeding tendency dominates the clinical picture. In the most severe cases, death may occur within a few hours due to acute renal failure, peripheral circulatory failure, or multiple organ failure.

## Investigations

Laboratory workup may reveal a variety of abnormalities, mostly nonspecific. These include leukocytosis, increased hematocrit, hypoglycemia, hepatic and muscle enzyme abnormalities, renal dysfunction, hypocalcaemia, hypo- or hyperkalemia, and metabolic acidosis. Serum transaminases levels can rise to tens of thousands although complete recovery usually ensues if treatment is initiated quickly. Hypoprothrombinemia, hypofibrinogenemia, and thrombocytopenia may be present. ECG abnormalities occur frequently and include ST-T changes suggestive of myocardial ischemia.

## Diagnosis

Confronted with a hyperthermic patient several conditions enter into differential diagnosis **(Table 12.1)**. Most valuable diagnostic aspects are a thorough history and the circumstantial evidence leading to hyperpyrexia. A real challenge to diagnosis is the possibility of cerebral malaria. History of living in or travel to endemic areas, examination of peripheral blood film, and rapid tests for malaria antigen can be of help. However, in any doubtful case, parenteral antimalarial therapy should be instituted as described in the section on "Cerebral Malaria" (*see* Chapter 8).

## Management

Immediate goal of treatment should be *rapid cooling* and cardiovascular support. The aim should be to achieve a core temperature of 39°C/102°F within 1 hour.

**Table 12.1:** Differential diagnosis of hyperthermia.

| Diagnosis | Etiology/common precipitating factors | Diagnostic features |
|---|---|---|
| Malignant hyperthermia | General anesthesia muscle relaxants | Muscle rigidity, hypotension, hypercarbia |
| Neuroleptic malignant syndrome | Neuroleptic medication (e.g., haloperidol, phenothiazines) | Extrapyramidal and autonomic dysfunction |
| Delirium tremens | Ethanol withdrawal | Agitation, tremors, heightened autonomic activity |
| Status epilepticus | Stoppage or sudden decrease in antiepileptic drugs | Tonic-clonic movements, rigidity |
| Cerebrovascular accidents (usually hemorrhage) | Severe hypertension, atherosclerosis | High fever following coma, CT brain scan diagnostic |
| Meningitis | Acute bacterial infection | Comparatively lower fever, neck rigidity, lumbar puncture |
| Sepsis | Compromised host, indwelling catheters, overwhelming infection | Appropriate clinical setting, usually high white cell count with shift to left |
| Thyroid storm | Poorly treated thyrotoxicosis with superadded acute surgical stress/medical disorders | Thyrotoxic features, high BP, agitation, thyroid tests diagnostic |
| Pheochromocytoma | Adrenal medulla and chromaffin tumors | Hypertension, increased vanillylmandelic acid (VMA)/ metanephrines |
| Cerebral malaria | *Plasmodium falciparum* infection | High index of suspicion in malaria prone subjects, positive blood film |

- ❖ **Airways and ventilation:** An adequate airway and ventilation should be maintained, and arterial blood gas levels monitored. Supplemental oxygen at high flow rates by mask or nasal cannula is beneficial.
- ❖ **Temperature reduction:** *Immediate measures* should aim at lowering of body temperature by *physical means* (not antipyretics). Conventional method is *"evaporative cooling"* which implies moving the patient to the nearest cool place, under a revolving fan, and removing most of the clothing. The *body should be placed in the lateral decubitus* (to expose maximal skin surface to the air), loosely wrapped in a cool wet sheet and frequently sprinkled with cold water (20°C). Additionally, ice packs should be applied to the head and the limbs, and the skin massaged with ice wrapped in cloth. The latter prevents cutaneous vasoconstriction (thereby accelerating heat loss), and also increases circulation between

the cold peripheral blood and overheated brain and other viscera (helping to reduce internal "core" temperature).

If the above measures fail to lower temperature rapidly, a more *intensive approach* will be required. Immersion in ice-water bath is probably the best way but may not be practical. Ice-water gastric lavage and/or peritoneal lavage with cold potassium-free dialysate, 2 L every 10–15 minutes are very effective to reduce core temperature.

When the rectal temperature drops to 39°C (102.2°F), temperature lowering measures should be discontinued to avoid hypothermia. Since hyperthermia may recur due to thermoregulatory instability, temperature should be monitored for 24 hours. Care should also be taken to prevent excessive hypothermia which may result in collapse.

Advanced techniques to reduce core temperature are based on "intravascular heat exchange" principle, and involve either hemodialysis or heat exchange catheters.

- **Drugs:** Hypothalamic set-point is not elevated in heat stroke (or environmentally induced hyperthermia) and, therefore, aspirin and acetaminophen have not been found to be helpful. They may even worsen coagulopathy and liver damage. Shivering is sometimes a problem, and can be controlled with benzodiazepines.

**Preserving renal function:** Adequate urine output should be maintained (30–50 mL/h) by proper hydration with ***rapid IV fluid administration.*** Massive fluid therapy is, however, not required and in most patients 1000–1500 mL over first 12 hours should be adequate. Urine output should be monitored by an indwelling urinary catheter, and if insufficient, mannitol infusion should be considered.

Blood pressure should stabilize with IV infusion of crystalloid solutions but some cases may require inotropic agents (CVP monitoring can be very helpful). Alpha-adrenergic drugs are contraindicated because they produce vasoconstriction and decrease heat exchange; therefore dobutamine may be preferable to dopamine as an inotropic agent because it does not have the alpha-adrenergic renal effects at rapid rates of infusion. ***Corticosteroids*** have been recommended with a view to reduce cerebral edema often present in such cases, but are best avoided. If oliguria is persistent, ***hemodialysis*** may be required.

In favorable cases the patient recovers completely. ***Indicators of bad prognosis*** are extreme hyperpyrexia (rectal temperature >42°C/107.6°F, persistent coma after cooling, markedly elevated hepatic transaminases, renal failure, and hyperkalemia associated with extensive rhabdomyolysis.

### Complications
- Acute renal failure
- Hepatic circulatory failure
- Brain cell damage, usually cerebellar
- Rhabdomyolysis
- Disseminated intravascular coagulation

- ❖ Cardiac arrhythmias
- ❖ Myocardial infarction

# HYPOTHERMIA

## ETIOLOGY

Systemic hypothermia is defined as a state in which the **core temperature is <36°C**. It is an uncommon medical emergency that occurs when external cold challenge overwhelms the body's capacity to generate and conserve heat. Hypothermia may result either from accidental exposure to very low ambient temperature (20°C or less) or when there is altered homeostasis such as in patients with acute cerebrovascular lesions, myocardial infarction, cirrhosis liver, pneumonia, renal failure, hypoglycemia, and severe infections.

Other risk factors include old age, chronic alcoholism, debilitating illness, hypopituitarism, myxedema, and administration of large amounts of refrigerated stored blood without rewarming. Alcohol indulgence and use of sedative-hypnotic or antidepressant drugs are some other predisposing factors.

## CLINICAL FEATURES

Harmful effects of hypothermia can start appearing when the core temperature (usually measured as rectal temperature) drops below 36°C. Such low temperatures alter many physiological functions with consequent decrease in oxygen consumption and slowing of gastrointestinal motility, peripheral nerve conduction, and respiration. Myocardial repolarization is altered (with ST-T changes), and cardiac arrhythmias may occur. The severity of symptoms is related to the intensity of hypothermia.

In a **mild case** [temperature between 34 and 36°C (93.2–96.8° F)] patients will exhibit tachycardia, tachypnea, and shivering. When hypothermia is **moderate** (rectal temperature between 30 and 34°C), circulation slows down leading to tissue hypoxia and capillary damage, thereby causing leakage of plasma, and hemoconcentration. The **hematocrit** increases by 2% for every 1 degree decline in temperature. Varying degree of **metabolic acidosis** is invariable, and is due to multiple factors such as lactate generation from decreased tissue perfusion and shivering, impaired hepatic metabolism, and impaired acid excretion. **Coagulopathy** often develops, and hypercoagulability may result in thromboembolism at multiple sites. In **more severe** hypothermia, (temperature <30°C) patients may appear to be dead to where with fixed dilated pupils, loss of other reflexes, and coma.

## DIAGNOSIS

Because lowered body temperature is the sole finding in these patients, and clinical presentation may be diverse, the diagnosis often depends on awareness of such a complication. It is mandatory to record rectal temperature by a chemical (or preferably electronic) thermometer whenever hypothermia is suspected. However certain laboratory investigations are unique to hypothermia and can be of great help. These include hypoglycemia, hypomagnesemia, and hypophosphatemia. **Metabolic acidosis and hemoconcentration** have been mentioned already. White cell count may not increase (and fever may be absent) even in the presence of infection since migration of neutrophils, and bacterial phagocytosis are impaired in hypothermia.

Alterations in *serum potassium* are common, and therefore potassium levels should be checked periodically (ECG changes of hypo- and hyperkalemia are often masked by hypothermia). Blood glucose is usually within normal range, and persistent hyperglycemia should suggest pancreatitis or diabetic ketoacidosis.

ote

> For this reason a hypothermic patient should not be declared dead until aggressive rewarming procedures have been employed and body temperature elevated to 36°C. Hence the motto "no one is dead until warm and dead". Survival is possible even after prolonged hypothermia because cardiac and cerebral functions may be long protected in this state.

## MANAGEMENT

*Principles of management* of hypothermic state are—(1) cardiopulmonary resuscitation, (2) correction of fluid, electrolyte and glucose abnormalities, (3) rewarming, and (4) treatment of underlying conditions. As a first aid measure the victim of hypothermia should be wrapped in dry, warm blankets at the scene of discovery, and transported to the nearest hospital.

- **Cardiopulmonary resuscitation:** Patency of airways, adequate ventilation should be ensured and oxygen administered at high flow rates. Cardiac status should be assessed by checking pulse for at least 1 minute. If cardiac rhythm is irregular, attempt should be made to correct arrhythmia by drugs or cardioversion. Attempts at defibrillation are usually unsuccessful at temperatures below 30°C (86° F).
- **Restoration of fluid, pH and electrolyte balance:** All patients of hypothermia with altered sensorium should receive IV thiamine 100 mg, naloxone 2.0 mg, and glucose 25 g. Since damage to capillaries by hypoxia allows escape of plasma into the tissue with consequent hemoconcentration and risk of multiple arterial thromboses, blood volume should be expanded with IV infusions of D5W, isolytes and plasma expanders such as low molecular weight dextran. Ringer's solution should be avoided because lactate is not metabolized efficiently by cold liver. If hypotension persists dopamine infusion in low doses is indicated.

Metabolic acidosis is common, and is in fact an important determinant of overall prognosis. When acidosis is marked (pH <7.0) 50-100 mL of 7.5% (45-90 mEq) of sodium bicarbonate should be given IV. Further doses are administered according to results of serial arterial blood gas studies. Both hypo- and hyperkalemia may occur, and serum potassium levels need regular monitoring.

❖ **Rewarming:** The sheet-anchor of treatment of hypothermia is "rewarming", but its aggressiveness will depend upon the intensity of hypothermia. When mild (rectal temperature >34-36°C) and the patient previously healthy, *"passive external rewarming"* is all that may be required. This comprises nursing the patient in a warm (34-36°C) room, providing a warm bed, blankets, and may be additional warm packs.

Patients with ***more severe hypothermia*** (core temperature <34°C) require ***"active rewarming"*** since they do not have the thermoregulatory shivering mechanism.

***Active rewarming can be external or internal.*** The former comprises exposing the patient to forced hot air (37-42°C) or radiant heat, and providing heating blankets. Heat should be applied to thorax only, and extremities left vasoconstricted to prevent sudden vasodilatation and drop in blood pressure. ***Active internal (core) rewarming*** is necessary in patients with more severe hypothermia, and can be achieved by several measures—(i) rewarming of the airways by humidified warm air/oxygen (~ 40°C) through a face mask or endotracheal tube, (ii) peritoneal dialysis with warm fluid (40-45°C), (iii) heated-fluid irrigation of the colon or stomach, (iv) administration of warm infusions (~ 40°C) especially when massive fluid replacement is required, and (v) extracorporeal warming (arteriovenous, cardiopulmonary, or venovenous bypass) which is the most efficient means of rewarming.

Since active rewarming may worsen hypovolemia and organ perfusion by shifting large amounts of blood to the periphery, it is important that adequate intravascular volume, cardiac support, acid-base balance, and proper oxygenation are established before attempts at raising body temperature.

❖ Appropriate measures should be instituted to treat and control the basic disease. Antibiotics are generally not required unless there is evidence of past infection, or pressing situations exist (e.g., elderly subjects, trauma, serious comorbidities such as diabetes, immunocompromised state). Corticosteroids can also be useful and should be given as hydrocortisone 100 mg IV every 4-6 hours for first 24 hours.

## MEDICAL EMERGENCIES IN THE AIR

### INTRODUCTION

During the past few decades air travel has become an increasingly common, and often advice is sought regarding fitness to undertake air journey. Factors affecting safety of air travel include not only the nature of subject's illness, but also the duration of flight, pressurization, and availability of supplementary oxygen. All these factors as well as other related medical aspects of air travel are discussed hereunder.

Most commercial aircraft cruise at altitudes between 22,000 feet (6,706 m) and 44,000 feet (13,411 m) on domestic as well as international flights. If unprotected, the occupants would become unconscious within 30 seconds and dead 6–8 minutes later due to lack of oxygen. However, this does not happen since all modern aircraft cabins are pressurized between 5,000 and 7,000 feet. While this ensures sufficient protection against acute severe hypoxia, nevertheless, the passengers and the crew are still exposed to reduction in $PaO_2$ to about 70 mm Hg (oxygen saturation about 92%) because of fall in atmospheric pressure. *Pressurization of the cabins to sea level would eliminate the problem of hypoxia, but this is not cost-effective.*

Two types of adverse factors operate during air travel—(1) hypoxia, and (2) alteration in body pressures from altitude.

## ADVERSE EFFECTS OF ALTITUDE HYPOXIA

Earliest effect of hypoxia (which may manifest even at 5,000 feet) is depression of functions of rods in the retina, resulting in decreased proficiency of night vision. **Acute altitude hypoxia,** however, principally affects cardiopulmonary system and the brain. *Hyperventilation is the primary physiological response* resulting in tachypnea, respiratory alkalosis, and decreased resting $PaO_2$ of 50–60 mm Hg (arterial saturation 80–90% at 8,000–10,000 feet). Such a degree of hypoxia significantly *increases pulmonary arterial pressure* and may push predisposed patients into right heart failure. Cerebrovascular features are minimal, generally subtle (between 5,000 and 8,000 feet), and comprise altered perception, impaired judgment and increased fatigability. Sometimes, headache, nausea, insomnia, altered personality, and even seizures may occur.

**Aggravating factors:**
- In the presence of *pre-existing cardiopulmonary disorders,* acute altitude hypoxia may induce increased airway resistance thereby further worsening hypoxia. This will be enhanced by any exertion at altitude since it will increase oxygen demand. Consequently, any pre-existing cardiac dysfunction or pulmonary hypertension is likely to worsen resulting in arrhythmias and right ventricular strain.
- **Smoking** in any form increases carboxyhemoglobin levels in the blood with consequent decrease in oxygen carrying capacity of circulating hemoglobin, further worsening hypoxia. Likewise alcohol (ethanol metabolism) results in low respiratory quotient which further decreases $PaO_2$.
- **Other factors:** Anemia, sedation, antihistamines, and deep sleep, all tend to increase hypoventilation and ventilation-perfusion mismatch resulting in further hypoxemia at high altitude.

# ADVERSE EFFECTS OF PRESSURE CHANGES

At an altitude of about 6,000 feet, all gases in the body increase in volume by about 30% because of reduced atmospheric pressure. Air trapped within any of the body cavities also undergoes such a physical change. This may be of little consequence in normal persons, but patients with certain diseases (e.g., acute otitis media, acute sinusitis, pneumothorax), or those recovering from major thoracic or gastrointestinal surgery, or patients who have air trapped within the cranium (e.g., following air encephalography) are particularly at risk. They should not be permitted air travel for at least 2 weeks after the episode.

# CLINICAL CONSIDERATIONS

Air travel is permitted for most ambulatory non-hospitalized persons with stable chronic disease. However, during jet travel, even normal people are likely to experience an *"in-flight syndrome"* due to certain degree of hypoxia. This syndrome comprises dizziness, fatigue, headache, tinnitus, nausea and lethargy, and may last up to 12 hours after landing. Some of the predisposing factors for this syndrome include old age, poor physical conditioning, fatigue, recent insomnia, and emotional stress.

The most common in-flight emergencies relate to cardiovascular, respiratory and nervous systems. Such emergencies tend to occur during air travel (especially during lengthy flights) because of certain predisposing factors such as hypoxia, immobility, stress and exhaustion imposed by air travel, problems with documentation and baggage at airports, and sometimes, prolonged period of waiting at air terminals. Some of the important diseases likely to be adversely affected by air travel **(Table 12.2)** are as follows:

- ❖ **Cardiovascular diseases:** As a rule, patients with acute myocardial infarction or unstable angina should avoid air travel for 3-4 weeks. However, in emergency situations, travel can be permitted with supplemental oxygen facility unless patient is in shock, or has unstable rhythm or heart failure. Such patients should have cardiac functions assessed by echocardiography, and air journey preferably deferred if left ventricular ejection fraction is very poor (< 25%).
- ❖ **Respiratory diseases:** Patients of chronic obstructive pulmonary disease (COPD) with vital capacity <50% of predicted value, and maximum voluntary ventilation <40 L/min should avoid long air journeys especially if their arterial $PaO_2$ is <67 mm Hg at sea level. If traveling is a must, they should have supplemental oxygen while flying. More stringent testing comprises a preflight hypoxia-altitude simulation test (HAST). In this test the subject breathes a hypoxic breathing mixture (containing 15% oxygen) to simulate an anticipated altitude hypoxia (about 8,000 feet) while blood oxygen levels are monitored serially by oximetry. Such tests cannot, however, be employed routinely in clinical practice. As a practical guideline, patients with COPD should be permitted air travel only if they

**Table 12.2:** Important contraindications for air travel.

| 1. | Cardiovascular diseases | • Congestive heart failure (>grade II/IV)*<br>• Recent myocardial infarction (within 3 weeks)<br>• Post CABG (within 3 weeks)<br>• Unstable angina<br>• Uncontrolled tachyarrhythmia<br>• Severe valvular heart disease<br>• Uncontrolled severe hypertension |
|---|---|---|
| 2. | Cerebrovascular diseases | • Recent (within 2 weeks) cerebral infarction<br>• Intracranial hemorrhage |
| 3. | Pulmonary | • Pneumothorax<br>• Pulmonary cysts<br>• Severe emphysema/hypoxemia of any etiology |
| 4. | Miscellaneous | • Recent surgery on eye, thorax or abdomen (within 2–3 weeks)<br>• Deep venous thrombosis<br>• Agitated or psychotic patients<br>• Severe anemia (hemoglobin < 8g/dL)<br>• Pregnancy (unless < 8 months) |

(CABG: coronary artery bypass grafting)
*New York Heart Association classification

are able to walk at least 100 m without becoming breathless. Presence of pneumothorax is an absolute contraindication for air journey.

Patients with bronchial asthma adequately controlled can fly without restriction but should carry with them their usual requirement of medicines including handheld inhalers and a nebulizer (preferably battery-operated).

- **Neurological diseases:** Patients with recent cerebral infarction should avoid air travel till about 4-6 weeks after the stroke. Elderly patients with severe atherosclerosis may suffer a setback in their mental faculties, resulting in confusion and irrational behavior. In general, patients who become confused or agitated during night are likely to develop similar symptoms during air travel. Such patients should preferably be accompanied by a relative or friend.

  *Epileptics are more liable to seizures during flight* because of such factors as hypoxia, fatigue and stress associated with air journey. Long flights involving several time zones may disrupt their drug schedule. They should be advised to adhere to their home schedule and take their medicines regularly till they reach the destination. Poorly controlled epileptics should be accompanied by a companion, and have their medication increased temporarily, beginning about 24 hours before the flight. They must avoid alcohol immediately before and during air journey.

- **Diabetes mellitus:** Diabetic patients on antidiabetic drugs often need advice regarding their therapy during air travel, especially if the journey is long. Such patients should generally stay on their home schedule both in respect of diet as well as medication. Air hostesses may be informed in advance regarding their meal time. They should adjust to the local, time only after reaching the destination. As a matter of additional safety, they should carry a glucometer with them to assess blood sugar level in an emergency situation.

❖ **Other conditions:** *Severe anemia* (hemoglobin <8.0 g/dL) is generally a contraindication to flying. If blood has been transfused, 48 hours should elapse before air travel is undertaken. It may be best to avoid flying when in advanced stage of *pregnancy* since problems related to delivery may arise unexpectedly during flight. From the point of newborn also, flying during first 48 hours of life is not safe since all the alveoli will not have expanded at birth. A degree of ventilation-perfusion inequality will then be present which would be worsened by high cabin altitude.

Many patients are prone to develop *travel/motion sickness*. This can be largely prevented by antiemetics administered orally 3–4 hours before the flight, and repeated at suitable intervals thereafter, if required.

**General measures:** Since smoking aggravates hypoxemia, smokers should avoid smoking a few hours before air journey. In fact a heavy smoker may already be at an equivalent altitude of several thousand feet while walking to the aircraft. Ethanol ingestion also worsens hypoxemia. Air carriers must be intimated in advance about possible oxygen requirement of such patients.

ote

> Patients on regular medicines should be advised to remember to carry their emergency medicines in their hand luggage so that they are not embarrassed in the flight to find that their medicines are locked up in the cargo hold.

# NEAR DROWNING

## GENERAL CONSIDERATIONS

*Near drowning* implies sudden asphyxiation following immersion in a liquid medium (invariably water). Additionally, there are important hemodynamic and biochemical disturbances which contribute to morbidity and mortality from drowning.

Consequent upon submersion, breath holding occurs for a variable length of time till the accumulating $CO_2$ stimulates the respiratory center sufficiently enough to force an inspiration resulting in inhalation of large quantities of water. Aspiration invariably seems to be present; ***"dry drowning"*** probably occurs with pre-aspiration cardiac arrest or with post-aspiration shifts of the aspirated fluid from the alveoli into the circulation. Pulmonary edema and electrolyte disturbances occur in both fresh water and sea-water drowning though mechanisms differ in the two situations.

**Chapter 12:** Environmental Emergencies

**Comorbidities** leading to drowning include intoxication, trauma (especially in shallow water and high-speed injuries), coronary artery disease, arrhythmias, seizures, hypoglycemia, and hypothermia.

## CLINICAL FINDINGS

Cases with near drowning may be awake, semiconscious, or unconscious. Consciousness may return spontaneously or following brief cardiopulmonary resuscitation, and both situations predict a good prognosis. Tachypnea, cyanosis, and wheezing are invariable, and there may be pink froth coming out from nose and mouth indicating pulmonary edema. Cardiovascular abnormalities are common and include tachycardia, arrhythmias, and hypotension. Circulatory collapse and cardiac arrest are not unusual.

### Laboratory Investigations

In patients surviving the immediate onslaught there may be acidosis, both metabolic and respiratory, and electrolyte abnormalities affecting levels of potassium, calcium, and magnesium. Chest X-rays will initially show aspiration of fluids and pneumonitis, but later films may reveal extensive pulmonary edema and acute respiratory distress syndrome.

Surviving patients may be left with hypothermia which should always be anticipated. Rewarming the patient with forced air heating is quite effective. Hypothermia associated with cardiac arrest is an indication for extracorporeal rewarming and cardiopulmonary resuscitation. Such efforts should be continued even when the patient has fixed dilated pupils, especially in infants and children in whom the brain is protected by hypothermia.

## MANAGEMENT

The victim should be immediately brought out of water in prone position, laid supine upon the ground, and mouth-to-mouth respiration started, without wasting even a second (after quickly clearing the oropharynx manually). Time should never be wasted in trying to drain water from the lungs (as this is not possible), or in loosening the clothes, or in examining the pulse and heart to determine whether the patient is alive or not. Such measures may, however, be resorted to if the help of another person is available. Uninterrupted mouth-to-mouth breathing must continue till the patient is transported to the nearest hospital, even if the patient appears to be virtually dead. If there is associated circulatory arrest, it should be managed simultaneously (see section on "Cardiac Arrest", Chapter 1).

In the hospital, the airway should be cleaned and proper ventilation ensured by early intubation. Oxygen therapy at high flow rates and positive end-expiratory pressure ventilation should be started to maintain $PaO_2$ >90. $FiO_2$ should not exceed 0.6 to prevent barotrauma and oxygen toxicity. If the patient is recovering, fluid and electrolyte disturbances should be assessed and suitably corrected. Hypovolemia should be corrected by IV infusions under CVP monitoring. When hemolysis is the predominant feature (as in fresh-water drowning), packed cells or whole blood should be transfused. Hypotension, if marked, will warrant vasopressors; IV corticosteroids may also be required. Furosemide 60–80 mg IV is the drug of choice if pulmonary edema is suspected. In all cases, it is also essential to administer broad-spectrum antibiotics for the prevention and treatment of aspiration pneumonia.

## ELECTRICAL INJURIES

### INTRODUCTION

Electric shock implies flow of current through the body while voltage represents the pressure behind the current flow. The severity of electric injury is influenced by the type of current as well as the degree of voltage involved, its duration, and the pathway of the current through the body. Direct current is less dangerous than alternating current (AC) used in most houses. AC results in tetanic muscle contractions that may lead to inability of the victim to separate from the source, prolonging contact.

Electric shock may produce momentary or prolonged loss of consciousness. The most serious effects occur in low resistance pathways such as muscular and vascular pathways. The maximum brunt is on the heart and the central nervous system. Ventricular fibrillation and asystole are the most serious cardiac effects, but ectopic beats and atrial fibrillation may also be observed. Neurological features include seizures, deafness, blindness, and aphasia. Even acute bulbar paralysis may occur with cardiac and/or respiratory arrest. Major thermal burns at the points of entrance and exit (of the current) follow a powerful shock, and the striated muscles in the pathway of the current are damaged leading to compartment syndromes. Rhabdomyolysis is a possibility. Instantaneous death often occurs when voltage is over 350.

If the patient survives the immediate impact of electric shock, he may be found in a state of confusion and disorientation. Orthopedic complications are not uncommon. Complete recovery may finally ensue or the patient may be left with bizarre neurological deficits and also visual disturbances.

### MANAGEMENT

The contact between the victim and the current should be snapped immediately, but the rescuer must be protected. The simplest method is to switch off the current quickly when possible, or sever the wire by a dry wooden-handled axe. If neither is immediately possible, the victim should be carefully dragged away with a dry wooden pole. If possible, this should be done by quickly padding the hands with thick layers of dry cloth or paper (non-conductive material). No attempt should ever be made to pull or push the patient manually as this often leads to death of the rescuer.

The rest of the treatment is largely resuscitative and symptomatic. If the victim is not breathing, basic cardiopulmonary resuscitation should be started at once, and continued till spontaneous ventilation is restored or the patient reaches hospital. In the hospital, intensive resuscitation measures may be required including assisted ventilation, fluid and electrolyte regulation, and treatment of shock (if present) by vasopressors. Antibiotics should be given to combat infection in the burnt areas; these will also require surgical measures for proper management.

## HIGH ALTITUDE SICKNESS

High altitude sickness, also called *"acute mountain sickness (AMS)"*, is a broad group of disorders which affect unacclimatized persons acutely exposed to low partial pressure of oxygen at high altitudes. At one end of the spectrum is air travel in *unpressurized aircraft* when it may manifest at altitude as low as 5,000 feet though in *pressurized aircraft* most people can ascend to 8,000 feet (2,400 meters) without difficulty. At the other extreme is rapid exposure to altitudes above 18,000 feet (5,500 meters) reached by expedition trekkers, or hike to a high altitude mountain resort, or during rapid transport/ascent of army personnel to such high altitudes during wars.

It is hard to determine who will be affected by altitude sickness, but *predisposing factors* include physical deconditioning, obesity, elderly persons, chronic smoking, and history of asthma. *Contributory factors* include rate of ascent, altitude attained, and amount of physical activity at high altitude as well as individual susceptibility.

## ■ CAUSES

With increasing altitude there is progressive decrease in available amount of oxygen required for physical and mental alertness. Though the percentage of oxygen in air, at 21%, remains almost unchanged up to 69,000 feet (21,000 meters), air density drops *(air is thinner)*, and so oxygen availability decreases. Consequently, there is increase in ventilation (low $PaCO_2$). This causes headache, the most common symptom of high altitude sickness.

## ■ CLINICAL FEATURES

Though individual susceptibility differs, symptoms of acute altitude sickness can begin to appear at around *6,600 feet (2,000 meters) above sea level* (*see* also section on "Medical Emergencies in the Air" as discussed earlier). Symptoms usually manifest 6-10 hours after ascent, and include, besides headache, malaise, anorexia, dizziness, and sleep disturbance. In most of these cases, the symptoms are temporary and abate within a day or so as altitude acclimatization occurs.

At higher altitudes, 11,500–18,000 feet (3,500–5,500 meters) oxygen saturation falls below 90% and $PaO_2$ below 60 mm Hg. Extreme hypoxia may occur resulting in lightheadedness, vomiting, paresthesia and confusion, shortness of breath on exertion, orthostatic hypotension, and drowsiness.

**Severe symptoms** may follow at this or higher altitudes with rapid ascent, so much so no permanent habitation occurs above 20,000 feet (6000 meters). At these altitudes AMS may progress to high altitude pulmonary edema (HAPE) or high altitude cerebral edema (HACE) which is potentially fatal. The former is due to generalized vasoconstriction in pulmonary circulation (normal response to hypoxia) which increases pulmonary capillary pressures resulting in outpouring of fluid into alveoli.

Exact mechanism of cerebral edema (HACE) is not clear. Possibly this is related to cerebral vasodilatation in response to hypoxia, resulting in greater cerebral blood flow and capillary pressure.

## PREVENTION

- ❖ **Preacclimatization:** Warning prospective mountaineers about possibility of serious complications at high altitude coupled with education and training to develop tolerance to low oxygen concentration greatly reduces the risk of developing serious forms of acute mountain sickness.
- ❖ **Other measures:** It may be possible to prevent altitude sickness using medicine(s) in advance, and adopting following precautions— (i) acetazolamide (Diamox) 250 mg twice daily and/or ibuprofen 400 mg three times a day before ascent to high altitude, (ii) prophylaxis with steroids (dexamethasone, 8 mg IV followed by 4 mg every 6 hours) is uncertain but these are helpful in the treatment of pulmonary or cerebral edema, (iii) spending a night at medium altitude before going higher reduces risk of altitude sickness, (iv) avoid large meals, alcohol, and drink plenty of non-caffeine liquids, and (v) avoid strenuous exercise for 1–2 days after arrival at high altitudes.

## TREATMENT

Once symptoms of AMS develop, treatment and stabilization of the patient at high altitude itself is fraught with danger unless good medical facilities are available. In all other situations (especially when high altitude cerebral edema is suspected), the only reliable treatment is to descend to an altitude about 4,000 feet (1,200 meters).

Oxygen should be administered to maintain saturations above 90%, and along with medicines, suffices to control symptoms in mild to moderate cases (below 12,000 feet, i.e., 3,700 meters). Portable hyperbaric chamber, when available, can reduce the effective altitude by about 5,000 feet (1,500 meters).

Hospitalization is generally recommended if symptoms persist for more than a few hours after return to lower altitudes.

# FROSTBITE

The term frostbite denotes tissue damage from exposure to extreme cold. It is an uncommon condition, seen mostly amongst military casualties during wars at high altitudes. However, frostbite may also occur in urban settings when physical disability, homelessness, substance abuse, and psychiatric disease result in cold exposure that threatens life and body parts.

The naming and classification systems are based on clinical examination alone and/or supplemented by sophisticated methods such as computed tomography and nuclear scanning of bone.

## PATHOPHYSIOLOGY

Two types of pathophysiological changes are seen in cold injury:
1. **Direct cellular damage** from freezing with resulting injury to the cell membrane coupled with intracellular metabolic derangements.
2. **Ischemic cellular damage** follows disruption of the microcirculation with vasoconstriction and small-vessel thrombosis.

The severity of frostbite injury is assessed by the degree to which frozen tissues are reperfused on thawing.

## MANAGEMENT

Frostbite being an uncommon condition, only principles of management are described here.

Awareness of the condition, training, and availability of proper equipment are necessary for satisfactory management. The earliest symptoms (motor and cognitive impairment) are subtle and likely to be missed. Rewarming before the freezing of the body parts leads to good results. Probably the best drugs to be used infield care are nonsteroidal anti-inflammatory agents. Thrombolytic intervention should be considered inappropriate cases. In other cases conservative treatment is perhaps the best. This comprises pain control, elevation of the injured extremity, topical wound care, excision of clearly necrotic tissue, wound closure, and rehabilitation.

# 13 CHAPTER

# Miscellaneous Emergencies

## GENERALIZED ANXIETY AND PANIC DISORDERS

### Classification

Anxiety reactions are ubiquitous phenomena of normal human life. However, anxiety becomes pathological when it interferes with day to day social, occupational, or recreational functioning. Earlier described as psychoneurotic disorders or reactions, and anxiety neurosis, these are now classified into generalized anxiety disorder (GAD) and panic disorder.

### *Generalized Anxiety Disorder*

This is defined as excessive anxiety and worry about several (more than one) life circumstance, which is difficult to control, highly variable, and lasts for 6 months or more. It is a "blend of thoughts and feelings characterized by a sense of uncontrollability and unpredictability over potentially aversive life events". As per the American Psychiatric Association's Diagnostic and Statistical Manual of Mental Disorders, 5th Edition (DSM 5), the diagnosis of GAD requires the presence of:

- Excessive anxiety and worry for more days and can last for a long time.
- The individual finds it difficult to control the worry.
- The anxiety and worry are associated with ≥3 of the following symptoms:
  - Restlessness or feeling on edge
  - Easily fatigued
  - Difficulty concentrating or mind going blank
  - Irritability
  - Muscle tension
  - Sleep disturbance
- Anxiety, worry, or physical symptoms cause distress or impairment in social, occupational, or other important areas of functioning.
- The disturbance is not attributable to the physiological effects of a substance or medical condition.
- The disturbance is not better explained by another mental disorder.

**Physical symptoms may be:** Inability to relax, feeling of shakiness, trembling, and being easily startled, palpitation, sweating, dry mouth, lightheadedness, frequent urination, epigastric discomfort, stomach upsets, and diarrhea. Difficulty in concentration, insomnia, irritability, apprehension, and impatience are **features of vigilance and scanning.**

*Mild depressive features may also be associated.* Many variants exist, and in some, *social phobias* may predominate.

Such symptoms are nearly always insidious and chronic, and hence these are not the type of cases to present as medical emergencies, and hence further discussion of GAD is more appropriate for an outpatient medical review text.

## Panic Disorders

### Definition

A panic attack is characterized by *a period of intense anxiety or fear, which is relatively short lived* (usually less than 1 hour), and accompanied by several physiologic/somatic manifestations. Such attacks are often recurrent, discrete, and usually occur spontaneously/unexpectedly. A common associated symptom is **agoraphobia,** which comprises anxiety/fear about being in places or situations from which escape may be difficult/embarrassing, or in which help may not be readily available in case of some unforeseen event. Such fears typically involve characteristic *situations* such as being outside the home alone, standing in a line, being in crowded places, and in closed vehicles such as subways, buses, and airplanes. Such situations are avoided by agoraphobics (traveling may be restricted), or are endured with marked anxiety and distress, or else require the presence of a companion.

Agoraphobia differs from *social and simple phobias* in that the former is characterized by a *"fear of some situations"* that includes being trapped, or being unable to escape in the event of having an unexpected panic attack or panic-like symptoms. "Social" and "specific" phobias, on the other hand, are limited to avoidance of "social situations", or only a few "specific situations". *Panic disorder and agoraphobia may coexist,* or either may be seen independent of the other.

### Clinical features

Panic attacks usually occur randomly and spontaneously. The patient may be engaged in a routine activity (such as driving a car, eating in a restaurant, listening to music, or sitting in a cinema hall) when he suddenly experiences an overwhelming fear, intense apprehension, and a sense of impending doom. While most of such attacks occur spontaneously without any obvious precipitating factor, there are several important events that may be associated with a higher risk of panic attacks. These include thyroid disorders (both hypo- and-hyper-thyroid), postpartum period, sexual activity, emotional trauma, automobile accident, and substance abuse. However, panic attacks may continue to occur spontaneously even long after such incidents (car accident or postpartum period), or after correction/control of other stress factors. Nocturnal attacks that awaken such patients from sleep are not uncommon.

The **major psychological symptoms** are *external fear and a sense of impending death and doom.* However, on repeated questioning, the patient is unable to name the reason or source of his/her fear. *It is a nameless terror, comes from nowhere, and the patient does not know when it will stop, if ever.* The patients may feel confused, have difficulty in concentrating, and often

> **Box 13.1: Classical symptoms of a panic attack.**
>
> - Palpitation, tachycardia, or pounding of heart
> - Trembling or shaking
> - Perspiration
> - Shortness of breath, suffocation, choking, or smothering
> - Chest discomfort or pain
> - Nausea and/or epigastric distress
> - Lightheadedness, dizziness, unsteadiness, or fainting
> - Paresthesia
> - Chills or hot flushes
> - Fear of losing control or going crazy
> - Fear of impending doom or death
> - Derealization (feeling of unreality such as being tossed out of bed, hit by an earthquake) and depersonalization (being detached from oneself)

try to leave whatever situation they are in. The classical symptoms of a panic attack are given at **Box 13.1**. In a typical attack, at least four of these features are present, and **develop abruptly, usually reaching a peak within 10 minutes.** However, many people report signs and symptoms of panic attack without meeting the requisite criteria of panic disorder.

**Examination of the patient during a panic attack** may reveal difficulty in speaking, and an impaired memory with features of depression or depersonalization. The symptoms may disappear quickly or gradually. After the episode is over, patients often have *anticipatory anxiety* about experiencing another or repetitive attacks, with somatic concern of death from a cardiac or respiratory problem. The resulting fearfulness and autonomic hyperactivity in the interval between panic attacks is variable, but may approximate the level experienced during the panic attack itself (making difficult differentiation from GAD).

Such patients often describe being demoralized as a result of such attacks, as also by personality changes arising from restriction of their activities (sometimes resulting in refusal to accept positions involving greater challenge and responsibility). The most serious outcome of panic disorder is the development of *phobic avoidance,* which may progress to the full agoraphobic syndrome. The course of the illness (without treatment) is highly variable. There are periods of waxing and waning, and long remissions followed by a new outburst are not uncommon.

*Associated symptoms*

Panic disorder is frequently associated with other clinical disorders such as *depression,* and many patients report a suicidal ideation. The two disorders may occur at the same time, or panic disorder may occur before depression. Unlike depressed patients they have a normal desire to engage in activities, but avoid them because of their phobias. *Patients with panic disorder often have a variety of gastrointestinal symptoms (such as abdominal pain, bloating, and diarrhea),* which are typically associated with irritable bowel syndrome. Alcohol or other substance abuse is also common in patients with panic disorder.

## Diagnosis

Panic disorder, like anxiety states, is more common in women than men. The patient is usually a young adult, though the disorder is not uncommon in fifth and sixth decades. Unexpected panic attacks are the hallmark of panic disorder. The condition needs to be differentiated from both psychiatric and medical disorders. The former include malingering, hypochondriasis, anxiety disorders due to general medical conditions and substance withdrawal, depressive disorders, post-traumatic stress, and psychosis.

A large number of **medical conditions** enter into differential diagnosis of panic disorder (**Table 13.1**). However, *it cannot be overemphasized that panic disorder is essentially a diagnosis of exclusion,* and any possible organic illness must be carefully excluded in such cases by a detailed clinical history and relevant investigations. The association between mitral valve prolapse and panic disorder is controversial. The two may coexist, so the diagnosis of panic disorder should be made independently of mitral valve prolapse.

## Course and prognosis

Panic disorder is generally a chronic disorder, which has an onset usually during the late adolescence or early childhood. However, the onset may be delayed, especially in women in whom symptoms may first appear

**Table 13.1:** Differential diagnosis of panic and (certain) medical disorders.

| Medical disorder | Possible clinical features in panic disorder |
|---|---|
| **Cardiovascular** | |
| Angina pectoris, myocardial infarction, hypertension, PSVT, mitral valve prolapse | Chest pain, pressure or discomfort, perspiration, feeling of choking, palpitation, dyspnea, suffocation |
| **Respiratory** | |
| Asthma | Sensation of shortness of breath, hyperventilation |
| **Gastrointestinal** | |
| Acid-peptic disease, colitis, | Abdominal distress, bloating, nausea, irritable bowel syndrome, vomiting, diarrhea |
| **Neurological** | |
| TIAs, seizure disorder, syncope, migraine, Meniere's disease | Lightheadedness, faintness, dizziness, shaking, paresthesia, derealization |
| **Endocrinal** | |
| Pheochromocytoma, thyroid disorders, hypoglycemia | Episodic palpitation and elevated blood pressure, headaches, fainting |

(PSVT: paroxysmal supraventricular tachycardia; TIAs: transient ischemic attacks)

near menopause. Patients of panic disorder run a high risk of developing depression (along with suicidal ideation), alcohol dependence, and obsessive-compulsive disorder.

The course of the illness is highly variable, and there is no reliable way to predict which patient will develop agoraphobia. Remissions and relapses are common. *The long-term prognosis is generally good* with about one-third of the cases becoming symptom free, and another 50% having only mild symptoms that do not affect their lives significantly. About 10–20% of patients continue to have significant symptoms marked by new outbursts. At the extreme end are patients who become completely house bound for decades. The prognosis is better in patients without any associated premorbid condition, and in those with infrequent panic attacks, and brief duration of symptoms.

## *Management*

Once the diagnosis of panic disorder is established, treatment should be aimed at: (1) blocking the occurrence of the spontaneous attack at any point in the course of the illness, and (2) correcting catastrophic thinking. The former is achieved by pharmacological measures and the latter by cognitive-behavioral therapy. Combining the two modes of therapy is more effective than either one alone.

1. **Pharmacotherapy:** Two groups of drugs are available for panic attacks:
   i. *Benzodiazepines:* Most commonly prescribed drug in this group is *alprazolam*. The effective dosage varies, but is likely to be 2-4 mg daily. It acts quickly and has few immediate side effects. Prolonged use may result in addiction, and patients becoming physically dependent on it (*see* also benzodiazepine toxicity, Chapter 9). However, the tolerance usually does not develop to the antipanic effects of the drug. Furthermore, the problem of dependence can be countered by slow tapering of the drug, which is possible when the second group of drugs (antidepressants) start becoming effective.
   ii. *Antidepressant drugs:* Tricyclic group of drugs as well as selective serotonin reuptake inhibitors (SSRIs) have been found to be useful in the management of panic disorder. However, these drugs can cause overstimulation in the initial stages of treatment, and therefore must be started in small doses, and then gradually titrated upward **(*start low and go slow*).** So far as drug therapy is concerned, *antidepressants have been found to be superior to benzodiazepines in the long-term management of panic disorder.*
2. **Cognitive and behavioral therapies:** Cognitive therapy involves explaining to the patient that panic attacks are self-limited and not life-threatening. Such procedures may help the patient in recognizing various body sensations (such as palpitation and breathlessness) as normal phenomena, and avoid their catastrophic misinterpretation. These therapeutic approaches fall in the domain of an experienced psychiatrist who should always be involved in the management of such cases.

## Summary

❖ General anxiety and panic disorders are common medical/psychiatric illnesses. Panic disorder often presents as an acute problem in emergency rooms.
❖ Distinction between GAD and panic disorder is not difficult, if the patient has frequent spontaneous panic attacks and agoraphobic symptoms. When patients with GAD have occasional panic attacks, they should be considered as having GAD.
❖ The clinical features of panic disorder mimic those of other organic illnesses. Therefore, *panic disorder is a diagnosis of exclusion.*
❖ Panic disorder can be managed by a combination of antidepressants and high-potency anxiolytics. *The principle of appropriate medication is* **"start low and go slow".**

# SYNCOPE

Syncope is a relatively common medical problem and implies a *sudden, transitory, and reversible loss of consciousness and postural tone.* Though often benign, some forms of syncope can herald a serious medical disorder.

## Etiology

A very large number of conditions can result in syncope, ranging from simple vasovagal faint to serious cerebrovascular and cardiac disorders **(Box 13.2)**.

---

**Box 13.2: Causes of syncope.**

- **Vasomotor abnormalities** *(neutrally mediated):*
  - *Vasovagal faint:* Emotional upset, pain or fear of pain, prolonged motionless standing, trauma
  - Acute hypovolemia (e.g., gastroenteritis, massive blood loss), intoxication (e.g., alcohol), micturition syncope, cough syncope carotid sinus syncope
- **Orthostatic hypotension:**
  - *Drugs:* Phenothiazine's antidepressants (tricyclic), antihypertensive, nitrates, alpha, blockers, diuretics, ACE inhibitors/receptor blockers, calcium channel blockers
  - Severe hypovolemia, autonomic neuropathies, surgical sympathectomy
- **Abnormalities of cardiac function:**
  - Cardiac arrest due to any cause acute myocardial infarction, tachyarrhythmias/bradyarrhythmias, mitral valve prolapse, sick sinus syndrome
  - Inadequate filling (e.g., pericardial disease, left atrial myxoma, tension pneumothorax)
  - Cardiac outflow obstruction (aortic stenosis, pulmonary stenosis, and hypertrophic obstructive cardiomyopathy)
  - Severe pulmonary hypertension, acute pulmonary thromboembolism
- **Cerebrovascular:** Transitory ischemic attacks, basilar artery insufficiency, subclavian steal syndrome, migraine

Basic to all these varied causes is a sudden impairment of brain metabolism due to inadequate blood flow and oxygen delivery from vasomotor or cardiac abnormalities.

## Clinical Features

A detailed description of either the mechanisms or clinical features of various types of syncope is beyond the scope of this book.

The most *common type of syncope is vasovagal attack,* which can be considered as prototype of the whole syndrome. Only a brief mention is made of the other types of syncope.

- **Vasovagal syncope:** Vasovagal disorders account most of the episodes of syncope. Syncope is often precipitated by a sudden emotional upset or confrontation with stress, which is inescapable (e.g., during venipuncture or dental procedure). Such situations trigger intense parasympathetic stimulation which combined with depression of vasomotor center produce central nervous system (CNS) hypoperfusion and subsequent syncope. Hot crowded environments, anemia, fever, and poor physical condition increase the risk of such syncope.

  Vasovagal episodes begin in *standing or sitting position,* and only rarely in a supine position. *Warning (prodromal) symptoms* last from 10 seconds to a few minutes and include nausea, sinking sensation, dizziness, sweating, blurred vision, and even vomiting. If the patient manages to sit or lie down, further progress of symptoms may cease, otherwise unconsciousness follows and even convulsions may occur. This is associated with partial or total lack of awareness of the surroundings. Examination of the patient in this state (which is seldom possible) reveals impaired consciousness, pallor, dilated pupils, bradycardia, and a slow, weak pulse (vagal-induced sinus bradycardia). Blood pressure is usually maintained.

  *Postsyncopal findings:* The onset of unconsciousness is the nature's way to restore autonomic balance, and this coupled with recumbent posture (which eliminates gravity) immediately establish adequate cerebral blood flow. A quick recovery therefore ensues without any postictal confusional state or neurological deficit. However, nervousness, nausea, headache, and dizziness may persist for hours.

- **Orthostatic syncope:** This is another common type of syncope, especially in the elderly, in diabetics, in states of hypovolemia (e.g., gastrointestinal losses, hemorrhage), and in patients on certain drugs (**Box 13.2**).

  *Combination of such drugs* (not uncommon in clinical practice) *can be hazardous* especially in the elderly in whom a normal vasoconstrictive response to assuming upright posture is often impaired.

  *Orthostatic vital signs* should be recorded though this may be contraindicated in the presence of supine hypotension, shock, or altered mental status. Pulse and BP should be recorded initially after the patient has been supine for 3 minutes and then again after the patient stands for 1 minute. Orthostatic hypotension is confirmed if, on assuming upright posture, pulse rate increases by 30 beats per minute or more, or systolic pressure decreases by 20 mm Hg or to <90 mm Hg. Occurrence of dizziness, blurring of vision, or syncope also indicate a positive test. The episode is however brief in duration, and the patient recovers rapidly and completely when put in supine position (elevation of legs to 30° for 1/2 to 1 minute).

- **Cardiac syncope:** Loss of consciousness in cardiac disease is most often due to an abrupt decrease in cardiac output with subsequent cerebral hypoperfusion producing symptoms identical to those of fainting. Such cardiac dysfunction may result from acute myocardial infarction, sudden rhythm disturbances (brady-or-tachyarrhythmias), cardiac inflow or outflow obstruction, or acute pulmonary embolism (**Box 13.2**).
Cardiovascular origin of syncope is suggested when it occurs during recumbency, during or following physical exertion, or in a patient with known heart disease. Cardiac inflow obstruction (e.g., atrial myxoma) should be suspected, if syncope is related to change in position. Physical examination in such cases will reveal engorged neck veins, weak pulse, or hypotension. The cause of syncope in such cases is usually obvious from clinical details, physical examination, and a 12-lead electrocardiogram will often reveal cardiac origin of the syncope, but many patients will require special investigations, such as exercise testing, cardiac imaging, and 24–72 hour Holter monitoring, or electrophysiological studies.

- **Cerebrovascular syncope:** *Transient ischemic attack(s)* (TIAs) due to ischemic stroke is not uncommon. However, it is nearly always associated with temporary neurological deficits referable to the involved territory (of the brain affected by arterial insufficiency). A special form is the **"drop attack"** in which the patient suddenly loses postural tone and "falls", but does not actually become unconscious nor develops any neurological deficit (for further details *see* section on "Ischemic Stroke", Chapter 4).

- **Other causes of syncope:** *Micturition syncope* is associated with distinctive situation, and is seen mostly in middle-aged and elderly males especially those with enlarged prostate. The risk of unconsciousness is greatest at night during or immediately following micturition. It is possibly due to enhanced vagal tone and rapid emptying of the bladder resulting in reflex vasodilatation with rapid drop in blood pressure and decreased cerebral perfusion. Contributory factors include drinking alcohol before going to bed (vasodilatation) and straining during voiding *(Valsalva effect)* both of which decrease the venous return with consequent cerebral hypoperfusion.

A similar mechanism accounts for *cough syncope,* which can occur after a prolonged episode of cough. Intrathoracic pressure increases with resultant fall in cardiac output *(Valsalva effect).* Other situations, which can result in syncope due to similar mechanisms, are *breath holding in children, defecation, weight lifting, and trumpet blowing.* Duration of syncope in all such cases is brief, and patient recovers rapidly and completely on assuming supine position.

An unusual type of syncope sometimes occurs in elderly people with a *hypersensitive carotid sinus* (**carotid sinus syncope**). It results from pressure on an abnormally sensitive carotid sinus as in buttoning a tight collar or turning the head to one side, as in backing a car. Baroceptors (located in carotid sinus) are stimulated triggering vagal and vasodepressor reflexes, which lead to marked bradycardia ending in syncopal attack. There may be history of multiple previous episodes with the same type of activity. The syndrome can be reproduced by pressure on the carotid sinus for a few seconds under ECG monitoring. However, before performing this provocative test, it should be assured patient does not have an occluded carotid artery.

## Diagnosis

This can be challenging. Syncope should be differentiated from dizziness, presyncope, or vertigo, all of which do not result in temporary loss of consciousness. *Typically,* syncopal attacks are very brief, lasting no longer than 20 seconds, followed by almost complete restoration of orientation and appropriate behavior.

Other causes of loss of consciousness, such as seizure, hyperventilation, hypoglycemia, and intoxication, can be differentiated by a *detailed history* (of each and every episode), interrogation of witnesses, and routine investigations including a 12-lead ECG. Depending upon the possible etiology, further investigations should then be planned, which may include 24–72 hour Holter monitoring, echocardiogram, carotid Doppler, brain MRI, and EEG. When the cause of syncope (especially if recurrent) still remains obscure, patient should be referred to a specialized center for further investigations such as *autonomic testing with a tilt table and electrophysiological studies* to assess sinus node dysfunction and atrioventricular (AV) node conduction.

## Treatment

This will vary according to the cause of syncope. Invariably, a vasovagal attack would be over by the time medical aid arrives. Any patient with imminent fainting episode should be promptly laid flat, clothes around the neck loosened and the tongue prevented from falling back. Subjects who are prone to these attacks should be advised to avoid standing immobile for prolonged periods especially in hot weather and stuffy environments.

In recurrent carotid sinus syncope, ephedrine 15 mg three times a day may be effective, while in cases with postural hypotension, attack may be prevented by sympathomimetic drugs, use of abdominal binders, elastic crepe bandages below the knees, use of common salt in excessive amount (3–5 g over and above daily consumption), or periodic injections of desoxycorticosterone acetate (DOCA), or fludrocortisone. When a definite cardiac or cerebrovascular cause is discovered, specific management will be required, so that syncopal attacks do not recur.

# PROPHYLACTIC IMMUNIZATION IN INFECTIOUS DISEASES

## General Principles

Every individual (adult or child) should have and maintain adequate protection (**immunity**) against infectious diseases to prevent development of the disease and, in some cases, reduce the risk of secondary transmission to other susceptible persons. Such defense mechanisms of the body can be **innate** (nonspecific) or **acquired** (specific) systems.

*Innate immunity* is present from birth, and includes physical barriers (intact skin and mucus membranes), chemical barriers (gastric acidity), and phagocytic cells and complement system. *Acquired immunity* is generally specific to a single organism or on the way to a group of closely related organisms.

Immunity can be acquired by two mechanisms: (1) **active,** and (2) **passive.** Active immunity is provided by individual's own immune system, and is usually long-lasting. It can be acquired by natural disease or by **vaccination.** The latter generally provides immunity similar to that provided by natural infection but without the risk from the disease or its complications. It includes *National Immunization Program* (recommended in India) with its aim to provide protection in infants and children against common infectious diseases prevalent in the country.

Passive immunity is provided either by the transfer of antibodies from immune individuals, most commonly across placenta, or by administration of immunoglobulins (a blood product). The transplacental transfer of antibodies is more effective against some infections (e.g., tetanus and measles) than others (polio, whooping cough). However, such *protection is often temporary,* commonly only for a few weeks or months.

## Pre-exposure Prophylaxis (PrEP)

From infants to children and adults, anyone can be affected by infectious disease(s) prevalent in the country. These can to a large extent be prevented by **active immunization** at the time of birth or in early years of life by adopting a National Immunization Program as recommended by Indian Medical Council. Nevertheless, there may have been a lapse or the immunization status uncertain, when certain individuals may have to be protected from a particular infectious disease on **an emergency basis** under certain conditions **(Table 13.2):**

- ❖ Outbreak of an epidemic, or projected visit (e.g., pilgrimage) to a place of possible epidemic
- ❖ Close contacts of serious infectious disease, e.g., hepatitis B
- ❖ If the infectious disease is likely to be acquired at an inappropriate time (e.g., during pregnancy, examinations, etc.), and it is desired to at least delay the occurrence of the disease.
- ❖ Immunodeficient subjects who have come in contact with a patient suffering from serious disease, and in whom the disease may run a progressive course.

**Table 13.2:** Active immunization schedule *(Recommended by Indian Medical Association).*

| Sl. No. | Age | Disease | Vaccination |
|---|---|---|---|
| 1. | At birth | Hepatitis B | Hepatitis B vaccine (1) |
| 2. | At birth | Polio | Oral polio vaccine (1) |
| 3. | Birth to 6 weeks | Tuberculosis | BCG (intradermal) *(insertion of left deltoid)* |
| 4. | 4–6 weeks | Hepatitis B | Hepatitis B vaccine (2) |
| 5. | 6 weeks | DPT*, polio | DPT vaccine (1); oral polio (2) |
| 6. | 10 weeks | DPT* | DPT vaccine (2) |
| 7. | 14 weeks | DPT, polio | DPT vaccine (3); oral polio (3) |
| 8. | 24 weeks | Hepatitis B | Hepatitis B vaccine (3) |
| 9. | 9–12 months | Polio | Oral polio vaccine (4) |
| 10. | 12–15 months | Mumps/measles/rubella | †MMR vaccine |
| 11. | 4–5 years | DPT, Polio | DPT booster; oral polio (5) |

*DPT: Diphtheria, pertussis, tetanus
†MMR: Mumps, measles, rubella

**Caution:** (1) Most vaccines should be given **IM** rather than deep SC, since former are less likely to cause local reactions; (2) in infants, most appropriate sites are anterolateral aspect of thigh or deltoid region to avoid, and not in buttocks to avoid damage to sciatic nerve or blood vessels; (3) if two or more injections are to be given at the same time, these should preferably be given in different limbs, or if in the same limb, at least 2.5 cm apart.

### *Contraindications to Vaccination*

- All vaccines are contraindicated, if there is history of a confirmed anaphylactic reaction to a previous dose of vaccine containing the same antigen.
- Live vaccine is contraindicated in pregnancy, in patients who are immunosuppressed, or on immunosuppressive or high dose steroid therapy.
- Immunization should be **deferred** if (1) the individual is acutely unwell to avoid wrongly attributing any new symptom or progression of symptoms to the vaccine. Minor illnesses without fever or systemic upset are not a reason for deferral, (2) when there is an evolving neurological condition.
- Live vaccines should be avoided at least 3 weeks before or 3 months after an injection of immunoglobulin since the latter may interfere with the immune response to live vaccine viruses.

## Post-exposure Prophylaxis (PoEP)

The risk of acquiring an infectious disease after exposure can be decreased by either age-appropriate immunization (as in measles, mumps, rubella, varicella, pertussis, and hepatitis B virus infections), by antibiotics or by immune globulins and antiviral medications. PoEP should be given as soon as possible following a high-risk exposure (**Tables 13.3 and 13.4**).

**Table 13.3:** Post-exposure prophylactic regimens for various blood-borne viral infections.

| Infection | Index patient's disease status | Status of exposed person | Regimen |
|---|---|---|---|
| Hepatitis B virus | Hepatitis B surface antigen +ve | Unvaccinated or inadequate vaccination | Hepatitis B immune globulin 0.6 mL/kg IM within 24 hours of exposure, followed by hepatitis B vaccine series |
| Hepatitis C virus | Anti-hepatitis C +ve with detectable Hepatitis C virus RNA | Hepatitis C –ve | None available |

**Note:** HIV infections has been omitted because of frequent changes in recommended treatment.

**Table 13.4:** Post-exposure prophylaxis regimens for common viral and bacterial diseases.

| Infection | Source patient's infectious status | Status of exposed person | Regimen |
|---|---|---|---|
| Hepatitis A virus | Serologically +; within incubation period until one week after onset of jaundice | Unvaccinated | A single dose of hepatitis A vaccine within two weeks of exposure |
| Influenza | From 1d before onset of symptoms until 1 day | *High-risk group | Influenza vaccine (in unvaccinated persons |
| Measles virus | From 2 days before onset of rash till all lesions have crusted | Unvaccinated | Specific immune globulin (Ig) 0.25 mL/kg IM within 5 days of contact; if specific Ig is not available, gamma globulin 0.1–0.2 mL/kg may be used. †MMR at 12–15 months |
| Rabies | Bites or scratches from a suspected rabid animal | Previously unvaccinated | ‡Rabies vaccine as early as possible + human rabies immune globulin (HRIG) –20 units/kg in a single dose |

*Contd...*

*Contd...*

| Infection | Source patient's infectious status | Status of exposed person | Regimen |
|---|---|---|---|
| Tetanus | After a tetanus-prone injury | Unvaccinated or last dose of tetanus toxoid >5 years ago | Tetanus toxoid vaccine + a single dose of tetanus Ig, 250 units IM (except after minor and clean wounds) |
| Varicella-zoster virus | From 1–2 days before onset of rash until all lesions have crusted | Nonimmune (nonvaccinated) and no history of disease | Varicella vaccine within 5 days of exposure; pregnant women, neonates, and immunocompromised persons: Ig 400 mg per kg IV or specific Ig 125 units per 10 kg IM as soon as possible (up to 10 days postexposure) |

*High-risk group: Patients with serious comorbid states, immunocompromised, adults >65 years, children <2 years, and pregnant or postpartum women

†MMR: measles, mumps, and rubella

‡Rabies treatment: For details, *see* section on Rabies, Chapter 8.

## GENERAL

- All wounds, bites, and licks should be cleaned thoroughly with water; antiseptics not especially useful; after mucosal exposure to blood or body fluids also, the exposed area should be irrigated with water copiously.
- The planned PoEP should be safe, effective, and affordable.
- For best results PoEP should be started as early as possible. However, for infections such as tetanus and rabies, prophylaxis can be given up to several months after exposure because incubation period can variable, and long.
- The PoEP can be an antiviral agent, a vaccine or immunoglobulin, or a combination of these.
- Live vaccines are contraindicated in immunocompromised persons and pregnant women.
- Certain infections cannot be prevented by PoEP despite the risk of transmission to an exposed person. These include hepatitis C virus, mumps, and rubella.

## APPENDIX

### Dopamine IV Drip Chart

**Drug concentration: 400 mg in 250 mL D5W (1.6 mg/mL)**

| Weight (kg) | 50 | 55 | 60 | 65 | 70 | 75 | 80 | 85 | 90 | 95 | 100 |
|---|---|---|---|---|---|---|---|---|---|---|---|
| (lb) | 110 | 121 | 132 | 143 | 154 | 165 | 176 | 187 | 198 | 209 | 220 |

*Contd...*

*Contd...*

| µg/kg/min | Flow rate (mL/hr) | | | | | | | | | |
|---|---|---|---|---|---|---|---|---|---|---|
| 2 | 4 | 4 | 5 | 5 | 5 | 6 | 6 | 6 | 7 | 7 | 8 |
| 3 | 6 | 6 | 7 | 7 | 8 | 8 | 9 | 10 | 10 | 11 | 11 |
| 4 | 8 | 8 | 9 | 10 | 11 | 11 | 12 | 13 | 14 | 14 | 15 |
| 5 | 9 | 10 | 11 | 12 | 13 | 14 | 15 | 16 | 17 | 18 | 19 |
| 6 | 11 | 12 | 14 | 15 | 16 | 17 | 18 | 19 | 20 | 21 | 23 |
| 7 | 13 | 14 | 16 | 17 | 18 | 20 | 21 | 22 | 24 | 25 | 26 |
| 8 | 15 | 17 | 18 | 20 | 21 | 23 | 24 | 26 | 27 | 29 | 30 |
| 9 | 17 | 19 | 20 | 22 | 24 | 25 | 27 | 29 | 30 | 32 | 34 |
| 10 | 19 | 21 | 23 | 24 | 26 | 28 | 30 | 32 | 34 | 36 | 38 |
| 15 | 28 | 31 | 34 | 37 | 39 | 42 | 45 | 48 | 51 | 53 | 56 |
| 20 | 38 | 41 | 45 | 49 | 53 | 56 | 60 | 64 | 68 | 71 | 75 |
| 25 | 47 | 52 | 56 | 61 | 66 | 70 | 75 | 80 | 84 | 89 | 94 |

**Dose:** 2–25 µg/kg/min [2–5 µg/kg/min—renal dose (increases perfusion); 5–20 µg/kg/min-beta—1 agonist; >20 µg/kg/min—alpha agonist, vasoconstriction]

## Dobutamine IV Drip Chart

### Drug concentration: 250 mg in 250 ml D5W (1 mg/mL)

| Weight (kg) | 50 | 55 | 60 | 65 | 70 | 75 | 80 | 85 | 90 | 95 | 100 |
|---|---|---|---|---|---|---|---|---|---|---|---|
| (lb) | 110 | 121 | 132 | 143 | 154 | 165 | 176 | 187 | 198 | 209 | 220 |
| µg/kg/min | Flow rate (mL/hr) | | | | | | | | | | |
| 2 | 6 | 6 | 8 | 8 | 8 | 10 | 10 | 10 | 10 | 12 | 12 |
| 3 | 10 | 10 | 10 | 12 | 12 | 14 | 14 | 16 | 16 | 18 | 18 |
| 4 | 12 | 14 | 14 | 16 | 16 | 18 | 20 | 20 | 22 | 22 | 24 |
| 5 | 16 | 16 | 18 | 20 | 22 | 22 | 24 | 26 | 28 | 28 | 30 |
| 6 | 18 | 20 | 22 | 24 | 26 | 28 | 28 | 30 | 32 | 34 | 36 |
| 7 | 22 | 24 | 26 | 28 | 30 | 32 | 34 | 36 | 38 | 40 | 42 |
| 8 | 24 | 26 | 28 | 32 | 34 | 36 | 38 | 40 | 44 | 46 | 48 |
| 9 | 28 | 30 | 32 | 36 | 38 | 40 | 44 | 46 | 48 | 52 | 54 |
| 10 | 30 | 34 | 36 | 40 | 42 | 46 | 48 | 52 | 54 | 58 | 60 |
| 15 | 46 | 50 | 54 | 58 | 64 | 68 | 72 | 76 | 82 | 86 | 90 |
| 20 | 60 | 66 | 72 | 78 | 84 | 90 | 96 | 102 | 108 | 114 | 120 |
| 25 | 76 | 82 | 90 | 98 | 106 | 112 | 120 | 128 | 136 | 142 | 150 |

**Dose:** 5–20 µg/kg/min: start at 5 µg/kg/min and increase by 2.5 µg/kg/min every 10–15 minutes as required.

# Index

Page numbers followed by *b* refer to box, *f* refer to figure, *fc* refer to flowchart, and *t* refer to table.

## A

Absolute neutrophil count  261, 262
Absorption  218
Acetaminophen  137, 327
Acetazolamide  408
Acetoacetic acid  331
Acetylcholine, overabundance of  344
Acetylcholinesterase  344, 347
Acetylcysteine  146, 327
Acid  339
　metabolites, retention of  222
Acid-base
　abnormalities  207, 329
　balance  332
　disorders  220, 221*t*
　disturbance  223, 223*t*
　equilibrium  207
　homeostasis  237
　studies  385
Acidosis  199, 125, 220
　severe  222*t*
Acquired immune disorder  249
Active immunization  312, 419
　schedule  420*t*
Acute attack  202
　treatment of  288
Acute bacterial meningitis  182
　empiric treatment of  187*t*
Acute chest pain  11
　diagnostic evaluation of  7*fc*
Acute confusional state  153, 155, 155*t*
　causes of  154*t*
Acute coronary syndrome  4, 5, 7*fc*, 9*fc*
　diagnosis of  7*t*
　pathogenesis of  6*f*
Acute diarrhea  124
　diagnosis of  126*t*
　diseases  124
Acute exacerbation, grade severity of  97
Acute hepatic failure  137, 336
　causes of  137*t*
Acute left heart failure  96, 359, 363
Acute mountain sickness  407
Acute myocardial
　infarction  10, 279, 417
　ischemia  32
Acute pancreatitis  146, 150*b*
　causes of  146*t*
　complications of  148*b*
　severity of  150*t*
Acute percutaneous coronary intervention  26
Acute renal failure  39, 228, 237*t*, 243, 305, 332, 342, 387, 397
　complications of  234*t*
　staging criteria of  229*t*
Acute respiratory distress syndrome  110, 116, 118, 298, 320, 325, 349, 387, 394, 405
Addison's disease  270
Addisonian crisis  270
Adenosine  65, 86
Adenovirus  125
Adrenal crisis, acute  270
Adrenal function tests  271
Adrenaline  362, 368
　hydrochloride  374
Adrenergic discharge, features of  284
Adrenergic stimulants, mechanism of action of  98*f*
Adrenocortical insufficiency
　acute  270
　primary  270
　secondary  270
*Aedes aegypti* mosquito  290, 293, 294
Agitation, control of  337
Agoraphobia  411
Air
　embolism  358
　encephalography  402
　medical emergencies in  400
Airway  82, 327, 396
　breathing, circulation, and drugs  326
　disease  102
　obstruction  388
　prevention of  90
　patency of  399
Alcohol  146, 204, 334, 415
　intoxication  154
　　clinical features of  335*t*
　smells of  336
　withdrawal  194
Aldosterone  270
Alkaline diuresis  331
Alkalinization  331
Alkalis  339
Alkalosis  220
　severe  222*t*
Allergic reactions  24, 362, 371, 374

# Index

Allergy 371
Allopurinol 369
Alprazolam 414
Alteplase 21, 50
Altitude hypoxia, adverse effects of 401
Aluminum phosphide poisoning 348
   salient features of 349$t$
Amebiasis 322
Amebic liver abscess 322
Amidopyrine 371
Aminocaproic acid 258
Aminoglycosides 369
Amino-penicillins 109
Amiodarone 20, 56, 57, 59, 69, 72, 73, 86, 87, 265, 369, 375
   interactions of 60$t$
Ammonia 140
Amnesic dementia 156
Amnesic episodes 329
Amoxicillin 369
Amphetamine 328, 351
Ampicillin 186, 302, 369
Amrinone 42
Analgesics 18, 342
   headaches 200
Anamnestic reactions 302
Anaphylactic reactions, treatment of 389
Anaphylactoid
   purpura 254
   reaction 362, 387
      treatment of 389
Anaphylaxis 371, 380, 387
   cause of 390
   hallmark of 388
Androgens 270
Anemia 234, 315, 334, 401, 416
   acute hemolytic 243
   classification of 242$t$
   hemolytic 245$t$
   progressive severe 242
   severe 241, 242, 404
Anesthetics agents 356
Aneurysm, localization of 178
Anginal pain, duration of 2
Angiography 136, 178
Angiomas 129
Angiotensin-converting enzyme 363, 367
   inhibitors 25, 32, 39, 229
Angiotensin-receptor blockers 229
Anion gap, increased 331
Anopheles mosquito 314
Anorexia 407
Antiarrhythmic 19, 27
   agents 369
   drugs
      classification of 57$t$
      site of action of 56$t$
   therapy 56

Antibacterial therapy 386$t$
Antibiotics 99, 129, 151, 154, 185, 308, 324, 356, 363, 369
   fever 375
   regimen 187
   therapy 108, 186
      duration of 187
Anticancer drugs 371
Anticholinergic syndrome 326
Anticoagulant therapy, duration of 49
Anticoagulation 31, 48
Anticonvulsants 198
   drugs 196$t$
Antidepressant drugs 326, 414
Antidiarrheal agents 127
Antidote 327, 327$t$, 330
   specific 333
   use of 339
Antiemetics 124
Antiepileptics 370
Antifibrinolytic agents 258
Antigen-based rapid diagnostic test 320
Antihistamines 326, 352, 362, 390, 401
Antihypertensive 154, 415
Anti-ischemic drugs 31
Antimalarial drugs 317
Antimicrobial therapy 238$t$, 305
Anti-platelet 31, 32
   agents 18
   drugs 28
   therapy 168
Antirabic treatment, complications of 314
Antithrombotic therapy 9, 20
Antithyroid drugs 265
Antitoxin 309
Antitubercular therapy 190
Antivenin 341
Antiviral medicines 297
Anxiety 31, 329
   anticipatory 412
   neurosis 410
   reactions 389, 410
   states 413
Aortic dissection 52
Aortic stenosis 415
Aphasia 406
Aplastic anemia 112, 245
   causes of 245$t$
   hallmark of 246
   severity of 246$t$
Apomorphine, use of 328
Appendix 86
Appropriate insulin therapy 275
Arbovirus 290
Aresenic compounds 352
Arrhythmia 67, 392, 405
Arterial blood gas 98, 111

Arterial pH 304
Arterioles 179
Artery supplying brain 171f
Artesunate 317, 370
Arthralgia 291, 294, 306, 374
Arthritis
   acute 287
      gouty 287
Artificial ventilation 332
*Ascaris lumbricoides* 125
Aseptic meningitis 191, 192, 299
Askin test 374
*Aspergillosis* 112
Asphyxia 307
   asthma, sudden 94, 100
Aspiration 324, 349
   pneumonia 199, 279, 307, 358
      treatment of 406
Aspirin 9, 16, 18, 28, 31, 33, 249, 253, 375
   therapy 16, 17fc
Asthma 358, 368
   acute 97t
      severe 93
   bronchial 403
   cardiac 36
   exacerbation
      slow-onset 95
      sudden onset 96
   history of 374
Asthmatic attack, acute 97
Ataxia 174, 335
Ataxic hemiparesis stroke 169
Atelectatic lung, perfusion of 359
Atenolol 57, 370
Atrial fibrillation 61, 68, 68f, 264, 350
Atrial flutter 61, 67, 69, 69f
Atrial myxoma, left 415
Atrial premature beats 62
Atrial tachycardia 61, 62, 62f
   multifocal 63, 67
Atrioventricular block 75
Atropine 75, 86, 347
   poisoning 326
Attack
   prolonged 203
   repetitive 412
   vasovagal 416
Attention deficit 153
Automated external defibrillators 83
Autonomic effecter cell 344
Autonomic ganglion cell 344
A-V nodal re-entrant tachycardia 63f
Avomine 124
Azithromycin 369
Azotemia 232
   prerenal 232, 304

# B

Babinski's sign 142
Bacteremia 382
Bacterial diseases 421t
Bad prognostic signs 320
Balloon tamponade 135
Barbiturates 326, 334
Barium 352
Barotrauma 405
Basophils 388
Behavior, aggressive 329
Behavioral therapies 414
Belching 4
Belladonna alkaloids 352
Benzene 245
   phosphorus 137
Benzodiazepines 326, 327, 329, 330, 363, 369, 414
   acute overdose of 329
   doses of 329
   overdose, diagnosis of 330
   superior to 414
   toxicity 414
      symptom of 329
Beta-2 agonists 98
Beta-adrenergic blocking agents 31, 58
Beta-blockers 9, 24, 28, 31, 32, 56, 58, 73, 154, 327, 350, 368, 370
Betadine 311
Beta-propiolactone 313
Bicarbonate 222, 278
   depletion 222
Bigeminy 70
Bi-level positive airway pressure 111
Bite
   location of 340
   physical activity after 340
Bladder 28
   care of 28
Bleeding
   cessation of 90
   disorders 241
   esophageal varices 134
   peptic ulcer 132
   rate of 88
   time 250
Blindness 406
Blocks platelet adenosine receptors 18
Blood 377
   borne viral infections 421t
   cultures 107
   loss
      acute 242
      massive 415
   pressure 376, 384, 397
      classification of 86t
      regulation of 207

redistribution of 380
salicylate levels 331
smear, parasites in 320
systems 360
transfusion 360, 361, 363
urea nitrogen 151
volume, restoration of 243
Body's capacity 398
Bone marrow
 disorders 252, 261
 suppression 290
Booster doses 313
Boric acid 328
Bowel, care of 28
Bradyarrhythmias 60, 74, 377, 417
Bradycardia 19, 60, 416
Brain 316
 anoxia 333
 cell damage 397
 samples 311
Brainstem 171f
 functions 163
 lesions 158
Breath, shortness of 295, 297, 408
Breathlessness 414
Bretylium 57
Broad-spectrum antibiotics 306
Bronchial obstruction 96, 122
Bronchodilators 38
 ipratropium bromide 99
Bronchoscopy 89
Bronchospasm 346, 362, 388
 acute 389
 sudden 389
Brucellosis 362
Brudzinski sign 183
Buccal mucosa 338
Budd-Chiari syndrome 137
Buffers 220
Burns 380, 383
 severe 280
Butazolidine 371

## C

Calcium 236, 255, 327
 abnormalities 215
 channel blockers 25, 25t, 31, 59, 65, 327, 370, 377, 415
 gluconate 87, 214
*Campylobacter jejuni* 125
Cancer 102
 chemotherapy 112
Captopril 51, 55, 154, 369
Carbamate 343
 inhibition with 344
 insecticides 346
 poisoning 344

Carbamazepine 196, 245, 369, 370, 375
Carbenicillin 186
Carbohydrate metabolism 331
Carbolic acid 354
Carbon
 monoxide 327, 333
 tetrachloride 137, 328
Carbonate 352
Carbonic acid 220
Carboxyhemoglobin 333
Carcinoma 129
 bronchogenic 107
Cardiac arrest 79, 415
Cardiac arrhythmias 55, 263, 359, 398
 control of 350
 treatment of 67t
 types of 60
Cardiac failure, congestive 266
Cardiac function, abnormalities of 415
Cardiac massage, effectiveness of 81
Cardiac output 40
Cardiac pain 1
Cardiac specific troponins 15
Cardiac tamponade, acute 84
Cardiac valve hemolysis 243
Cardiomyopathy
 alcoholic 336
 hypertrophic obstructive 415
Cardiopulmonary disorders, pre-existing 401
Cardiovascular abnormalities 139
Cardiovascular disease 88, 402, 403
Cardiovascular emergencies 1, 86t, 87t
Cardiovascular system 316
Cardioversion 65, 70
Carotid
 external 171f
 sinus 418
  massage 65
  syncope 415, 418
Catabolic state 309
Catastrophes, cerebrovascular 164
Cathedral ceiling syndrome 205
Cefotaxime 302
Ceftazidime 109
Ceftriaxone 109, 302
Cefuroxime 109
Cell
 hibernation 384
 stunning 384
Cellular toxicity 298
Central nervous system 182, 216, 218, 264, 298, 344, 345, 356, 388, 416
Central neurological dysfunction 268
Central venous
 catheter 212
 pressure 139, 264
Cephalosporins 154, 186, 369

Cerebellum 171f
Cerebral
  artery
    anterior 170
    middle 170
    posterior 170
  circulation 380
  cortex 344
  dysfunction 299, 394
  edema 181
    high altitude 408
    mechanism of 408
    treatment of 143
  embolism 172
  infarction 169
  malaria 319, 320, 395, 396
  perfusion pressure 164
  stroke 335, 336
  thrombosis 168, 279
  vascular episode 305
  venous thrombosis 181
Cerebrospinal fluid 298, 320, 356
Cerebrovascular accident 280, 389, 396
Cerebrovascular diseases 403
Cerebrovascular lesion 392, 398
Cervical vertigo 205
Chemicals 262
Chemotaxis, defective 112
Chemotherapeutic agents 302, 369
Chemotherapy 127, 245
Chest
  pain 1, 295
    development of 299
    evaluation of 1
    intensity of 11
  radiograph 89
  X-ray 264
Cheyne-Stokes respiration 41
Chikungunya 294
  fever 293, 294
    confirmation of 294
  virus 293, 295
*Chlamydia pneumoniae* 106
Chloramphenicol 186, 245, 368, 369, 371, 375
Chloride 352
  resistant metabolic alkalosis 225
Chlorophenothane 343
Chloroquine 317, 321, 370
  phosphate, dosage of 321
Chlorpromazine 354
Cholera 303, 304
  clinical manifestations of 304
Choleric stools 305
Cholestyramine 344
Cholinergic over activity, signs of 346
Cholinergic syndrome 326

Cholinesterase 344, 346
  inhibitors, primarily 343
Chronic obstructive pulmonary disease 101, 114, 226, 368, 402
Cilnidipine 25
Cimetidine 154
Ciprofloxacin 302, 370
  resistant Salmonella typhi 302
Circulatory collapse 338
Circulatory overload 359, 363
Cirrhosis liver 398
Citrate intoxication 363
Clonidine 154, 309, 326, 370
Clopidogrel 9, 28, 31, 33, 168
*Clostridium tetani* 307
Coagulation tests 361
Coagulopathy 138, 144, 234, 398
Cobra bite 340
Cocaine 194
Codeine 332
Cognitive-behavioral therapy 414
Colchicine 288
Cold
  extremities 378
  injury 409
Colitis, dysenteric 322
Colonoscopy 136
Coma 160t, 274, 279, 343
  causes of 158b
  diabetic 272
  hypoglycemic 272, 272t
  prolonged 335
Complete blood count 138, 241
Compressions 81
Computerized tomographic scan 156
Confusion 153, 234, 335
Confusional state 156
Connective tissue diseases 102
Consciousness
  loss of 418
  state of 161
Continuous positive airway pressure 116
Conversion reaction 155
Convulsions 189
Convulsive, generalized 197
Coombs test, positive direct 361
Copper
  salts 352
  sulfate-blue vitriol 352
Cor pulmonale
  acute 46
  chronic 115
Coronary artery
  bypass grafting 403
  complete thrombotic occlusion of 10
  disease 1, 2, 7, 405
Coronary atherosclerosis 10

Coronary heart disease  5
Coronary thrombus  10
Coronavirus disease (COVID-2019)  325
    symptoms  325
    treatment  325
    complications of  325
Corrosive poisoning  338
Cortex  153
Cortical dementia  156
Corticosteroids  154, 172, 190, 244, 251, 266, 267, 269, 271, 289, 342, 397
    concomitant administration of  132
    doses of  339
Cortisol  270
Costochondritis  4
Cotrimoxazole  369
Cough
    development of  299
    syncope  95, 415
    variant asthma  95
Cranial nerve palsies  183
    multiple  191
Creatine phosphokinase  15
Creosote  354
Crescendo angina  8, 29
Cresol  354
Critical allergic reactions  376, 381, 387
Crotalidae  339
Cyanide  327, 348, 352
    toxicity  349
Cysticercosis  194
Cytochrome oxidase, inhibitor of  348
Cytomegalovirus  112
    infection  362
Cytotoxic brain edema  140

## D

Da Costa syndrome  4
D-dimer estimation  48
Deafness  406
Death  279
    cause of  346
Decerebrate state  162
Decontamination, gastrointestinal  330
Decorticate posture  162
Deep coma  170
Deep venous thrombosis, treatment of  49
Dehydration  199, 360
    moderate to severe  331
Dehydroemetine  322
Dehydroepiandrosterone  270
Delirium  155, 155*t*, 329, 337
    tremens  336, 396
Dementia  155, 155*t*
    frontal  156
    multi-infarct  156
    subcortical  156
    syndrome  156*t*
Dengue  300
    fever  290, 291
    hemorrhagic fever  290
    infection, primary  292
    shock syndrome  290, 291
    virus  290
Dental procedure  416
Depression  156, 412
Desmopressin  258
Desoxycorticosterone acetate, injections of  418
Dexamethasone  370, 408
Dextropropoxyphene  295
*Dhatura*  332
Diabetes mellitus  9, 26, 112, 403
Dialysis  237, 328, 332, 338
Diarrhea  305, 344, 349, 362, 388, 410, 412
    acute infective  125*b*
    mild  303
    secretory  125
    watery  124
Diazepam  302, 309
Diet  27, 143
Digitalis
    dosage of  368
    quinidine  154
Digoxin  60, 327, 370
Dihydroergotamine  203
Diltiazem  57, 60, 65, 87
Diphtheria  420
Direct lung injury  119
Disopyramide  56, 57, 369
Disseminated intravascular coagulation  122, 243, 248, 250, 259, 279, 387, 397
    causes of  259*t*
Diuresis  328
Diuretics  38, 172, 338
Diverticular disease  129
Dizziness  297, 335, 337, 343, 392, 407, 417
Dobutamine  42, 43, 87, 370
Dobutrex  87
Doll's eye movements  162
Donor blood  362
Dopamine  42, 43, 87, 370, 381, 385
    high-dose  229
Doxycycline  318, 369
Dramamine  124
Drop attack  417
Drugs  66, 137, 261, 327
    antiallergic  363
    antidiabetic  403
    interactions  363, 367
        mechanism of  367
    side effects of  371
    therapy  65, 77, 156, 324

Dual infections 293
Duloxetine 375
Dysentery 124
Dysphagia 307
Dyspnea 4

# E

*Ebola* 295
  virus
    disease 295
    human-to-human transmission of 296
Echocardiogram 16
Echocardiography 37, 47, 346
Eclampsia 52, 54, 194
Eczema, history of 374
Edema
  acute pulmonary 35, 54, 359
  high altitude pulmonary 408
  severe pulmonary 348
Ejection fraction 33
Electrical injuries 406
Electrocardiogram 2, 12, 47, 64, 264, 350
Electroencephalogram 193
Electrolyte 70, 207, 332
  abnormalities 207
  balance 207, 329, 337, 338
  control of 236, 278
  disorder 154
  imbalance 329
    correction of 275
  regulation 407
  therapy 282
Embolism 45
Embolus, size of 45
Emergency
  drug-induced 363
  endocrinal 263
  environmental 391
  gastrointestinal 123
  hematological 241
  hypertensive 51, 54, 54*t*
  personal prophylaxis 310
  surgery 90
  treatment 163
Emetine 322
Enalapril 369
Encainide 57
Encephalitis 154, 156, 291, 293, 310, 314
  acute 192, 307
  type of 311
Encephalopathy 137, 141, 138, 179, 183, 194, 303
  post-traumatic 156
End-expiratory pressure ventilation 405

Endocrine
  disorders 216, 218
  drugs 367
Endoscopic retrograde cholangiopancreatography 151
Endoscopic therapy 135
Endoscopy 132
Endothelium, capillary 340
Endotoxin 298, 362
Endotracheal intubation 110
Enterotoxin 303
Enterovirus 125
Enzyme 344
  cyclooxygenase, inhibition of 16, 18
  hepatic 301
Eosinophilia 375
Epididymo-orchitis 306
Epigastric discomfort 410
Epilepsy 154, 194
Epinephrine 42, 87, 227, 342, 344, 390
Episode 392, 418
Epistaxis 291
  severe 52
Ergots 203
Erythromycin 186, 369
Erythropoietin, synthesis of 207, 233
*Escherichia coli* 109
  enteroinvasive 125
  enteropathogenic 125
  enterotoxigenic 125
Esmolol 25, 266
Esophageal disorders 3
Esophageal gastric-duodenal endoscopy 132
Esophagitis 129, 132
Estrogen therapy 306
Ethambutol 186, 190, 370
Ethanol 137, 249, 326
  metabolism 401
Ethionamide 369
Ethyl alcohol, administration of 338
Ethylene glycol 137
Exacerbations 97
Excessive heat production, disorders of 394
Exercise 121
Exogenous surfactant therapy 121
Exophthalmos, malignant 263
Expiration 103*f*
External cardiac massage, method of 82*f*
Extracellular fluid 210
Extrinsic coagulation pathway 255*fc*
Eye movements 160, 162

# F

Falciparum malaria 293, 316, 321
  clinical syndromes of 316*t*
Famotidine 370

Fansidar 318
Febrile
　illness 183
　reaction 359, 361
　　risk of 361
Fentanyl 332
Fenthion 343, 346
*Fetor hepaticus* 142
Fever 264, 374, 385, 416
　enteric 300, 301
　high 394
　high grade 294
Fibrillation 67
Fibrin degradation products 260
Fibrinolysis 23, 28
　dosage schedule of 50*t*
Fibrinolytic agent, choice of 21
Fibrinolytic therapy 21, 22, 32, 49
　complications of 24
Flaccid paralysis, acute symmetrical 267
Flagellate 297
Flail chest 226
Flecainide 57, 60
Flu 311
Fludrocortisone 418
Fluid 332
　administration 121
　aggressive replacement of 275
　balance 163, 207, 329, 338
　challenge 235
　compartments 377*f*
　hypotonic 379
　large amount of 305
　loss 377
　management of 139, 235
　overload 234
　replacement 304
　replenishment 130
　therapy 139, 275, 282, 293
　types of 127, 275, 305
Flumazenil 327, 330
Fluorescent antibody test 311
Fluoroquinolones 302
Focal neurological
　deficit 176, 184
　signs 320
Fondaparinux 49
Food poisoning 124
Foramen magnum 357
Forced diuresis 332, 336
Foreign body airway obstruction 91
Formaldehyde 337, 353
Formaline 353
Free fatty acids 273
Frostbite 409
Full blown syndrome 389
Furosemide infusion 235

## G

Gallstones 146
Gamma-aminobutyric acid 141
Gastric
　acidity 419
　aspiration 329
　contents 129
　distension 303
　injury 93
　intubation 357
　lavage 328, 331, 337, 339, 350, 357
　symptoms 297
Gastritis, erosive 129, 132
Gastroenteritis 415
　acute 124, 377
Gastrointestinal bleeding 129*b*, 280, 336
　acute 129
　lower 129, 135
Gastrointestinal disorders 3, 223
Gastrointestinal loss 304, 416
Gastrointestinal symptoms 218, 412
Gastrointestinal tract 380
Generalized anxiety disorder 410
Gentamicin 186
*Giardia lamblia* 125
Glasgow coma
　scale 330
　score 177
Glitazones 26
Globus hystericus 389
Glomerular filtration rate 209
Glomerulonephritis 231
Glucagon 286
Glucocorticoids 99, 270
Glucose 393
　containing solutions 379
　primary
　　overutilization of 285
　　underproduction of 285
　transfusion of 359
Glutamine 140
Gold salts 245, 249, 369
Gram stain 185, 191
Gram-negative
　bacteria 383
　organisms 362
　sepsis 280
Gram-positive bacteria 383
Granulocyte 246
　colony stimulating factor 113, 247
　transfusions 262
Granulomatous disease, chronic 112
Graves' ophthalmopathy 267

# H

*Haemophilus influenzae* 108
Hageman factor 255
Halofantrine 318
Halogen 137
Halothane 375
Hand-held inhalers 96
Hands, position of 82f
Hashimoto's thyroiditis 268
Head injury 336
Headache 170, 320, 337, 343, 356, 407
  acute
    gouty 199
    severe 201fc
  chronic 200
    cluster 204
  cluster 203
  etiological classification of 199t
  mild to moderate 357
  recurrent 200
Heart 2
  block
    complete 76f
    second degree 75
  disease 417
    ischemic 5
  failure 33, 54, 263, 377
    advanced chronic 35
    congestive 34, 154, 226, 243
    diastolic 34
    left 34
    right 34
    severe congestive 110
    types of 34
  rate 79
Heat
  collapse 393
  cramps 391, 392
  dissipation, disorders of 394
  edema 391
  exhaustion 391, 392
  hyperpyrexia 393
  illness 391
  loss, accelerating 396
  reactions, acute 391
  stroke 280, 391, 393, 394, 397
    develop 395
  syncope 391, 392
Heimlich maneuver 91, 92f, 93f
  principle of 91
Hematemesis 89, 132, 134
Hematuria 291
Hemiplegia 174, 284, 320
Hemoconcentration 399
Hemodialysis 280, 330, 397

Hemoglobin 319
  lesser amount of 334
  low 384
Hemoglobinuria 361
Hemogram 241
Hemolysin 298
Hemolysis, severe 340
Hemolytic anemia 245t
  causes of 243t
Hemolytic crisis, acute 244
Hemolytic reaction 360
Hemolytic uremic syndrome 243
Hemoperfusion 330
Hemophilia 255
  A 257
  B 257
  treatment 257t
Hemorrhages 184, 292, 331, 416
  acute intracerebral 54
  gastrointestinal 291
  intestinal 303
  intracerebral 165, 173, 174
  multiple 291, 299
  severe 342
  subarachnoid 165, 174, 175
Hemorrhagic manifestations 291, 340
  treatment of 342
Hemostasis 243
  conventional tests for 248t
Hemostatic disorders 247
Henoch-Schonlein purpura 254
Heparin 20, 28, 48, 249, 253
  therapy 260
Hepatic circulatory failure 397
Hepatic disease 368, 369t
Hepatic dysfunction 299
Hepatic encephalopathy 130, 135, 140
  clinical grading of 142t
Hepatitis 306
  A virus 421
  autoimmune 137
  B 419
    virus 362, 421
  C virus 362, 421
Hepatorenal syndrome 144, 299
Hepatosplenomegaly 246
Herniation
  syndromes 160, 161
  types of 160
Heroin 332
Herpes simplex virus 112, 191, 192
Heterologous therapeutic sera 381
Hiccup 170
High cervical spinal cord injury 381
Histamine 374
Hodgkin's lymphoma 112

Hormone
    action blockers  265
    adrenocorticotropic  270
    release blockers  265
    synthesis blockers  265
Human activated protein C  386
Human body temperature  391
Human diploid cell vaccine  312
Human immune system defect  112
Human rabies immunoglobulin  312
Huntington's chorea  156
Hydantoins  371
Hydralazine  370, 374
Hydration status  126
Hydrocephalus  156, 183, 191
Hydrocortisone  362
    hemisuccinate  374
    injections  342
Hydrocyanic acid  352
Hydrophobia  311
Hydroxide  352
Hyperbaric oxygen  334
Hyperbilirubinemia  298, 299
Hypercalcemia  217
    causes of  218t
    clinical manifestations of  218t
    treatment of severe  219b
Hypercapnia  114
Hypercapniac respiratory failure  115
    causes of  114b
Hyperglycemia  45, 276, 386
    triad of  274
Hyperkalemia  199, 212, 399
    causes of  213t
    degree of  214
    mild  214
    progressive  214
Hypernatremia  194, 207
Hyperosmolality  272
Hyperosmolar hyperglycemic nonketotic coma  279, 280t, 281
Hyperparasitemia  319
Hyperparathyroidism, primary  217
Hyperphosphatemia  217, 233, 234
Hyperpnea  331
Hyperpyrexia  188, 194, 199, 265, 266, 336, 391
Hypersensitive carotid sinus  418
Hypertension  26, 52, 174, 178, 234, 238
    control of  172
    malignant  51
Hypertensive crisis  51, 179, 180
Hypertensive encephalopathy  179
    mechanism of  179
Hyperthermia  154, 391, 393, 397
    cause of  394b
    classic  393
    differential diagnosis of  396t
    exertional  393
    malignant  396
Hyperthyroid states  263
Hyperthyroidism  154
Hypertonic glucose infusion  215
Hyperventilation  283, 389, 401, 418
Hypoaldosteronism  213
Hypocalcemia  194, 215-217, 234, 363
    causes of  216t
    clinical manifestations of  216b
    severe  217, 350
Hypocalcemic crisis  215
Hypofibrinogenemia  260
Hypoglycemia  154, 269, 272, 284, 319, 320, 392, 398, 399, 405, 418
    fasting  285
    principle causes of  285b
Hypoglycemic agents  273
Hypokalemia  211, 212b, 399
    causes of  211b
Hypomagnesemia  217, 350, 399
Hyponatremia  139, 194, 208, 210, 234, 269
    dilutional  392
    hypervolemic  209
    hypovolemic  209
    severe  269
Hypophosphatemia  218, 399
Hypoproteinemia  233
Hypoprothrombinemia  331
Hypotension  19, 60, 274, 331, 362, 385, 405
    component of  381
    control of  350
    severe  349, 384
Hypothalamic functions, disorders of  394
Hypothermia  154, 268, 333, 384, 386, 398, 399, 405
    harmful effects of  398
    severe  398, 400
Hypothyroid state  263
Hypothyroidism  154
Hypoventilation, alveolar  114
Hypovolemia  125, 349, 384
    acute  415
    control of  350
    correction of  43
    severe  348, 415
    states of  416
Hypovolemic shock  291, 303, 378, 380, 389
    management of  380
Hypovolemic vascular collapse  271
Hypoxemia  102, 113, 114, 385, 401, 404
    reversal of  120
Hypoxia  199, 390, 408
    acute altitude  401
    altitude simulation test  402
    problem of  401

## I

Iatrogenic emergencies 356
Idiopathic thrombocytopenic purpura 249, 250
Idiosyncratic reactions 375
Imipenem 111, 369
Immune
   globulin 245
   system defenses 112*t*
   thrombocytopenia 249
   thrombocytopenic purpura, drug-induced 253
Immunity 419
   acquired 419
   defective cell-mediated 112
   lower 315
Immunization, passive 312
Immunotherapy 308
Inadequate venous return 392
Indomethacin 249
Infarction, actual 335
Infections 88, 102, 138, 139, 154, 238, 259, 262, 357, 382
   bacterial 122
   control of 120
   fever of 391
   hospital-acquired 104
   human 298
   secondary 292, 339
   severe 398
Infectious diseases 419
Inflammatory colitis 129
In-flight syndrome 402
Influenza 297, 299, 300, 421
   A 296
      virus 296
Inhaled allergens 95
Innate immunity 419
Inotropic drugs 42*t*
Insecticide poisoning 245, 342
Insomnia 329
Inspiration 103*f*
Insulin 215
   regular 276
   therapy 276
      advantages of small-dose 276
Intact skin 419
Intensive care unit 212, 330
Intentional drug 368
Intermediate syndrome 346
Internal mammary artery hemorrhage 359
Interstitial compartment 377
Interstitial fluid 391
Interstitial lung disease 102
Interstitial nephritis drugs 231
Interventional therapy 49
Interventricular septum 27
Intestinal obstruction 357
Intestinal perforation 303
Intoxication 415, 418
   acute alcoholic 335
   degree of 336
Intra-abdominal sepsis 386
Intra-aortic balloon counter pulsation 41, 43
Intracranial diseases 154
Intracranial pressure 54, 164
Intraluminal thrombus 6
Intramuscular regimen 276
Intrarenal failure 230
Intrathecal therapy 190
Intravascular volume 229, 376
Intravenous drugs 54*t*
Intravenous fluids 150
Intravenous heparin 20
Intravenous nitroglycerine 19
Intravenous pyelography 233
Intrinsic acute renal failure, causes of 231*b*
Intubation 130
Iodine 265
   tincture 353
Iron
   preparations 353
   therapy 374
Irritable bowel syndrome 413
Ischemic cellular damage 409
Ischemic colitis 129
Ischemic encephalopathy 156
Ischemic stroke 165, 167, 417
Isoniazid 137, 154, 186, 190, 194, 369, 370, 375
Isoproterenol 42, 87
   infusion 77
Isosorbide dinitrate 16, 370
Isotonic saline 380

## J

Jaundice 315
Joint tissues 287

## K

Kanamycin 186
Kernig sign 183
Ketoacidosis 272
   alcoholic 275
   diabetic 154, 273, 380
Ketoacidotic coma 272, 272*t*
Ketoconazole 369, 375
Ketosis 274
   causes of 275
Kidney 52, 316
   function 295
Kinin system 374

*Klebsiella pneumoniae* 109
Kneel astride 92
Korsakoff syndrome 156
Kussmaul respiration 274, 281

## L

Labetalol 370
Labyrinthitis 205, 206
Lactic
　acid 283, 331
　acidosis 272, 279, 282
　dehydrogenase 149
Lactulose 143
Lacunar stroke 169
Lamotrigine 375
Landry Guillain-Barré syndrome 307
Large artery cerebral thrombosis 169
Laryngeal edema 388, 389
Larynx 311
Lead poisoning 194
Left ventricular
　ejection fraction 8
　failure 122
　hypertrophy 79
*Legionella pneumoniae* 106
*Leptospira*
　genus 297
　*icterohemorrhagica* 299
Leptospiremia 298
Leptospires 300
Leptospirosis 293, 297, 298, 300
　cases of 301
　diagnosis of 300
　transmission of 298
Leukemia
　acute 112
　chronic lymphocytic 252
Leukocytosis 319
Leukopenia 291
　presence of 320
Leukotriene 374
　modifiers 100
Levofloxacin 111
Levothyroxine 269
Liberal oral fluids 302
Lidocaine 20, 56, 57, 72, 87, 154, 194, 369
Life-threatening hemoptysis 88
　causes of 88*t*
Liothyronine 269
Lipase 298
Lisinopril 369
Liver
　failure
　　acute 293
　　causes of 139
　flap 141

function 295
　tests 324
Lomotil 127
Loperamide 127
Low cardiac output 229
Lower limbs 391
Low-molecular weight heparin 9
Lumbar compartments 357
Lumbar puncture 356, 357
Lung 316
　auscultation of 12, 37
　injury 118
　　indirect 119
Lymphadenopathy 246
Lysergide 353
Lysol 354
Lysosomal enzymes 374

## M

Macrolides 109
Magnesium 236
　sulfate 99
Malaise 407
Malaria 194, 300, 314, 362, 314
　antigens, detection of 316
　cases of severe 318
　chemoprophylaxis for 321
　infection 321
　parasite, species of 316
　severe 317, 319
　symptoms of 315
　types of 315
Malignancy 217, 259
Mallory-Weiss
　syndrome 123, 133
　tear 129
Mannitol 357
Masseter muscles 307
Massive pulmonary embolism 46, 47*f*
Measles 419
　virus 421
Mechanical thrombectomy 171
Mechanical ventilation 116, 117, 309, 334
Meckel's diverticulum 136
Mediastinitis 339
Medical disorder 413
　differential diagnosis of 413*t*
Medication errors 368
Medicine, contemporary 301
Mefloquine 154, 317, 318, 320, 321, 370
Melena 132
Memory, lapses of 329, 367
Meniere's disease 205
Meniere's syndrome 206
Meningeal inflammation 183
Meninges, tubercular infection of 188

Meningitis 154, 194, 306, 357, 396
  acute 200
  bacterial 187t
  types of 184, 184t
Meningoencephalitis 306
  causes of 311
Mental alertness 407
Mental status, altered 385
Mercaptans 141
Mercury 353
Meropenem 111
Metabolic acidosis 125, 221-223, 273, 274, 331, 337, 349, 379, 398-400
  causes of 223t
Metabolic acids, overproduction of 222
Metabolic alkalosis 221, 223, 224
  causes of 224b
Metabolic coma 163
Metabolic disorders 158
Metabolic emergency 263
Metabolic waste, removal of 207
Methicillin 186
Methimazole 369
Methoxamine 42
Methyl alcohol poisoning 337
Methyldopa 137, 154, 369, 370, 375
Methylprednisolone 267
Metoclopramide 154
Metoprolol 57, 87, 370
Metronidazole 154, 308, 322, 324, 371
Mexiletine 56, 57
Microbial toxins, liberation of 382
Microcirculatory obstruction 315
Microscopic agglutination test 300
Micturition syncope 415, 417
Migraine 201
Migrainous vertigo 206
Mineralocorticoids 270
Miscarriage 321
Mitral valve prolapse 413
Mixing artesunate powder 318
Monoamine oxidase inhibitor 367
Monocytes 290
Monosodium urate crystals 287
Monotherapy 196
*Moraxella catarrhalis* 106
Morphine 332, 358
  sulfate 309
Motion sickness 404
Motor signs 160
Mouth-to-mouth ventilation 82f
  technique of 83f
Mucous membranes 334
Mucus hypersecretion 388
Mucus membranes 419
Multiorgan failure 137
Multisystem organ failure 382, 387

Mumps 305, 306
Muscarinic manifestations 345
Muscle
  contraction headaches 199
  necrosis 15
  spasms, control of 309
Muscular fasciculation 346
Musculoskeletal disorders 4
Mycobacteria 112
*Mycobacterium tuberculosis* 188
*Mycoplasma pneumoniae* 106
Myelitis 307, 314
Myeloid growth factors 262
Myocardial contractility 376, 377
Myocardial function 346
Myocardial infarction 13f, 54, 154, 280, 398
  complications of 26
  electrocardiographic localization of 15t
Myocardial ischemia 335, 384
  aggravate 43
Myocardial lesion 392
Myocardial necrosis 9
Myocardial repolarization 398
Myocarditis 306
Myocardium 341, 348, 359
Myoglobin, releasing 298
Myopathy 226
Myxedema 398
  coma 263, 268
  madness 268

# N

Naloxone 327, 333
Naphthalene 353
  balls 353
Narcotics 37, 115, 327
Nasogastric intubation 150
Natural death 79
Nausea 4, 234, 388
Near drowning 404
Nebulization 390
Nebulized corticosteroids 99
Neck stiffness 306
Necrotic gut 385
Negri bodies 311
*Neisseria meningitides* 183
Neoplasm 88
Neoplastic diseases 218
Nephrotic syndrome 181
Nephrotoxin exposure 230
Neuritis 306
Neuroanatomic syndromes 160t
Neurocirculatory asthenia 4
Neuroglycopenic symptoms 284
Neuroleptic malignant syndrome 396
Neurological diseases 403

Neurological disorder, acute 395
Neurological emergencies 153
Neurological signs, critical evaluation of 162
Neuroma, acoustic 205
Neuromuscular blocking agents 309
Neuromuscular disorders 114
Neuropathy 234
Neurotoxic 339
Neutropenia 112, 261
    causes of 261$t$
Never apply ice 341
New malaria vaccine 321
Nifedipine 369
Nightmares 329
Nitrates 9, 16, 25, 28, 31-33, 38, 354, 415
Nitrofurantoin 369
Nitroglycerine 87, 204
Nitroprusside test 274
Non-caffeine liquids 408
Noninvasive ventilatory assistance 116
Non-ketotic hyperosmolar diabetic state 154
Non-marrow disorders 252
Non-narcotic agents 328
Non-occlusive thrombus 29
Non-pitting edema, localized 388
Nonpoisonous snakes 339
Non-ST-elevated myocardial infarction 7, 10, 14$f$, 29
Nonsteroidal anti-inflammatory drug 191, 253, 265, 288, 292, 363, 367, 384
Non-ST-segment elevated myocardial infarction 7
Nonvolatile acids 220
Noradrenaline 87, 381, 385
Norepinephrine 42, 43, 229
Norfloxacin 371
Normovolemic hyponatremia 209, 210
Norphine 18, 358
Norwalk virus 125
Nutrition 121, 151, 163, 237

# O

Obesity, pathological 226
Obidoxime 347
Obstructive choledocholithiasis 151
Obstructive uropathy 230
Octreotide 133
Oculocephalic reflex 162
Offending dog 313
Oliguria 125, 271, 342
    progressive 349
Oliguric phase 235
Oophoritis 306
Opening airway, head-tilt neck-lift method of 82$f$
Opiate poisoning, acute 332

Opiate receptors 332
Opioid 326
    intoxication 333
Opisthotonus 307
Optic atrophy 337
Oral anticoagulants 363
Oral carbohydrates 268
Oral hypotensive drugs 180
Oral rehydration 392
    solutions 126
    therapy 304
Oral therapy 51
Orchitis 306
Organ failure, mechanism of 384
Organic headaches 199
Organochlorine
    insecticides 343
    poisoning 343
Organophosphate 344, 346, 347
    poisoning, clinical features of 345$t$
Organophosphorus insecticides 343
Oropharynx 405
Orthostatic hypotension 415, 416
Orthostatic syncope 416
Orthostatic vital signs 416
Oseltamivir 297
Osteomyelitis 386
Otitis media, acute 402
Oxacillin 375
Oxidizing agent, mild 350
Oximes 347
Oxygen
    delivery, reduced 333
    supplemental 28
    tension 350
    toxicity 405

# P

Packed red cells, transfusion of 361
Pain
    abdominal 274, 291, 297, 412
    character of 2
    epigastric 337
    relief of 150
Palpitation 414
Pancreatitis 280, 306, 380, 383
    degree of 150
    idiopathic acute 146
Pancytopenia 246
Panic attack 412, 414
    symptoms of 412$b$
Panic disorder 410-413, 415
    diagnosis of 414
    differential diagnosis of 413$t$
Papillary muscle 27
Paracetamol 295, 351

Paradoxical embolus 173
Paradoxical pulse 85
Paradoxical reactions 329
Paralysis 343
Paralytic complications, treatment of 342
Paralytic ileus 303
Paraplegia 320
Parathyroid hormone 215, 218
Parenchymal lung diseases 116
Parenteral fluid therapy 293
Paresthesia 343, 408
Parkinson's disease 156
Parkinsonism 335
Parotitis
    bilateral 306
    unilateral 306
Paroxysmal atrial tachycardia 63
Paroxysmal nocturnal hemoglobinuria 245
Paroxysmal supraventricular tachycardia 62, 67, 413
Partial thromboplastin time 20, 247, 250
    prolonged 248t
Pathogen, type of 383
Pedal edema 25
Pelvic inflammatory disease 386
Penetrating artery disease 169
Penicillin 154, 370, 374
    G 186, 308, 381
Pentazocine 371
Pentoxifylline 371
Peptic ulcer
    disease 129
    perforation of 128
Percutaneous coronary intervention 32
Perforation, gastrointestinal 128
Perhexiline 369
Pericardial disease 415
Pericardial pain 3
Pericardiocentesis 85, 86f
Pericarditis 2, 234
Peripheral blood film 241
Peripheral circulatory failure 128, 199, 243, 303, 336
Peripheral vasoconstriction, features of 41
Peritonitis 339
    generalized 128
Persistent hypotension 349
Perspiration 331
Pertussis 420
Pesticide poisoning 342
Pethidine 332
Petroleum distillates 354
Petting 310
Pharmacodynamic behavior 367
Pharmacodynamic profile 42t
Pharmacokinetic interactions 60

Pharmacologic agents 95, 134
Pharmacological therapy 180
Pharmacotherapy 414
Phenergan 18, 206
Pheniramine maleate 342, 359, 374
Phenol 354
Phenothiazine 354, 369
    antidepressants 415
Phenylbutazone 245
Phenytoin 56, 57, 87, 137, 196, 245, 328, 369, 370, 375
Pheochromocytoma 396
Phobic avoidance 412
Phosphoric acids 220
Phosphorus 236
Physostigmine 327
Pilgrimage 419
Piperacillin 111, 369
Placenta 321
Plasma
    thromboplastin 255
    volume 292
Plasminogen 374
*Plasmodium* 314
    *falciparum* infection 316
    *vivax* infection 315
Platelet 246, 247, 341
    aggregation 16
        control of 16
    count 247
    disorders 248
    infusions 260, 293
    transfusions 293
Platelet-activating factor 374
Pleural tapping 358
Pneumonia 112, 154, 226, 234, 280, 398
    acute severe 104
    atypical 106
    bacterial 109
    community-acquired 104, 105
    diagnosis of 106
    hospital-acquired 109
    postoperative 112
    primary atypical 106
Pneumothorax 122, 226, 358, 402
    primary 101
    recurrent 104
    secondary 101
        spontaneous 102, 102b
    spontaneous 101
Poison
    acute 326
    common types of 351t
    removal of 328
    severe 338
    systemic effects of 340
    systemically absorbed 328

types of  351
unabsorbed  328
Polio  419
Polymerase chain reaction  193
Polymorphonuclear leukocytosis,
    moderate  324
Polymyxin  186
Polyneuritis  307, 314
Polypharmacy  363
Polyps  129
Portosystemic encephalopathy  140
Positional vertigo  206
Positive airway pressure  116
Positive blood cultures  382
Positive end-expiratory pressure  120
Postexposure prophylactic treatment  311
Post-exposure prophylaxis  421
Post-ganglionic parasympathetic fibers  344
Postprandial hypoglycemia  285
Postrenal failure  230
Post-thoracentesis hypoxia  359
Posture  37, 163
Potassium  212, 236, 278
    abnormalities  210
    elimination  215
    permanganate  355
    supplementary  392
    supplements  367
Povidone iodine  311
Pralidoxime  347
Prazosin  370
Pre-aspiration cardiac arrest  404
Prednisolone  371
Predominant water deficit  208
Pre-eclampsia  54
Pregnancy
    advanced stage of  404
    fatty liver of  137
    medication in  372$t$
Prehospital fibrinolysis  23
Preinfarction angina  8
Premature labor  321
Prerenal failure  229
Pressure changes, adverse effects of  402
Procainamide  56, 57, 60, 87, 369
Proctoscopy  126
Prodromal symptoms  416
Prophylactic immunization  419
Prophylaxis  50
    indication for  310
    pre-exposure  419
Propoxyphene  369
Propranolol  57, 60, 135, 268, 370
Propylthiouracil  265
Prostaglandins  374
Proteinuria  233
Prothrombin time  138, 247, 250

Proton-pump inhibitors  132
Pseudocyst  148
Pseudodementia  156
Pseudohemoptysis  89
*Pseudomonas aeruginosa*  383
Psychiatric disorder  157, 413
Psychogenic chest pain  4
Psychoneurotic disorders  410
Psychosis, acute functional  155, 155$t$
Psychotic behavior  335
Pulmonary arterial pressure  401
Pulmonary aspiration  358
Pulmonary capillary wedge pressure  41
Pulmonary congestion  41
Pulmonary edema  349, 359, 363
    classification of  36$t$
Pulmonary embolism  3, 45
Pulmonary hypertension  401
Pulmonary stenosis  415
Pulmonary thromboembolism  45, 110, 122
Pulse
    imperceptible  349
    oximetry  97
    weak  416
Pump failure  27
Pupillary abnormalities  170
Pupillary size  161
Pupils  160
    dilated  416
Pure motor hemiplegia  169
Pure sensory stroke  169
Purpura, evaluation of  250$fc$
Pyelonephritis  386
Pyelonephrosis  386
Pyogenic meningitis  182
Pyonephrosis  385
Pyrazinamide  186, 190, 369, 370, 375
Pyrexia  293, 294, 301, 310, 323, 362
Pyridoxine  327
Pyrimethamine  318
Pyruvic acid  331

## Q

Qinghaosu  317
Quadriparesis  174
Quinidine  56, 57, 60, 249, 369, 375
Quinine  249, 317, 318, 370
Quinolones  109, 154, 370

## R

Rabies  310, 421
    paralytic form of  311
Radiculitis  314
Radiculopathy  4
Radiofrequency ablation  66

Radiography  106, 245
Ranitidine  154, 342, 371
Ranson's criteria  150b
Rashes  374
Rat paste  355
Reaction  363, 410
  types of  387
Red blood cell  242t, 320, 341
  hemolysis of  243
  scans, technetium-labeled  136
Red cell morphology  245t
Reflex spasms  307
Refractory anemia  245
Refractory hypoglycemia  286
Rehydration, rapid  304
Relapse rate  302
Renal damage  299
Renal disease  368
  drug therapy in  369t
Renal disorders  213
Renal dysfunction  299
Renal emergencies  207
Renal excretion  219
Renal failure  138, 144, 154, 199, 238t, 293, 304, 361, 398
  etiology of  233t
Renal function
  impairment of  218, 331
  preserving  397
Renal lesions  298
Renal tubules  341
Reperfusion  22
  arrhythmias  24
Replacement therapy  257
Reserpine  370
Respiration  160
  pattern of  161
Respiratory acidosis  221, 223, 226
Respiratory alkalosis  221, 223, 226, 330
  causes of  227b
Respiratory center, depression of  346
Respiratory depression  332
  progressive  333
Respiratory diseases  402
Respiratory distress  349, 374
Respiratory drive abnormality  114
Respiratory emergencies  88
Respiratory failure  113, 114, 379
  acute  97
Respiratory infections  95
Respiratory insufficiency  113
Respiratory problem  412
Respiratory processes  220
Respiratory support  116
Rest angina  30
Resuscitation
  cardiopulmonary  81, 399
  termination of  84

Reticulocytes  246
Retinopathy, hypertensive  52
Retrobulbar neuritis  337
Retro-ocular pain  291
Revascularization  44
Reye's syndrome  137
Rhabdomyolysis  397
Rheumatoid arthritis  294
Rib fracture  93
Rice-water stool  304
Rifampicin  137, 186, 190
Rifampin  369, 370
Ringer's solution  379, 399
Risus sardonicus  307
Rofecoxib  375
Rotavirus  125
  infection  125
Ryle's tube feeding  309

## S

Saddle back fever  291
Salbutamol  390
Salicylate  292
  poisoning  330
Salivary glands  345
Salmonella  126
Salsol  98
Schizontemia, peripheral  319
Sclerotherapy, endoscopic  135
Scrotum  306
Sedation  309, 401
Sedative hypnotic toxicity  329
Seizures  178, 183, 184, 188, 194, 195, 234, 405, 406, 418
  causes of  194t
  disorder  389
  generalized  195
Selective serotonin reuptake inhibitors  203
Self-save technique  92
Semiprone position  90
Semple vaccine  313
  dosage schedule for  313t
Senile dementia  156
Sensorium, altered  271
Sepsis  138, 234, 259, 381, 382, 396
  diagnosis of  384
  recognition of  385
  severe  382, 385
  syndrome  383, 387
    clinical feature of  384
Septic arthritis  386
Septic shock  381, 382, 386
  microbiology of  383t
Septic thrombophlebitis  386
Septicemia  279
Serodiagnostic methods  295

Serologic tests 324
Serological confirmation 292
Serratia marcescens 109
Serum
   ammonia 142
   enzymes 15
   glutamic oxalacetic transferase 149
   potassium 399
   transaminases 395
Sexual activity 411
Shock 129, 266, 291, 342, 359
   cardiogenic 39, 378, 380
   causes of 378*t*, 379
   component of 378
   distributive 381
   early stages of 378
   electric 406
   full blown 379
   hemorrhagic 379
   hypovolemic 291, 303, 378, 380, 389
   irreversible 279
   liver syndrome 384
   neurogenic 381
   obstructive 378, 381
   pathology of 377
   pleural 358
   powerful 406
   severe 379
   state of 376
   syndrome 291, 362, 376
      causes of 378
      types of 376, 378
   traumatic 381
   types of 378*t*, 380
   vasodilator 381
   warm 384
Short-chain fatty acids 141
Sick sinus syndrome 74
Sickle cell disease 181
Sickness, high altitude 407
Silver nitrate 355
Simple phobias 411
Sinus
   arrest 60
   bradycardia 74
      vagal-induced 416
   tachycardia 61
Sinusitis, acute 402
Skeletal muscles 298
Skin
   contamination 338
   rash 294
      presence of 184
   testing 342
Slurred speech 335
Smooth muscle cells 6
Snake bite 339, 340
   poisoning 339, 340

Social phobias 411
Sodium 236, 278, 393
   abnormalities 207
   bicarbonate 215, 327
   nitrite 327
   overload 208
   thiosulfate 327
   valproate 196
Somatostatin 134
Soreness, abdominal 93
Sotalol 56, 57, 370
Spasms
   involve pharynx 311
   recurrent 307
Special diagnostic tests 48
Spinal cord 344
Spinal roots 1
Splenectomy 244, 252
Spontaneous bleeding 256
Sputum 107
Stable chronic disease 402
*Staphylococcus aureus* 124
Starvation ketosis 275
Statins 9, 26, 28, 32
*Status asthmaticus* 94
   treatment of 99
Status epilepticus 197, 396
Status migraine 203
ST-elevated myocardial infarction 7, 9, 14*f*
Stemetil 206
Steroids
   anabolic 137
   prophylaxis with 408
Stokes-Adams
   attack 78
   syndrome 77
Stomach upsets 410
Stool 329
   examination 324
Stored blood 363
*Streptococcus pneumoniae* 106, 108, 183, 186, 188, 383
Streptokinase 21, 50
Streptomycin 186, 375
Stress, emotional 402
Strict aseptic technique 362
Stridor 390
Stroke 164
   acute ischemic 54
   classification of 165*b*
   clinical evaluation of 165
   embolic 172
   hemorrhagic 165, 173
   management 166
   syndrome 194
   syndrome, clinical manifestations of 170*b*
ST-segment elevated myocardial infarction 6, 10

Stupor  274
Subcutaneous heparin  20
Subcutaneous insulin  277
Subdural hematoma  154, 156, 336
Subendocardial infarction  13
Subocclusive coronary thrombus  32
Subocclusive intraluminal thrombus  7
Subtentorial lesions  157, 158
Sudden cardiac death  79
Sudden rhythm disturbances  417
Suicidal ideation  414
Sulfa-containing drugs  249
Sulfadoxine  318
Sulfamethoxazole  186
Sulfonamides  137, 186, 245, 328, 369, 374
Sulfuric acids  220
Sun-downing syndrome  154
Supratentorial mass lesions  157, 158
Supraventricular ectopic beats  67
Supraventricular tachyarrhythmias  61
Supraventricular tachycardia  57, 61, 350
Surgery, gastrointestinal  402
Sweat glands  345
Sweating, absence of  394
Swine flu  296, 297
Swine influenza  296
Sympatholytic syndrome  326
Sympathomimetic syndrome  326
Symptomatic carotid stenosis  168
Symptomatic hypocalcemia  217
Syncopal attacks  78
Syncope  359, 415, 417
    cardiac  417
    causes of  415*b*, 417
    cerebrovascular  417
    types of  416
Syphilis  362
Systemic bleeding  24
Systemic immune reaction  298
Systemic inflammatory response
    syndrome  377, 381, 382
Systemic lupus erythematosus  245, 250, 252, 374
Systemic vascular resistance  376, 381
Systolic dysfunction  33
Systolic heart failure  33

## T

Tachyarrhythmia  60, 266, 377, 417
    rapid control of  72
Tachy-Brady-arrhythmias  45
Tachycardia  8, 271, 274, 377, 384, 405
    diagnosis of  61*fc*
    nodal re-entrant  63
    re-entry  62, 63
    wide-complex  68

Tachypnea  41, 384, 385
Tamiflu  297
Tannic acid  354
Tazobactam  111
T-cell deficiency  112
Telephonic prescribing  368
Temperature reduction  396
Tension pneumothorax  102, 104, 415
Tentorium cerebelli  357
Tetanospasmin  307
Tetanus  307, 419, 420, 422
    immune globulin  308
    toxin  307, 308
Tetracycline  186, 318, 369, 370
Theophylline  194
Therapeutic test  316
Thiocyanates  328
Thiouracils  371
Thoracentesis  358
Thoracic deformity, severe  114
Thoracic ganglia  1
Thoracic surgery  402
Thrombocytopenia  252*t*, 260, 363
Thrombocytopenic purpura  306
Thromboembolism, prevention of  69
Thrombolysis  171
Thrombotic stroke  168, 194
Thrombotic thrombocytopenic purpura  243
Thyroid
    associated ophthalmopathy  266
    crisis  263, 266
    disorders  411
    emergencies  263*t*
    gland  263
    hormone  269, 367
    stimulating hormone  264
    storm  396
Thyroiditis  306
Thyrotoxic hypokalemic periodic
    paralysis  263, 267
Tissue
    damage activates  255*fc*
    injury, severe  259
    plasminogen activator  22
Tobramycin  186
Tocainide  57
Tolbutamide  245
Toluene  245
Torsades de pointes  60, 61, 72
Total body water  207
Total parenteral nutrition  151
Tourniquet test  291
Toxemia  301
Toxic
    agents  328*t*
    coma  163
    effects  337

mushrooms 137
myocarditis 348
reactions 343
Toxicity 367
Toxins 245, 262
Toxoplasmosis 194
Tracheal intubation, indications for 117
Tracheotomy 309
Tranquilizers 27
Transfusion hemosiderosis 363
Transfusion reactions, types of 360*t*
Transfusion syphilis, risk of 362
Transient bacteremia 382
Transient ischemic attack 167, 413, 417
Trauma 154, 383
    emotional 411
Travellers' diarrhea 125
Tremors 335
Tricyclic antidepressants 327
Trigeminal autonomic cephalgia 203
Trigeminy 70
Trimethoprim 186
Triphasic fever 291
Triptans 202
Troglitazone 375
Trophozoites 322
Tropical diseases 290
Troponins 7
Tubercular meningitis 188
Tubular disorders 230
Tubular necrosis, acute 128, 230, 279, 361
Typhoid 301
    state 301

# U

Ulcers
    acute 320
    chronic 128
Uncal herniation syndrome 162
Unpressurized aircraft 407
Unstable angina 7-9, 29, 54
Upper abdominal surgery 226
Upper gastrointestinal bleeding 129, 131
Upper respiratory catarrh 291
Urate lowering therapies 289
Uremia 232
Uric acids 220
Urinary tract 234
Urine 306, 329
    alkalinization of 328, 331
Urokinase 21, 22, 50
Urticaria 371, 389
    eruptions 388
    history of 374
Uveitis
    chronic 298
    recurrent 298

# V

Vagotonia 12
Valproic acid 249, 369, 370
Valsalva effect 417
Vancomycin 186, 370
Varicella-zoster virus 422
Vascular headaches 199
Vasculitis 374
    hypersensitivity 254
Vasoactive amines 374
Vasomotor abnormalities 415
Vasopressors 42
Vasospasm 178
Vasovagal faint 415
Vasovagal syncope 416
Vast capillary bed 376
Venipuncture 416
Venom injected, amount of 340
Venous stasis 391
Ventilation 48, 396
    impairment of 102
Ventilation-acquired pneumonia 112
Ventilation-perfusion abnormalities 114
Ventricular arrhythmias 8
Ventricular fibrillation 67, 73, 73*f*, 406
Ventricular premature beats 67, 70
Ventricular tachyarrhythmias 70
Ventricular tachycardia 60, 61, 67, 71, 71*f*, 350
Ventricular-free wall 27
Verapamil 56, 57, 87, 369
Vertebrobasilar arteries 170
Vertigo
    acute 204
    benign paroxysmal 206
Vessel vasculitis, small 231
Vestibular neuronitis 205, 206
*Vibrio cholerae* 303
Viper bite 340
Viper snakes 340
Viral agents 125
Viral aseptic meningitis 300
Viral diseases, transmission of 362
Viral encephalitis, type of 310, 311
Viral hepatitis 245, 293, 300
    serologies 138
Viral meningitis 300
Viral particles 312
Viral pneumonia 110
Viral syndrome 291
Virchow's triad 45, 51
Virus 112, 137, 305
    infection 296
Vision, blurring of 417
Visual disturbances 337, 406
Vital functions 385
Vital functions, maintenance of 326, 327

Vital life functions, maintenance of 347
Vital organ functions 385
Vital signs, support of 90
Vitamin $B_6$ 327
Volatile component 220
Vomiting 4, 93, 170, 234, 337, 362, 388, 408
    acute 123
    causes of 123
    severe 297

# W

Warfarin 60
Warning arrhythmias 70
Water depletion 392
Weil's syndrome 299, 300
Wernicke's encephalopathy 286, 337
West Nile virus 191
Wheeze 362, 390
Whipple's triad 285
Whole blood transfusion 361
Whooping cough 419
Widal test 302
Wilson's disease 137
Withdrawal syndrome, acute 336
Wolff-Parkinson-White syndrome 66, 67f
Worsening hypovolemia 384
Wound 312
    care of 309, 341
    cleaning of 311

# Y

Yellow phosphorus 355
*Yersinia enterocolitica* 125

# Z

Zanamivir 297
Zolpidem 329
Zoonotic infection 298

EU GSPR Authorised Reprsentative
Logos Europe, 9 rue Nicolas Poussin
1700, La Rochelle, France
Phone: +33 (0) 6 67 93 73 78
E-mail: contact@logoseurope.eu

www.ingramcontent.com/pod-product-compliance
Ingram Content Group UK Ltd.
Pitfield, Milton Keynes, MK11 3LW, UK
UKHW051912130725
2358IPUK00012B/33